Clinical Breast Imaging

Clinical Breast Imaging

Editor: Cody Perez

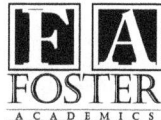

FA FOSTER
A C A D E M I C S

www.fosteracademics.com

www.fosteracademics.com

FA
FOSTER
ACADEMICS

Cataloging-in-Publication Data

Clinical breast imaging / edited by Cody Perez.
    p. cm.
Includes bibliographical references and index.
ISBN 978-1-63242-628-4
1. Breast--Imaging. 2. Breast--Radiography. 3. Breast--Diseases--Diagnosis.
4. Breast--Cancer--Diagnosis. I. Perez, Cody.
RC280.B8 C55 2019
616.994 49--dc23

Foster Academics,
118-35 Queens Blvd., Suite 400,
Forest Hills, NY 11375, USA

ISBN 978-1-63242-628-4 (Hardback)

Contents

Preface

This book has been an outcome of determined endeavour from a group of educationists in the field. The primary objective was to involve a broad spectrum of professionals from diverse cultural background involved in the field for developing new researches. The book not only targets students but also scholars pursuing higher research for further enhancement of the theoretical and practical applications of the subject.

The reproduction or representation of a breast's form is done for medical examination using breast imaging. There are several techniques of breast imaging, such as X-ray, ultrasound, magnetic resonance imaging (MRI) and scintimammography. X-ray techniques, particularly mammography, allow the early detection of breast cancer, while galactography helps to visualize the milk ducts and detect lesions. MRI serves as an alternative to mammography, for the detection of cancer. Ultrasound performs the imaging of the breast and may be used either as a diagnostic tool or a screening procedure. For mammograms with suspicious results, or for women with post-operative scar tissue, dense breast tissue or breast implants, scintimammography is used to detect cancer cells in breasts. This book traces the progress of breast imaging and highlights some of its key concepts and applications. Some of the diverse topics covered in this book address the varied breast imaging techniques. It is an essential guide for both experts and students alike.

It was an honour to edit such a profound book and also a challenging task to compile and examine all the relevant data for accuracy and originality. I wish to acknowledge the efforts of the contributors for submitting such brilliant and diverse chapters in the field and for endlessly working for the completion of the book. Last, but not the least; I thank my family for being a constant source of support in all my research endeavours.

Editor

Quantitative metric profiles capture three-dimensional temporospatial architecture to discriminate cellular functional states

Lindsey McKeen-Polizzotti[1†], Kira M Henderson[1†], Basak Oztan[2], C Cagatay Bilgin[2], Bülent Yener[2] and George E Plopper[1*]

Abstract

Background: Computational analysis of tissue structure reveals sub-visual differences in tissue functional states by extracting quantitative signature features that establish a diagnostic profile. Incomplete and/or inaccurate profiles contribute to misdiagnosis.

Methods: In order to create more complete tissue structure profiles, we adapted our cell-graph method for extracting quantitative features from histopathology images to now capture temporospatial traits of three-dimensional collagen hydrogel cell cultures. Cell-graphs were proposed to characterize the spatial organization between the cells in tissues by exploiting graph theory wherein the nuclei of the cells constitute the *nodes* and the approximate adjacency of cells are represented with *edges*. We chose 11 different cell types representing non-tumorigenic, pre-cancerous, and malignant states from multiple tissue origins.

Results: We built cell-graphs from the cellular hydrogel images and computed a large set of features describing the structural characteristics captured by the graphs over time. Using three-mode tensor analysis, we identified the five most significant features (metrics) that capture the compactness, clustering, and spatial uniformity of the 3D architectural changes for each cell type throughout the time course. Importantly, four of these metrics are also the discriminative features for our histopathology data from our previous studies.

Conclusions: Together, these descriptive metrics provide rigorous quantitative representations of image information that other image analysis methods do not. Examining the changes in these five metrics allowed us to easily discriminate between all 11 cell types, whereas differences from visual examination of the images are not as apparent. These results demonstrate that application of the cell-graph technique to 3D image data yields discriminative metrics that have the potential to improve the accuracy of image-based tissue profiles, and thus improve the detection and diagnosis of disease.

Background

Errors in the structural organization and function of tissues are a major cause of many devastating human diseases, including cancer. Currently, clinicians use diagnostic profiles to distinguish between varying degrees of tissue health and disease. These profiles typically contain a combination of quantitative (e.g., expression of molecular markers, epidemiology) and qualitative (e.g., image-based assessment) data. The primary means of diagnosing most cancers is histopathological examination of a biopsy, and the resulting diagnostic profile serves as the "gold standard" in almost all cases. This examination focuses on the following traits [1]:

1. *Nuclear atypia*: The morphological atypicality of a cell (such as polymorphism, multinucleated cells, and gigantic cells) often but not always implies cancer.

2. *Cytoplasmic changes*: Higher values of the ratio of the surface area of the nucleus to that of the cytoplasm may imply cancer.

* Correspondence: ploppg@rpi.edu
† Contributed equally
[1]Department of Biology, Center for Biotechnology and Interdisciplinary Studies, Rensselaer Polytechnic Institute, Troy, New York, USA
Full list of author information is available at the end of the article

3. presence of other changes such as increased vascularity and necrosis.

4. *Cellularity*: An increase in the number/density of cells within a tissue may indicate proliferation of a cancer, or simply an increase in inflammatory processes.

5. *Cell distribution*: The location and organization of cells relative to each other is used to identify cancer. For example, cancerous brain tissues have more randomly distributed cells, whereas areas of inflammation have more evenly distributed cells. The diagnostic profile for prostate cancer includes digital rectal examination, expression levels of prostate serum antigen (PSA), and numerous image-based approaches (e.g., magnetic resonance imaging, ultrasound, CT scan, conventional biopsy/Gleason score) (reviewed in [2]). Both the incidence and mortality of prostate cancer have declined in the US and UK since the addition of PSA levels to this profile, yet the diagnostic value of the PSA test is still debated [3]. Many other molecular markers for prostate cancer are now appearing in the literature [4], though the functional roles of many are unknown. A similar situation exists for diagnosing breast cancers, such that the rate of misdiagnosis varies widely between clinicians and is nearly 40% in some cases [5].

Much of the classification errors in diagnosing solid tumors stems from incomplete tumor profiles, i.e. understanding the relationship between the functional state of a tissue and its structural organization. For example, the imaging methods used to grade the severity of solid tumors rely largely on the observations of the pathologist and qualitative metrics such as the thickness of an epithelial cell layer, atypical cell morphology, and relative uptake of contrast agents [6]. Even expression of most molecular markers is measured qualitatively, e.g., by the degree of staining with an antibody [7]. While these methods can enrich diagnostic profiles, they largely fail to address the underlying structural malfunctions that form the basis for the disease. Development of quantitative tools for image analysis and predictive modeling is thus a rapidly expanding field, showing great promise for improving diagnostic accuracy [6,8,9].

We recently developed a graph theoretical-based method, called cell-graphs, for capturing structural characteristics of histopathological images that enabled distinguishing healthy, damaged, and cancerous states of brain, breast, and bone tissues [10-12]. Our earlier studies relied on modeling functional state via the spatial organization of cell nuclei within standard histological biopsy images, and achieved accuracy equivalent to current diagnostic standards. For example, despite the visual resemblance between damaged and diseased brain tissues (both display a high cell density), the features extracted from the cell-graphs were able to distinguish between them with greater than 95% accuracy[10].

Cell-graphs are generalizations of Delaunay Triangulations that were previously used to model the spatial distribution of cells in a tissue by encoding a pair-wise relationship between two vertices [13]. In a cell-graph, nodes (or vertices) represent the cell nuclei and pairs of nodes are connected by a link (or edge) based the chemical, physical or spatial, biological relationship between them. Distance-based construction of edges was most commonly used in previous studies [10-12,14-17]. Application of graph theory to these cell-graphs provides a rich set of computational metrics that represent the structural characteristics of the underlying tissue samples. Utilization of machine learning techniques then allows us to classify different functional states of tissues. We elected to use graph theory-based methods because they have an impressive record of modeling complex relationships in numerous contexts. Real-world graphs of varying types and scales have been extensively investigated [18] in technological [19-21], social [22-28] and biological systems [29-31]. In spite of their different domains, such self-organizing structures unexpectedly exhibit common classes of descriptive spatial (topological) features [17,18,21,23,32]. These features are quantified by definition of computable metrics.

The major novelties of this study include: 1) cell-graph analysis of three-dimensional tempero-spatial tissue samples with various origins and functional states, 2) differentiation between the tissue samples based on unique structural formations relative to functional state, 3) exploitation of multi-way analysis to identify the most influential signatures that capture most of the variation in the data, and 4) establishing a correspondence between cell-graph features for *in-vitro* and *in-vivo* histology samples. The previous cell-graph work was confined to two-dimensional histology samples stained with haematoxylin and eosin. In this study we expanded our analysis to temporal analysis of 3D hydrogel models of the three most common types of tissues that develop solid tumors (epithelial, connective, and neural), to explore additional temporospatial information currently inaccessible in conventional histology samples. 2D and 3D cell culture models form the foundation for virtually all drug screening regimens and remain valid in vitro representations of human tissues[33]. Furthermore, 3D cell culture is widely used in the fields of biology and medicine to study the organization of cells in native extracellular matrix (ECM) constructs [34-36]. Likewise, cell lines with varying molecular mechanisms and protein characteristics are often used to represent a range of functional health states. Although there are limitations to *in vitro* studies, the cell lines used in this study represent a range of tissue types allowing us to directly compare the structural profiles of various functional states through analysis of cell-graph metrics. The resulting sets of cell-graph metrics that evolved over time yielded a distinct profile for each cell/tissue type, and thus have potential to identify structure-function relationship changes in a three-dimensional cell culture system. The long term goal of this study is to further understand cancer models by interpreting changes in metrics in terms of underlying changes in molecular mechanisms of cancer progression. To uncover these mechanisms, it is necessary to simplify the model in order to isolate specific cell-collagen-I interactions.

Methods

Cell Culture Techniques

The different cell types and their respective culture conditions are listed in Table 1. The functional categories of each cell type are listed in Table 2.

Flourescence Imaging

Gels were fixed using 3% paraformaldehyde at 6 different time points (hours): 10, 16, 24, 72, 120, 168. Each was washed with PBS, then stained with nucleic acid dye (sytox green). Images of cells encapsulated within collagen-I hydrogels were captured using a Zeiss LSM 510 META confocal microscope with a 10X dry objective. Representative Z-stack images of 100 μm thickness with 900 μm × 900 μm cross-section area were collected for five samples of each time point.

Segmentation of Nuclei

To segment the cell nuclei, we first binarize the images. Binarization separates the image values into foreground and background classes. In our context, the foreground class represents the cell nuclei, whereas the background

Table 2 Cell Line Categories

	Connective	Epithelial	Neural
Non-tumorigenic	NHOst, hDFB	MCF10A, RWPE-1	NHA
Cancer	MG63	AU565, MDA-MB-231, MCF7, DU145	U118MG

class represents the combination of cells and extracellular proteins. Binarization is accomplished by comparing the image values against a threshold function. Considering the large number of images that need to be processed, we employ Otsu's simple but effective automatic threshold selection algorithm[37] that determines a global (single) threshold for the image based on the histogram of image values. Each connected component in the resulting binary image corresponds to a nucleus and the coordinates of the centroids of these nuclei are calculated to identify the coordinates of the node (vertex) set for cell-graph generation.

Generation of Cell-Graphs

After obtaining the set of vertices in the images, we construct the cell-graphs based on the pairwise nuclei distances [10-12,14-17]. We assume that a biological relation exist between two nuclei, i.e. a link (or edge) between two nodes is established, if the Euclidean distance between the corresponding centroids are less than a threshold D. We tested 3 thresholds: $D = 60, 75$, and 90 μm. The graphs corresponding to 60 and 90 μm turned out to be too sparse and dense, respectively. Therefore, we decided to use 75 μm as the threshold.

Figure 1 illustrates the steps involved in extracting cell-graph features in 3D. Figure 1a shows an example

Table 1 Cell Culture Conditions

Name	Cell Type	Media
MCF10A	Precancerous Human Breast Epithelial	Dulbecco's Minimum Essential Media (DMEM)/F12, 5%Horse Serum (HS), 1% Penicillin Streptomycin (PS), 20 ng/ml Epidermal Growth Factor (EGF), .05 μg/ml Hydrocortisone, 10 μg/ml Insulin-bovine, 100 ng/ml Cholera Toxin
AU565	Human Breast Cancer HER2+/ER-	Roswell Park Memorial Institute-1640 Medium (RPMI), 10%Fetal Bovine Serum (FBS), 1%Ps
MCF7	Human Breast Cancer HER2-/ER+	Minimum Essential Media (MEM)α, 10%FBS, 1%PS, 0.01 mg/ml Insulin- bovine
MDA- MB231	Human Breast Cancer HER2+/ER2+	DMEM, 10%FBS, 1% PS
hDFB	Human Dermal Fibroblasts	DMEM, 10%FBS, 1%PS
NHA	Normal Human Astrocytes	NHA media from Lonza
U118MG	Human Glioblastoma	DMEM, 10% FBS, 1%PS
NHOst	Normal Human Osteoblast	NHOst media from Lonza
MG63	Human Osteosarcoma	DMEM, 10%FBS, 1%PS
RWPE-1	Non-tumorigenic Human Prostate	Keratinocyte serum free media from Gibco
DU145	Human Prostate Carcinoma	DMEM, 10%FBS, 1%PS

The eleven human cell lines and the corresponding culture media used in our experiments are listed in Table 1. These cells were chosen to represent connective, epithelial and neural tissue shown in Table 2. All cells were grown in conventional 2D cell culture flasks at 37°C in a humidified incubator containing 5% CO_2. Upon reaching 80% confluency, cells were collected by treatment with trypsin-EDTA (SAFC Biosciences), washed in phosphate buffered saline (PBS), counted with a hemocytometer, and suspended in 1% collagen solution (1×10^6 cells/ml) to form hydrogels as described previously [14]. Gels were maintained under the same conditions as the 2D cultures.

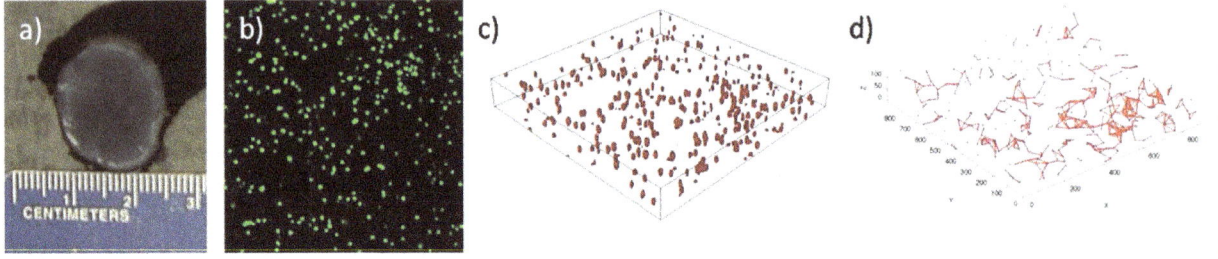

Figure 1 Cell-graphs uncover hidden tissue architecture generated from 3D *in vitro* collagen-I hydrogels. 1a shows a macroscopic image of an MG63 collagen I hydrogel following fixation. 1b displays a two-dimensional slice from 3D confocal image of hydrogel (green = nuclei). 1c is a computer generated representation of confocal image after application nuclei segmentation algorithm to identify cell location in 3D space. 1d shows how cell-graphs are built by applying graph theory to computer-generated confocal image representation.

of MG63 osteosarcoma cells, one of the eleven different types of cells representing various tissue functional states (listed in table 1), encapsulated in a collagen-I hydrogel at time 0. Figure 1b shows a two-dimensional slice of stained nuclei in a confocal fluorescence Z-stack from the hydrogel in Figure 1a. The nuclei were then identified with the application segmentation algorithm described earlier (Figure 1c) to establish nodes within the graph. We applied our cell-graph algorithm to define edges between nodes (Figure 1d) within a distance-based threshold of 75 μm resulting in a 3D cell-graph.

Calculating Features from Cell-Graph Metrics

On each cell-graph, G_i $(V_i(t), E_i(t))$, where $V_i(t)$ and $E_i(t)$ represents the list of vertices and nodes at time point t and i represents the index for the cell line, we calculated 20 metrics as listed in Table 3 based on the structural features of the graphs. We then conducted an analysis in the following section to determine the metrics that have the most discriminative power between the different tissue types over time.

Three-Way Data Modeling and Analysis of Feature-Time-Cell line Joint Relationships

The data is organized to a third-order tensor with features, time, and cell-line modes whose dimensions are I, J, and K, respectively. An entry $\underline{T}_{ijk}$ in the cube corresponds to the value of metric i at time point j for cell-line k where $i = 1,...,20$; $j = 1,..., 6$; and $k = 1, ..., 11$. Two common models in multi-way data analysis are Tucker3 [38-40] and Parallel Factor Analysis (PARAFAC) [41]. A three-way tensor $\underline{T} \in \mathbb{R}^{I \times J \times K}$, where $\mathbb{R}$ denotes the set of reel numbers, is decomposed using a *(P,Q,R)*-component Tucker3 model [42] as

$$\underline{T}_{ijk} = \sum_{r=1}^{R} \sum_{q=1}^{Q} \sum_{p=1}^{P} \underline{G}_{pqr} A_{ip} B_{jq} C_{kr} + \underline{E}_{ijk,}$$

where P, Q, and R indicate the number of components extracted from the first, second and third modes ($P \leq I$, $Q \leq J$, and $R \leq K$, respectively), $A \in \mathbb{R}^{I \times P}$, $B \in \mathbb{R}^{J \times Q}$, and $C \in \mathbb{R}^{K \times R}$, and are the component matrices, $\underline{G} \in \mathbb{R}^{P \times Q \times R}$ is the core tensor, and $\underline{E} \in \mathbb{R}^{I \times J \times K}$ represents the error term.

Parallel Factor Analysis (PARAFAC) [41] or Canonical Decomposition (CANDECOMP)[43] represents a tensor by the linear combination of rank-one tensors. An R-component PARAFAC model on a third-order tensor $\underline{T} \in \mathbb{R}^{I \times J \times K}$ is given by

$$\underline{T}_{ijk} = \sum_{r=1}^{R} a_r \circ b_r \circ c_r + \underline{E}_{ijk}$$

where a_r, b_r, and c_r are the rth columns of the component matrices $A \in \mathbb{R}^{I \times R}$, $B \in \mathbb{R}^{J \times R}$, and $C \in \mathbb{R}^{K \times R}$, respectively, $\underline{E} \in \mathbb{R}^{I \times J \times K}$ is the error term, and $\circ$ denotes the vector outer product.

Prior to the model fitting, the tensor is normalized by first *centering across* the time and cell-line modes and then *scaling within* the features mode by the standard deviations[44]. In order to capture most of the variation in data, we first unfolded the tensors in each mode and determined the number of principal components that explains at least 95% of the variation in the data. The Tucker3 model was fit with $6 \times 5 \times 8$ core tensor and the PARAFAC model was fit using 8-components to the normalized tensor where 93.7% and 89.6% of the variations in the data are captured, respectively. The analysis then focused on the feature mode in order to identify a subset of the cell-graph metrics that are more influential than the others to explain the variation in the three-way data. For this purpose, we used the Hotelling's T^2 statistics and the sum of squared residuals of each mode. The larger the value of these statistics, the easier it is to distinguish between the different metrics and, therefore, they are useful indicators of the influence of metrics as outliers to explain the variation in the data. These statistics are built in the MATLAB PLS Toolbox 4.0 and MATLAB Tensor Toolbox 2.4 [45]. Figure 2 shows the Hotelling's T^2 values versus the sum of squared residuals and Figure 3 shows only the Hotelling's T^2 values of each metric. From these figures, the most influential

Table 3 Cell-graph metrics, interpretations, and categories

Index	Metric Label	Metric Interpretation	Metric Category
1	Average Degree	Number of edges per node	Compactness
2	Clustering Coefficient C	Ratio of total number of edges among the neighbours of the node to the total number of edges that can exist among the neighbours of the node per node	Clustering
3	Clustering Coefficient D	Ratio of total number of edges among the neighbours of the node and the node itself to the total number of edges that can exist among the neighbours of the node and the node itself per node	Clustering
4	Clustering Coefficient E	Ratio of total number of edges among the neighbours of the node to the total number of edges that can exist among the neighbours of the node per node excluding the isolated nodes	Clustering
5	Average Eccentricity	Average of node eccentricities where the eccentricity of a node is the maximum shortest path length from the node to any other node in the graph	Compactness
6	Diameter	Maximum of node eccentricities	Compactness
7	Radius	Minimum of node eccentricities	Compactness
8	Average Path Length	Average distance between the nodes of a graph, where the distance between two nodes is the number of edges in the shortest path that connects them	Compactness
9	Hop Plot Exponent	Slope of the line fitted to the hop plot values in log-log domain, where the hop plot value for hop h is the number of node pairs for which the path length between the pairs is less than or equal to h	Compactness
10	Giant Connected Component Ratio	Ratio between the number of nodes in the largest connected component in the graph and total the number of nodes	Clustering
11	Number of Connected Components	Number of clusters in the graph excluding the isolated nodes	Clustering
12	Average Connected Component Size	Number of nodes per connected component	Clustering
13	Percentage of Isolated Points	Percentage of the isolated nodes in the graph, where an isolated node has a degree of 0	Compactness
14	Percentage of End Points	Percentage of the isolated nodes in the graph, where an isolated node has a degree of 1	Compactness
15	Number of Central Points	Number of nodes within the graph whose eccentricity is equal to the graph radius	Compactness
16	Percentage of Central Points	Percentage of the central points in the graph	Compactness
17	Average of Edge Lengths		
18	Standard Deviation of Edge Lengths		
19	Skewness of Edge Lengths	Statistics of the edge length distribution in the graph	Spatial Uniformity
20	Kurtosis of Edge Lengths		

metrics are chosen as number of central points, clustering coefficient D, percentage of isolated points, standard deviation of edge lengths, and number of connected components.

Two-Way Data Modeling and Analysis of Feature-Tissue Joint Relationships

Our histology data set contains 329 malignant and 210 benign brain samples, 128 malignant and 195 benign breast samples, and 49 malignant and 20 benign bone samples. The average of the 20 cell-graph metrics over the samples of each tumor-type is taken to construct 6 × 20 two-way data matrix. In order to determine the influence of a metric to describe the variations in the data, a singular value decomposition (SVD) -based technique is employed. First, the data is normalized by centering across the tumor-type and scaling within the features mode. Next, the data is decomposed into its *factor scores* and *loadings* using SVD. Finally, the influence of a metric is measured by the sum of absolute factor scores corresponding to the first K factor loadings where K is the number of principal components that explains at least 95% of the variation in the data. K is determined to be three, reflecting the number of different tissue types.

Results

We extended our previously published cell-graph method of feature extraction into three dimensional collagen-I hydrogel cultures that remodel over time. We extracted the set of 20 quantitative features (table 3) from the generated cell-graphs. We then applied tensor

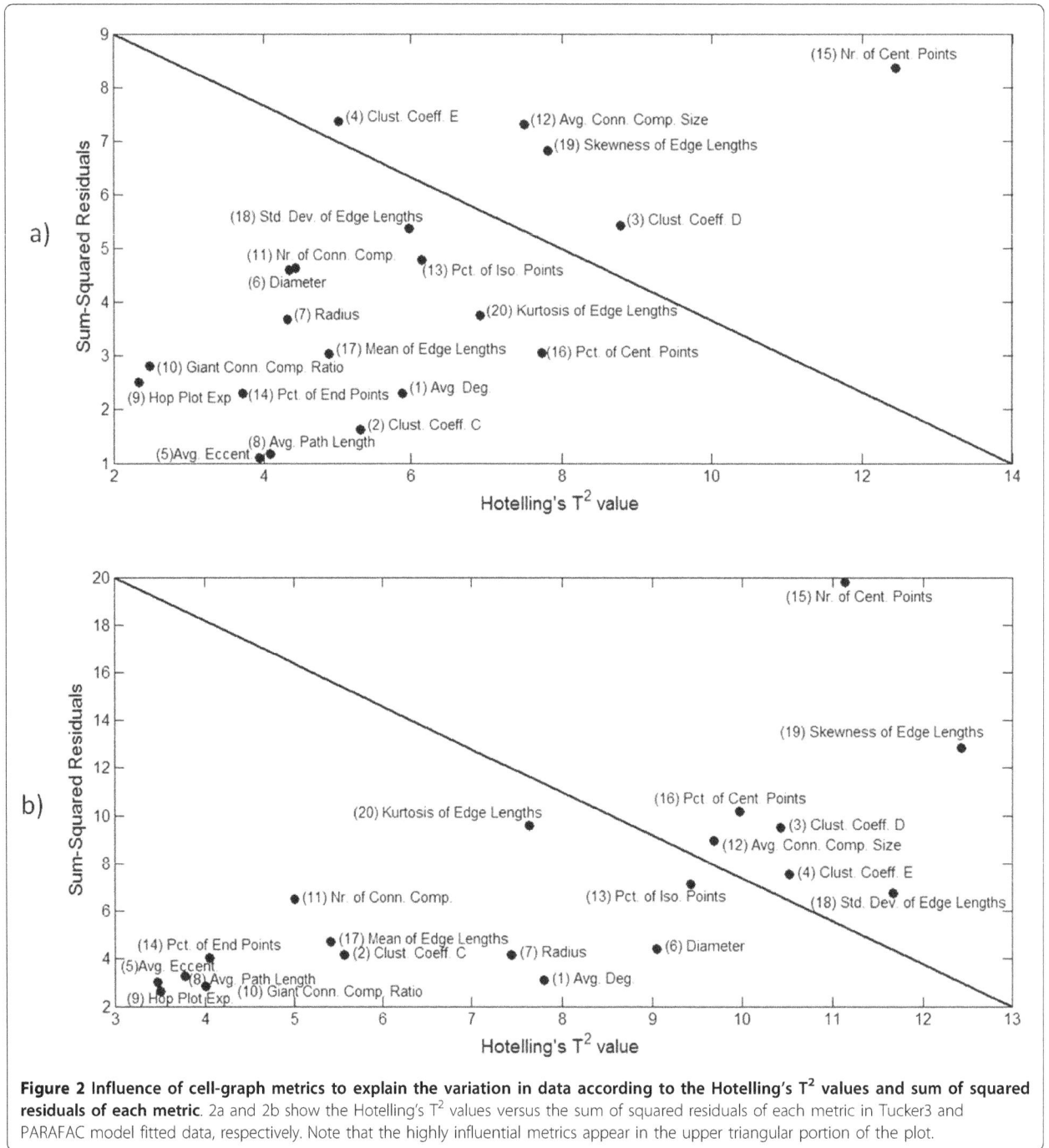

Figure 2 Influence of cell-graph metrics to explain the variation in data according to the Hotelling's T^2 values and sum of squared residuals of each metric. 2a and 2b show the Hotelling's T^2 values versus the sum of squared residuals of each metric in Tucker3 and PARAFAC model fitted data, respectively. Note that the highly influential metrics appear in the upper triangular portion of the plot.

analysis to the extracted features using Tucker3 and PARAFAC models to identify the features that contribute the most to discriminating between different cell/tissue temporospatial architectures over time. Figure 2a and 2b show the influence of each metric according to Hotelling's T^2 and sum of squared residuals scores for Tucker3 and PARAFAC models, respectively. The most important metrics are located in the upper right triangular region of these figures. Figure 3a and 3b shows

Hotelling's T^2 scores only for Tucker3 and PARAFAC models, respectively. The metrics are displayed in increasing importance from the lower left corner to the upper right corner in this figure. We determined the five most important metrics for distinguishing between different hydrogel architectures over time based on their nuclear organization using the combination of results from Figures 2 and 3: number of central points, percentage of isolated points, number of connected components,

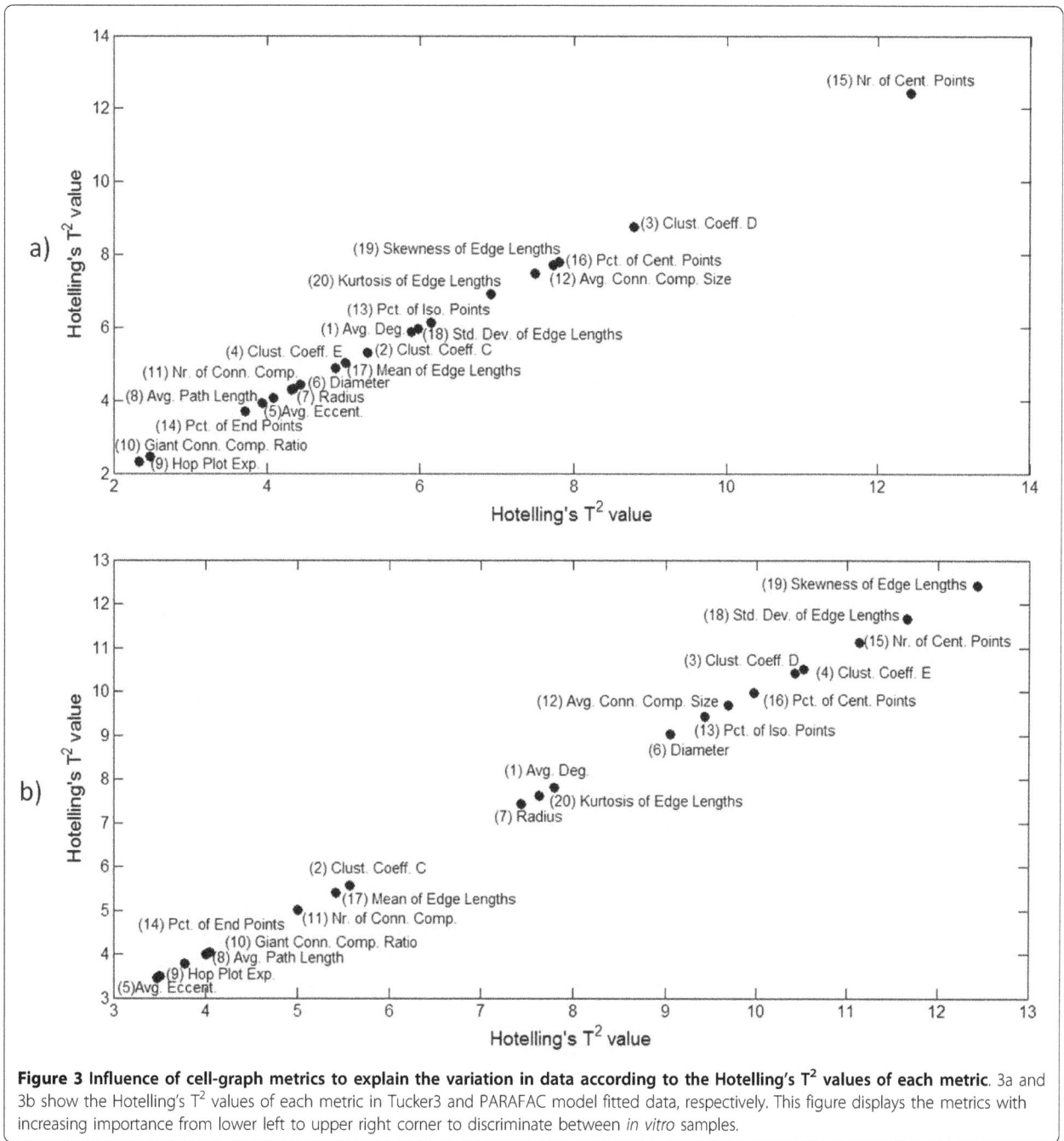

Figure 3 Influence of cell-graph metrics to explain the variation in data according to the Hotelling's T² values of each metric. 3a and 3b show the Hotelling's T² values of each metric in Tucker3 and PARAFAC model fitted data, respectively. This figure displays the metrics with increasing importance from lower left to upper right corner to discriminate between *in vitro* samples.

clustering coefficient D, and standard deviation of edge lengths.

To validate our findings, we used the cell-graphs for the histology data that we analyzed using a similar framework in our earlier studies [10-12]. The discriminatory power of the extracted cell-graph metrics was successfully shown for the malignant and benign histology samples of brain [10], breast [11], and bone [12] tissues. Since these samples were surgically removed histopathology samples no temporal information is available. Thus, our histology data has two modes: tissue samples and features extracted on these samples. These data sets are obtained from 2D imaging of tissue samples from pathology department archives thus they do not have the depth information. Figure 4 shows the influence of cell-graph metrics to describe the variations in the histology data.

Figure 5 shows the Venn diagram of the five most significant metrics for the histology and the *in-vitro* data. We found considerable overlap between the two sets of discriminative metrics as displayed by the Venn diagram in Figure 5c. This confirms that our 3D hydrogels

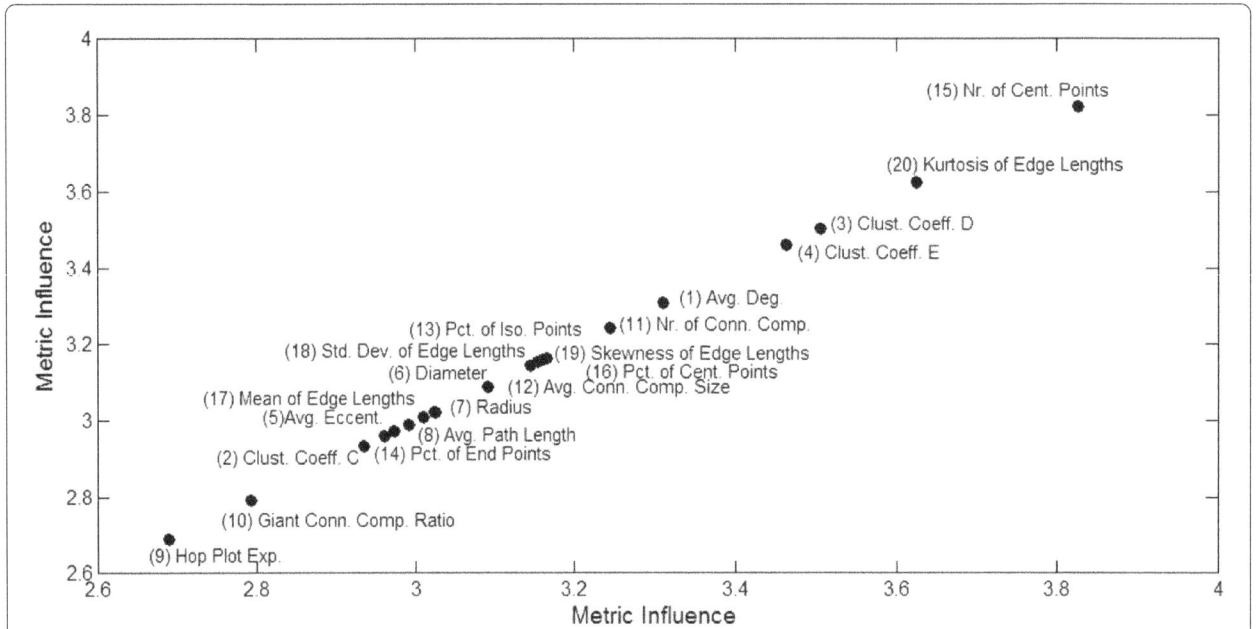

Figure 4 Influence of the cell-graph metrics to describe the variations in the histology data. This figure displays the metrics with increasing importance from lower left to upper right corner to discriminate between histology samples.

maintain important structural properties found in histological samples.

We grouped the metrics into subcategories that describe particular aspects of structural organization. The *percentage of isolated points* and *number of central points* reflect the overall compactness of a cell-graph, as shown in Figure 6. The compactness metrics can quantify changes in cell density over time that we represented in the biological images in the top right of Figure 6. The change in cell density from low to high results in higher

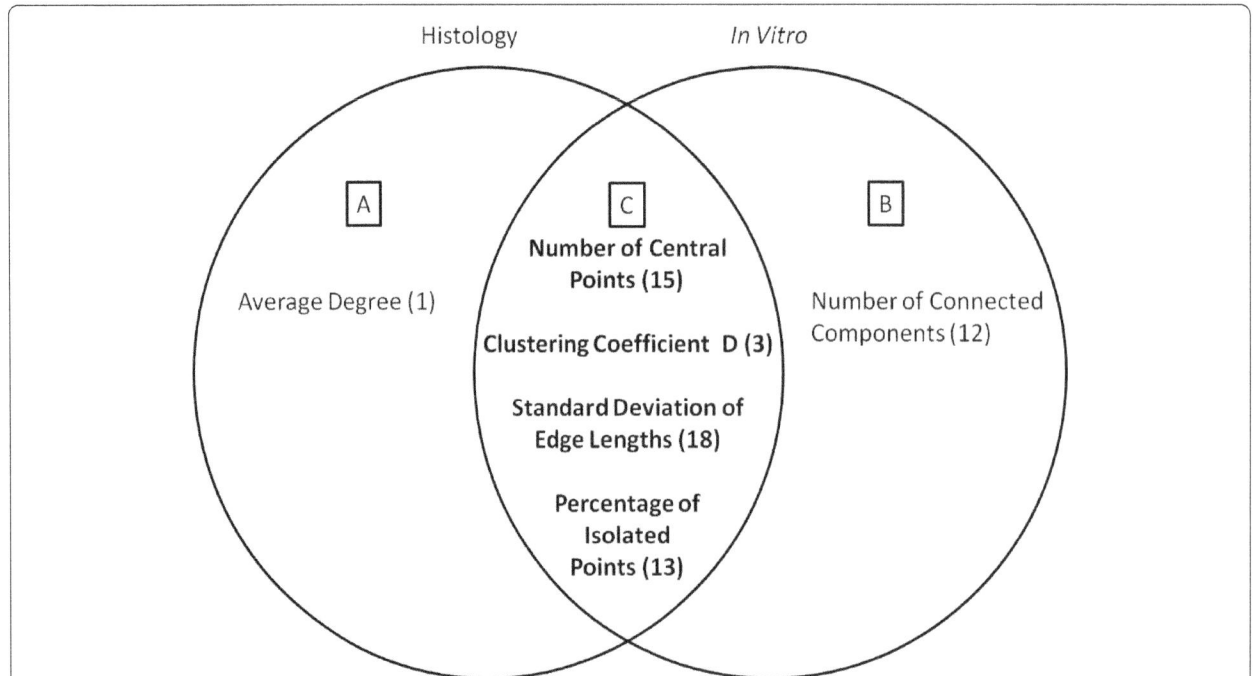

Figure 5 Histology and *In Vitro* tissue both have similar as well as unique metrics that can be used to distinguish between tissue types. The Venn diagram displays the most important metrics found by singular value decomposition and tensor analysis for the histology tissue and *in vitro* tissue images, respectively. The most discriminative metrics from the histology samples, *in vitro* samples and shared discriminative metrics are shown in figures 5a, 5b and 5c respectively. Numbers refer to feature numbers in Table 3.

	Sample Diagram of Cell Graph	Description of Metrics	Representative Biological Change
Compactness	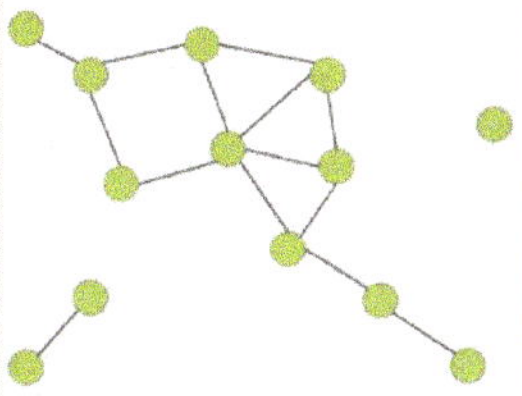	**Percentage of Isolated Points:** is the percent of isolated nodes in a graph. A node is isolated if it has no edges to neighboring nodes. In this sample there is one isolated node which is equivalent to 7.7% of nodes in the graph.	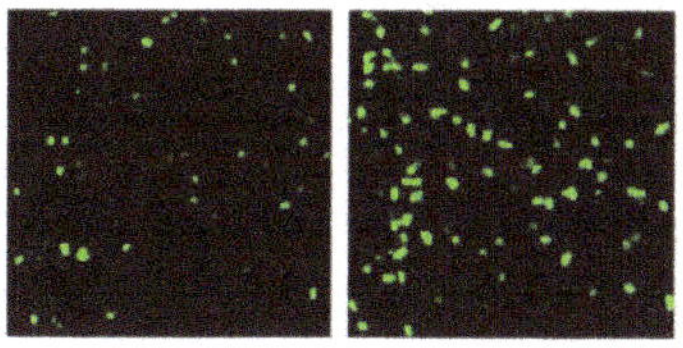
	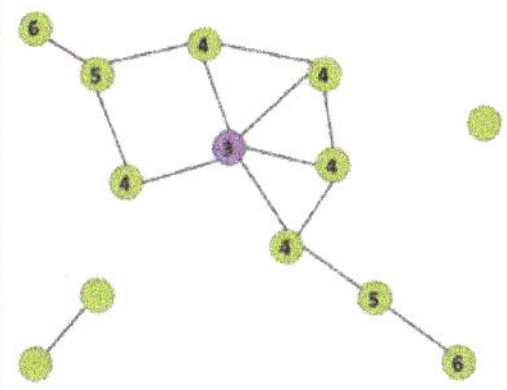	**Number of Central Points:** is the number of nodes within the graph whose eccentricity is equal to the minimum eccentricity of the graph(radius). Eccentricity of a node is the maximum shortest path length from the node to any other node in the graph. The central point nodes tend to be greater in graphs with discrete clusters or high density. In this sample there is only one node whose eccentricity is equal to the graph radius.	**Low Density**　　**High Density** *Larger Percent of Isolated Points*　　*Smaller Percent of Isolated Points* *Small Number of Central Points*　　*Large Number of Central Points*
Clustering	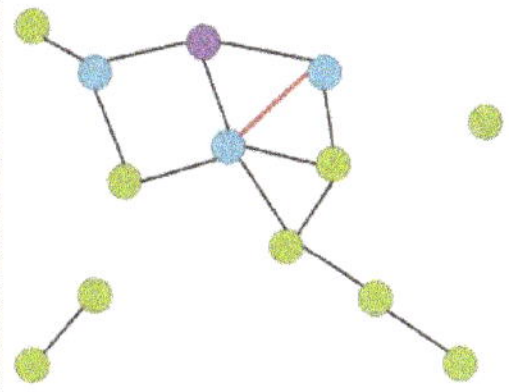	**Number of Connected Components:** A connected component is defined as at least 2 nodes connected by an edge. This sample has 2 connected components because the isolated node does not count. **Clustering Coefficient D:** represents the percentage of connections between the neighbors of the node and the node itself. The purple node has 3 neighbors(blue) and 2 of the neighbors are also linked(red) so this node would have a clustering coefficient of 2/3.	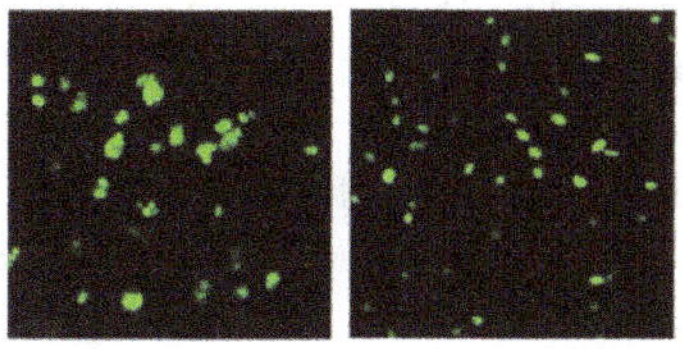 **Discrete Clusters　Uniform Distribution** *High Number of Connected Components*　*Low Number of Connected Components* *High Clustering Coefficient*　*Low Clustering Coefficient*
Uniformity	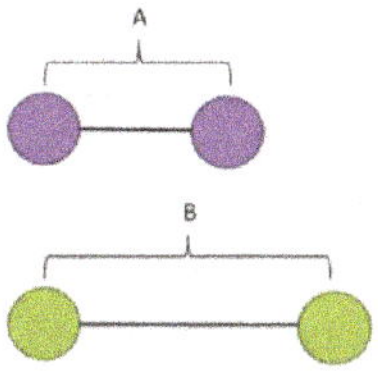	**Standard Deviation of Edge Lengths:** The edge length is defined as the spatial distance between the centers of two connected nuclei. Both the purple nuclei and the green nuclei are within the same pre-defined threshold to define an edge, however the actual distance of their edges varies and is captured by the edge length metric. This metric measures the standard deviation of the average edge length within a cell graph to characterize the uniformity of a sample.	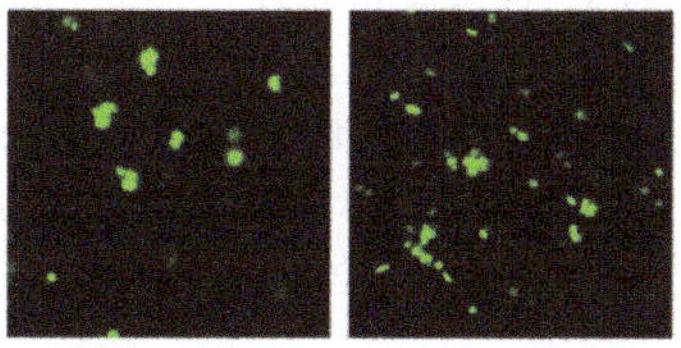 **Dense Cluster　　Disperse Cluster** *Low Standard Deviation of Edge Lengths*　*High Standard Deviation of Edge Lengths*
Visually Complex Patterns of Nuclei	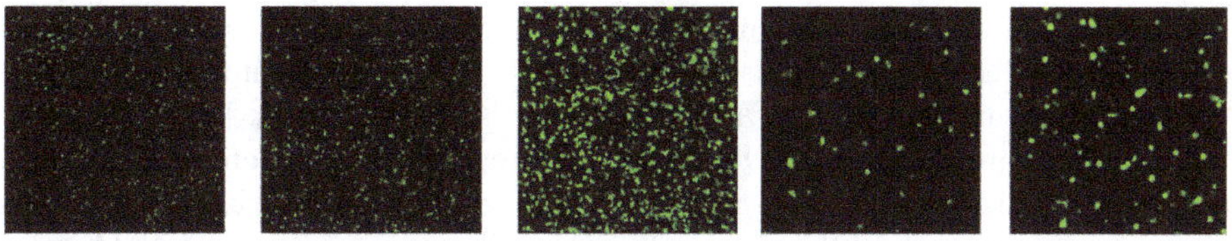		

Figure 6 **The most significant metrics determined from the normalized tensor analysis describe the compactness, clustering and uniformity properties of tissue structure**. The diagrams on the left illustrate the metrics described in the central column. Representative images in the right column show variation for the corresponding metrics from the left column. The final row gives examples of the images analyzed in this study to show how it is difficult to quantify the important metrics by eye.

compactness and is captured by an increase in number of central points and a decrease in the percent of isolated points.

The second subcategory of descriptive metrics, *number of connected components* and *clustering coefficient D*, capture the extent of cell clustering in a sample. As seen in the representative biological images in the clustering row of Figure 6, samples with discrete clusters have a high number of connected components and a high clustering coefficient. On the contrary, uniformly distributed cells (non-clustering) have a low number of connected components and a low clustering coefficient, i. e. a majority of the cells in the sample are connected within a single connected component. The *standard deviation of edge lengths* describes the consistency in the distance distribution between the nuclei, thus establishing the level of uniformity in the sample. A sample with uniform-dense clusters, as shown in the lower right of Figure 6, results in a low standard deviation edge of lengths and high uniformity. Alternatively, a sample with a disperse cell cluster distribution yields a high standard deviation edge of lengths and a lower uniformity.

The biological images from Figure 6 represent the extremes of the three subcategories of metrics, compactness, clustering and uniformity. In reality, the hydrogel architecture of different cell types typically lies between the extremes of each metric, and changes over time as the structure develops. The last row in Figure 6 gives examples of the variety of visually complex patterns of cell nuclei, from 5 different cell types, analyzed as part of this study. In these instances, visual inspection of hydrogel architecture images does not distinguish between the cell types and time points. Therefore, we used the cell-graphs and quantified the changes in metric values over time to differentiate the cell types from each other.

Figure 7 shows that the data trends from five cell-graph metrics are sufficient to distinguish between the hydrogel architectures formed by eleven different cell types. In Figure 7a, the raw data of the five metrics (determined by tensor analysis, Figures 2 and 3) were plotted for each cell type over time. Individual plots for each metric in Figure 7a can be found in Additional files 1, 2, 3, 4 and 5. To directly compare the metric trends between cell type architectures, we generated Figure 7b as a visual representation of the same data in Figure 7a. Figure 7b shows that the metrics for each cell type exhibit a distinct pattern of value changes over time. The patterns indicate both the direction of change (i.e. up arrow, down arrow or flat line) and relative magnitude (i.e. number of arrows). In addition, we performed two-sample Kolmogorov-Smirnov tests between pairs of cell-lines to investigate if the corresponding metrics belong to the same probability distribution

function. For each pair of cell-lines, the test is performed over the five most significant features. If the two cell-lines come from the same probability distributions, the result of the test is 0, and 1 otherwise. The results of the five tests are combined by logical *OR* operation. Figure 7c shows the results for the 11 cell lines used in our experiment at 10% significance level. It is clearly seen that most of the cell-lines belong to different probability distributions that the influential metrics are effective in distinguishing between the different cell-types. From this large set of data, only the data from the closely related AU565 and MB231 breast cancer cells to lack statistical significance. This data is capable of discriminating all cell lines from each other except between AU565 and MB231.

The first six cell types listed in Figure 7b are of epithelial origin (breast and prostate cells) representing a range of cancer grades from pre-cancerous to metastatic. Each has a unique metric profile. The standard deviation of edge lengths metric values distinguish the MCF10A (pre-cancerous) breast epithelial cells from the AU565 breast cancer cells because they trend in opposite directions over time. Like the AU565 cells, the MCF7 cells also show similar trends to the MCF10A cells for the percentage of isolated points and average connected component size metrics. However, in addition to the opposing standard deviation of edge lengths trend that distinguishes the AU565 from the MCF10A cells, the MCF7 cells also show an opposing decreasing trend in the number of central points. The metric trends for MB231 cells also differ from those for MCF10A. While the uniformity metric trends for MB231 cells resemble those for the MCF7 cells, the metrics that capture clustering and compactness show opposite trends. Compared to the other breast cancer cells, the percentage of isolated points and average connected component size for MB231 cells show opposite trends. Interestingly, the non-tumorigenic RWPE1 prostate cells and the MCF10A breast cells have nearly identical metric trends with only a slight difference in the magnitude of the average connected component size. Likewise, the metric changes between non-tumorigenic RWPE-1 prostate cells and metastatic DU145 prostate cells are similar to those seen between the non-tumorigenic MCF10A breast cells and the breast cancer lines.

The non-tumorigenic NHA cells and the cancerous U118 cells are glial cells from brain tissue origin. The brain hydrogels exhibit a pattern of metric trends which differentiates them from the hydrogels of other cell/tissue types in this study.

Although the pattern of metric trends is similar in both of the brain hydrogels, the NHA cells are distinguishable from their cancerous counterpart (U118) due to the opposite trend in the number of central points

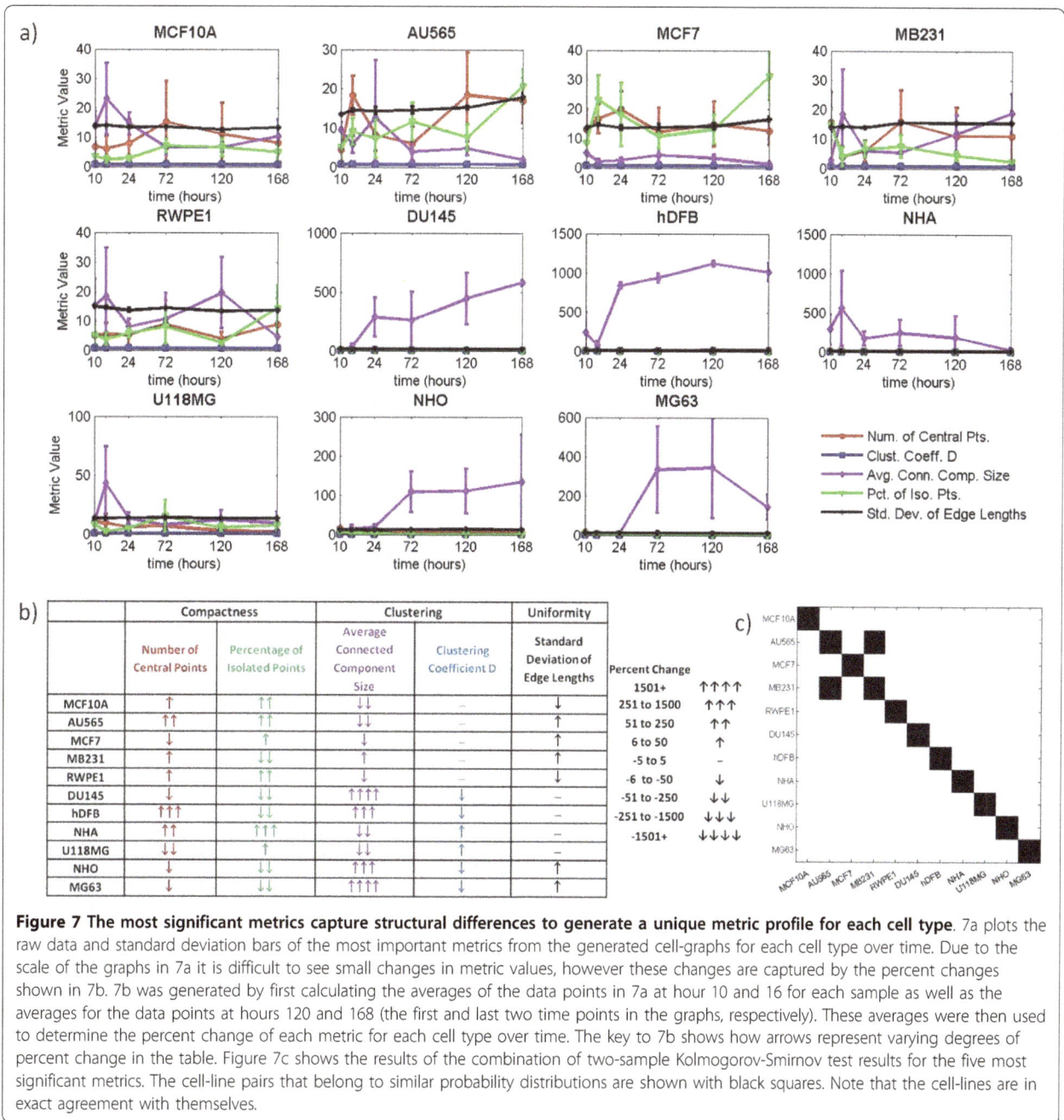

Figure 7 The most significant metrics capture structural differences to generate a unique metric profile for each cell type. 7a plots the raw data and standard deviation bars of the most important metrics from the generated cell-graphs for each cell type over time. Due to the scale of the graphs in 7a it is difficult to see small changes in metric values, however these changes are captured by the percent changes shown in 7b. 7b was generated by first calculating the averages of the data points in 7a at hour 10 and 16 for each sample as well as the averages for the data points at hours 120 and 168 (the first and last two time points in the graphs, respectively). These averages were then used to determine the percent change of each metric for each cell type over time. The key to 7b shows how arrows represent varying degrees of percent change in the table. Figure 7c shows the results of the combination of two-sample Kolmogorov-Smirnov test results for the five most significant metrics. The cell-line pairs that belong to similar probability distributions are shown with black squares. Note that the cell-lines are in exact agreement with themselves.

and the magnitude change in the percentage of isolated points. Both of the metrics that distinguish between the non-tumorigenic and cancerous brain cells are measures of compactness. Similar to the brain cells, the representative bone hydrogel architecture (NHOst and MG63) have a distinct set of metric trends, which differentiate them from the other tissue types in the study. The NHOst and MG63 are distinguishable from each other due to the magnitude of the average connected component size, a measure of clustering. Interestingly, the DU145 cells (metastatic prostate epithelial) show similarity between the bone cells (NHOst and MG63) and the fibroblasts (hDFB). The only variations between the DU145 and bone cells are the trends of the standard deviation of edge lengths. The DU145 compared to the hDFB only show different trends in the number of central points. Similarly, the MB231 cell line (metastatic breast epithelial) shows the same pattern of metric trends as the hDFB (fibroblasts), with differences in magnitude of change and slight variation in the clustering coefficient D and standard deviation of edge lengths.

Discussion

A hallmark of all complex tissues is carefully organized cell and ECM architecture. We believe this architecture is determined, at least in part, by a set of organizational "rules" that determine how cells orient with respect to each other. According to our model, both damaged and cancerous tissues exhibit architectures that deviate significantly from the non-tumorigenic state dictated by these rules, but it is very difficult to quantify changes in these rules by eye. Teasing out the characteristic differences between different functional states in a tissue thus benefits from identifying and understanding the biological foundation for these rules.

This study represents the first attempt at defining these rules, by assigning rigorous quantitative metrics to architectural properties of 3D hydrogels containing distinct cell types. 3D collagen-I hydrogels provide elements of tissue structure which are not obtainable in traditional 2D histology imaging. In this model system, cells from diverse tissue origins interact differently with the collagen-I ECM and each other, resulting in a range of tissue architectures over time. The features extracted from the cell-graphs of 3D confocal images of cell nuclei from the hydrogels are analyzed using Tucker3 model to extract signature graph features. While it is very difficult to quantify important metrics from our images by eye, our computational approach uncovers hidden relationships in these images to discriminate between cell types in 3D, over time.

Our method improves upon histopathological image analysis using nuclear distance-based cell-graphs [13] to include more aspects of tissue structure-function relationships. Comparison of the Singular Value Decomposition analysis of our 2D histology data and tensor analysis of our 3D *in vitro* feature sets revealed partial overlap of the most significant discriminating metrics. In Figure 5a, the *average degree* metric represents the connectivity and compactness of the 2D histology samples is the most significant for distinguishing between tissue types. The most significant metric in Figure 5b, *number of connected components*, characterizes the clustering of the sample. The overlapping metrics in Figure 5c show that histology and *in vitro* samples share metrics that characterize the compactness, clustering and uniformity of cellular structure organization in order to distinguish between tissue types.

With the metrics determined by tensor analysis, we were able to distinguish multiple functional states of tissues based solely on their nuclear organization in a 3D collagen-I hydrogel. Using the metric profiles for each cell type (Figure 7b), we are able to discriminate different grades of breast and prostate cancer due to a variety of characteristic differences in trends between cell types. The profiles also successfully distinguish non-tumorigenic

brain and bone tissue organization from their cancerous counterparts. However, it is only a change in magnitude of the average connected component size that is able to distinguish between the non-tumorigenic and cancerous bone cells. In the future, we will seek to identify new metrics that better distinguish the differences between mesenchymal tissues.

Our findings present an intriguing possibility, that the data in this study may be capturing features of the epithelial to mesenchymal transition (EMT). EMT is defined as a cellular change from epithelial phenotype to mesenchymal phenotype, involving a loss of adherens junctions, change in intermediate filament expression, and an increase in cell mobility [46-49]. These cellular changes tend to result in a more aggressive, metastatic cancer. While EMT is a characteristic of epithelial tumor progression, it is difficult to quantify using structural changes or molecular markers[50].

In this study, we have included cell types which represent varying stages of EMT, based on their protein expression profile. The breast cancer cell types (MCF10A, AU565, MCF7, and MB231) represent progressive cancer grades from precancerous to metastatic (respectively). Interestingly, our metric profiles capture differences in metric trends between each cell type. The first change between MCF10A and AU565 represents a change in uniformity of cell distribution. The AU565 and MCF7 cell organizations differ by a change in the trend for the *number of central points* metric, representing a change in the clustering of the cells within tissue architectures. MB231 are further discriminated from the MCF7 cells by an increase in the compactness of the tissue, as demonstrated by the change in *number of central points* and *percentage of isolated points*. MB231 also shows a change in *average connected component size* trend compared to the other breast cancer lines. In addition, the MB231 metric profile shares similar trends as the mesenchymal fibroblast cell line as opposed to it's' breast cancer counterpart, MCF10A. The DU145 cells show remarkably similar metrics to both the osteogenic (NHOst, MG63) and fibroblast cells, with a change in only one metric trend between them. The resemblance in trends between the MB231 and DU145 cells with the mesenchymal tissue organizations (particularly the osteogenic lines NHOst and MG63) may reflect the frequency with which breast and prostate cancer metastasizes to bone.

Conclusions

Collectively, our findings demonstrate that our three-dimensional cell-graph methodology is capable of discriminating between structural patterns of cellular organization in model tissues representing different grades of tumor progression and tissue origin that cannot be quantified by eye. The distinguishing features are based on three-mode tensor analysis of graph theoretical properties calculated for each cell type over time. By extending the sensitivity of image analysis and tissue modeling to uncover diagnostic, hidden, temporospatial relationships between cells in model tissues, we feel this is a significant step towards enriching diagnostic profiles for disease. Such enhanced profiles have the potential to improve diagnostic accuracy and identify hidden traits that may suggest new therapeutic interventions.

Additional material

> **Additional file 1: Figure S1- Raw data plots for the number of central points metric**. Shows the raw data for the number of central points metric plotted for each cell type individually over time.
>
> **Additional file 2: Figure S2- Raw data plots for the clustering coefficient D metric**. Shows the raw data for the clustering coefficient D metric plotted for each cell type individually over time.
>
> **Additional file 3: Figure S3- Raw data plots for number the average connected component size metric**. Shows the raw data for the average connected component size metric plotted for each cell type individually over time.
>
> **Additional file 4: Figure S4- Raw data plots for the percentage of isolated points metric**. Shows the raw data for the percentage of isolated points metric plotted for each cell type individually over time.
>
> **Additional file 5: Figure S5- Raw data plots for the standard deviation of edge lengths metric**. Shows the raw data for the standard deviation of edge lengths metric plotted for each cell type individually over time.

Acknowledgements
This work was partially supported by National Institutes of Health Grant #RO1 EB008016.

Author details
[1]Department of Biology, Center for Biotechnology and Interdisciplinary Studies, Rensselaer Polytechnic Institute, Troy, New York, USA. [2]Department of Computer Science, Rensselaer Polytechnic Institute, Troy, New York, USA.

Authors' contributions
LMP and KH carried out the generation and maintenance of cellular 3D collagen I hydrogel cultures, collected confocal fluorescent microscopy images, participated in the design of the study, generation of figures and tables, analysis and interpretation of data, draft, and revision of the manuscript. BO carried out the generation and analysis of 2D histology image and contributed to the revising of the manuscript. CB carried out the 3D fluorescent image segmentation, cell-graph generation, and metric extraction. BY carried out the tensor analysis and contributed to drafting the methods and revising manuscript. GP participated in the design of the study, analysis and interpretation of data, and draft of the manuscript. All authors read and approved the final manuscript.

Competing interests
The authors declare that they have no competing interests.

References

1. Burger P, Scheithauer B, Vogel FS: **Surgical Pathology of the Nervous System and Its Coverings.** New York: Churchill Livingstone;, Fourth 2002**Chapter 4.**

2. Humphrey PA, Andriole GL: **Prostate cancer diagnosis.** *Mo Med* 2010, **107**(2):107-112.

3. Albertsen PC: **The unintended burden of increased prostate cancer detection associated with prostate cancer screening and diagnosis.** *Urology* 2010, **75**(2):399-405.

4. You J, Cozzi P, Walsh B, Willcox M, Kearsley J, Russell P, Li Y: **Innovative biomarkers for prostate cancer early diagnosis and progression.** *Crit Rev Oncol Hematol* 2010, **73**(1):10-22.

5. Jensen AJ, Naik AM, Pommier RF, Vetto JT, Troxell ML: **Factors influencing accuracy of axillary sentinel lymph node frozen section for breast cancer.** *Am J Surg* 2010, **199**(5):629-635.

6. Weinmann AL, Hruska CB, O'Connor MK: **Design of optimal collimation for dedicated molecular breast imaging systems.** *Med Phys* 2009, **36**(3):845-856.

7. Jasani B, Douglas-Jones A, Rhodes A, Wozniak S, Barrett-Lee PJ, Gee J, Nicholson R: **Measurement of estrogen receptor status by immunocytochemistry in paraffin wax sections.** *Methods Mol Med* 2006, **120**:127-146.

8. Doyle S, Feldman M, Tomaszewski J, Madabhushi A: **A Boosted Bayesian Multi-Resolution Classifier for Prostate Cancer Detection from Digitized Needle Biopsies.** *IEEE Trans Biomed Eng* 2010.

9. Rosenkrantz AB, Kopec M, Kong X, Melamed J, Dakwar G, Babb JS, Taouli B: **Prostate cancer vs. post-biopsy hemorrhage: diagnosis with T2- and diffusion-weighted imaging.** *J Magn Reson Imaging* 2010, **31**(6):1387-1394.

10. Demir C, Gultekin SH, Yener B: **Learning the topological properties of brain tumors.** *IEEE/ACM Trans Comput Biol Bioinform* 2005, **2**(3):262-270.

11. Bilgin C, Demir C, Nagi C, Yener B: **Cell-graph mining for breast tissue modeling and classification.** *Conf Proc IEEE Eng Med Biol Soc* 2007, **2007**:5311-5314.

12. Bilgin CC, Bullough P, Plopper GE, Yener B: **ECM-Aware Cell-Graph Mining for Bone Tissue Modeling and Classification.** *Data Min Knowl Discov* 2009, **20**(3):416-438.

13. Gurcan M, Boucheron L, Can A, Madabhushi A, N. R, Yener B: **Histopathological image analysis: A review.** *IEEE reviews in Biomedical Engineering* 2009, **2**.

14. Lund AW, Bilgin CC, Hasan MA, McKeen LM, Stegemann JP, Yener B, Zaki MJ, Plopper GE: **Quantification of spatial parameters in 3D cellular constructs using graph theory.** *J Biomed Biotechnol* 2009, **2009**:928286.

15. Gunduz C, Yener B, Gultekin SH: **The cell graphs of cancer.** *Bioinformatics* 2004, **20**(Suppl 1):i145-151.

16. Demir C, Gultekin SH, Yener B: **Augmented cell-graphs for automated cancer diagnosis.** *Bioinformatics* 2005, **21**(Suppl 2):ii7-12.

17. Bilgin C, Shayoni R, Dayley W, Baydil B, Sequeira S, Yener B, Larsen M: **Cell-graph modeling of salivary gland morphology.** *IEEE International Symposium on Biomedical Imaging: From Nano to Micro* 2010.

18. Barabasi AL: **The New Science of Networks.** Perseus Books Group;, 1 2002.

19. Shavitt Y, Tankel T: **Big-Bang simulation for embedding network distances in Euclidean space.** *Ieee Infocom Ser* 2003, 1922-1932.

20. Gunduz C, Yener B: **Accuracy and sampling trade-offs for inferring Internet router graph.** Rensselaer Polytechnic Institute; 2003.

21. Faloutsos M, Faloutsos P, Faloutsos C: **On power-law relationships of the Internet topology.** *Comp Comm R* 1999, **29**(4):251-262.

22. Broder A, Kumar R, Maghoul F, Raghavan P, Rajagopalan S, Stata R, Tomkins A, Wiener J: **Graph structure in the Web.** *Comput Netw* 2000, **33**(1-6):309-320.

23. Albert RHJ, Barabasi A-L: **Diameter of the World-Wide Web.** *Nature* 1999, , **401**: 130-131.

24. Milgram S: **The small-world problem.** *Psychology Today* 1967, , **2**: 61-67.

25. Newman MEJ: **Who is the best connected scientist? A study of scientific coauthorship networks.** *Physics Review* 2001, **E64.**

26. Wasserman SKF: **Social network analysis:methods and applications.** Cambridge UK: Cambridge University Press; 1994.

27. Liljeros F, Edling CR, Amaral LA, Stanley HE, Aberg Y: **The web of human sexual contacts.** *Nature* 2001, **411**(6840):907-908.

28. Goldberg MPH, Magdon-Ismail M, Riposo J, Siebecker D, Wallace W, Yener B: **Statistical modeling of social groups on communication networks.** *Pittsburgh PA: First conference of the North American Association for Computational Social and Organizational Science* 2003.

29. Wuchty SER, Barabasi A-L: **The architecture of biological networks.** New York: Kluwer Academic Publishing; 2003.

30. Jeong H, Tombor B, Albert R, Oltvai ZN, Barabasi AL: **The large-scale organization of metabolic networks.** *Nature* 2000, **407(6804)**:651-654.

31. Jeong SPM, Barabasi A-L, Oltvai ZN: **Lethality and centrality in protein networks.** *Nature* 2001, , **411**: 41-42.

32. Watts D, Strogatz S: **Collective dynamics of small-world networks.** *Nature* 1998, , **393**: 440-442.

33. Hillisch A, Hilgenfeld R: **Modern methods of drug discovery.** Basel; Boston: Birkhäuser Verlag; 2003.

34. Justice BA, Badr NA, Felder RA: **3D cell culture opens new dimensions in cell-based assays.** *Drug Discov Today* 2009, **14(1-2)**:102-107.

35. Schindler M, Nur EKA, Ahmed I, Kamal J, Liu HY, Amor N, Ponery AS, Crockett DP, Grafe TH, Chung HY, *et al*: **Living in three dimensions: 3D nanostructured environments for cell culture and regenerative medicine.** *Cell Biochem Biophys* 2006, **45(2)**:215-227.

36. Yamada KM, Cukierman E: **Modeling tissue morphogenesis and cancer in 3D.** *Cell* 2007, **130(4)**:601-610.

37. Otsu N: **A thresholding selection method from gray-level histogram.** *IEEE Transactions on Systems, Man, and Cybernetics* 1979, **9(1)**:62-66.

38. Tucker LR: **Some Mathematical Notes on 3-Mode Factor Analysis.** *Psychometrika* 1966, **31(3)**:279-279.

39. Tucker LR: **Implicaitons of factor analysis to three-way matrices of measurement of change.** *Problems In Measuring Change* Madison: Madison: The University of Weisconsin Press; 1963, 122-137.

40. Tucker L: **The extension of factor analysis to three-dimensional matrices.** *New York* 1964.

41. Harshman RA: **Foundations of the PARAFAC procedure: Modesl and conditions for an explanatory multi-modal factor analysis.** *UCLA working papers in phonetics* 1970, **16**:1-84.

42. Golub GH, Van Loan CF: **Matrix computations.** Baltimore: Johns Hopkins University Press;, 3 1996.

43. Carroll JD, Chang JJ: **Analysis of Individual Differences in Multidimensional Scaling Via an N-Way Generalization of Eckart-Young Decomposition.** *Psychometrika* 1970, **35(3)**:283.

44. Bro R, Smilde AK: **Centering and scaling in component analysis.** *J Chemometr* 2003, **17(1)**:16-33.

45. **PLS Toolbox 4.0 for use with MATLAB.** [http://software.eigenvector.com].

46. Iwatsuki M, Mimori K, Yokobori T, Ishi H, Beppu T, Nakamori S, Baba H, Mori M: **Epithelial-mesenchymal transition in cancer development and its clinical significance.** *Cancer Sci* 2010, **101(2)**:293-299.

47. Weigelt B, Peterse JL, van 't Veer LJ: **Breast cancer metastasis: markers and models.** *Nat Rev Cancer* 2005, **5(8)**:591-602.

48. Polyak K, Weinberg RA: **Transitions between epithelial and mesenchymal states: acquisition of malignant and stem cell traits.** *Nat Rev Cancer* 2009, **9(4)**:265-273.

49. Yang J, Weinberg RA: **Epithelial-mesenchymal transition: at the crossroads of development and tumor metastasis.** *Dev Cell* 2008, **14(6)**:818-829.

50. Cardiff RD: **The pathology of EMT in mouse mammary tumorigenesis.** *J Mammary Gland Biol Neoplasia* 2010, **15(2)**:225-233.

Pre-publication history

The pre-publication history for this paper can be accessed here:
http://www.biomedcentral.com/1471-2342/11/11/prepub

2

Breast cancer detection using sonography in women with mammographically dense breasts

Jimmy Okello[1*], Harriet Kisembo[1], Sam Bugeza[1] and Moses Galukande[2]

Abstract

Background: Mammography, the gold standard for breast cancer screening misses some cancers, especially in women with dense breasts. Breast ultrasonography as a supplementary imaging tool for further evaluation of symptomatic women with mammographically dense breasts may improve the detection of mass lesions otherwise missed at mammography.

The purpose of this study was to determine the incremental breast cancer detection rate using US scanning in symptomatic women with mammographically dense breasts in a resource poor environment.

Methods: A cross sectional descriptive study. Women referred for mammography underwent bilateral breast ultrasound, and mammography for symptom evaluation. The lesions seen by both modalities were described using sonographic BI-RADS lexicon and categorized. Ultrasound guided core biopsies were performed. IRB approval was obtained and all participants provided informed written consent.

Results: In total 148 women with mammographically dense breasts were recruited over six months. The prevalence of breast cancer in symptomatic women with mammographically dense breasts was 22/148 (15%). Mammography detected 16/22 (73%) of these cases and missed 6/22 (27%). The six breast cancer cases missed were correctly diagnosed on breast ultrasonography. Sonographic features typical of breast malignancy were irregular shape, non-parallel orientation, non circumscribed margin, echogenic halo, and increased lesion vascularity (p values < 0.005). Typical sonofeatures of benign mass lesions were: oval shape, parallel orientation and circumscribed margin (p values <0.005).

Conclusion: Breast ultrasound scan as a supplementary imaging tool detected 27% more malignant mass lesions otherwise missed by mammography among these symptomatic women with mammographically dense breasts. We recommend that ultra sound scanning in routine evaluation of symptomatic women with mammographically dense breasts.

Keywords: Sonography, Breast cancer, BIRADS, Dense breasts

Background

Breast cancer is common in women and a leading cause of cancer mortality in women world wide [1]. In Uganda breast cancer is the third most common cancer in women after cervical cancer and Kaposi's sarcoma [2]. The incidence of breast cancer in Uganda has nearly tripled from 11:100,000 in 1961 to 31:100,000 in 2006 [3]. Breast cancer cases in sub Saharan Africa present in relatively young women, mostly late in stage III and IV, run an aggressive course and carry a low 5 year survival rate of 39% [4]. Reasons for the early nature of cancer presentation in Uganda is not wholly understood. However multiple factors presumably responsible for this nature of cancer presentation includes genetics, health seeking behaviour and short life span among others.

Mammography as the gold standard imaging method for breast cancer screening in unison with advances in treatment has resulted in reduced breast cancer mortality in the western societies; however this has not been appreciated in resource limited countries like Uganda where access to functioning mammography units and trained personnel is limited. Dense breast tissue has been proven to be the most important inherent limitation

* Correspondence: okellojimmy@hotmail.co.uk
[1]Department of Radiology and Radiotherapy, Mulago National Referral and University Teaching Hospital, Kampala, Uganda
Full list of author information is available at the end of the article

of mammography in the diagnosis of breast cancer as some cancers are missed, often requiring ultrasound to complete the breast imaging assesment [5]. In addition dense fibroglandular tissue per se is associated with increased risk of breast cancer and also lowers the sensitivity of mammography to as low as 30-48% [6].

Methods

Design

A cross sectional descriptive study.

Setting

We conducted this study between 1st February to 30th August at Mulago Hospital, the National Referral and a Teaching Hospital for Makerere University located in Kampala, Central Uganda. It has a capacity of 1,500 beds. Mulago Hospital Radiology Department has one functional mammography unit which is uses computed radiography technology to produce digital mammographic images, its open from Monday from Friday and receives patients referred from breast clinics within Mulago as well as the other private hospitals within and outside the city. About 5 diagnostic mammograms were performed daily. The hospital has a functional pathology department offering diagnostic laboratory services managed by experienced pathologists. A female mammographer with a-15-years experience performed the mammograms. The mammograms, breast ultrasound scans and image interpretation as well as US guided core biopsies were performed by a team of consultant radiologists and residents in accordance with the BI-RADS atlas.

Inclusion criteria

Women 25 years and above with mammographically dense breasts who consented to participate in the study were included. However, women taking hormone replacement therapy were excluded.

Sampling and data collection

Women referred for mammography were x-rayed in accordance with the cut off age spelt in the Uganda breast cancer clinical guidelines. Those with mammographically dense breasts were consecutively recruited upon obtaining an informed written consent to participate in the study.

Data was collected using a pre-coded and pre tested questionnaire. Study variables included;

Socio-demographic data such as Age, gender, menopausal status, indication for mammography, mass lesion visibility on mammogram, Sonographic BI-RADS descriptors, BI-RADS final assessment categorization as well as histological diagnosis.

The mammograms were performed using Phillips Mammogram diagnost UC model 2000 with a dual focal spot 0.3/0.1 mm acceptable for both diagnostic and screening purpose. 18 × 24 cm imaging plates with a single intensifying screen for computed radiography. Philips Computed Radiography computer system with its laser printer.

A Philips HD7 2009 model manufactured by Philips and Neusoft Medical systems Co. Ltd, Shenyang, China, with a 7. 5 to12 MHz broad band linear probe were used to scan the patients.

US-guided core biopsies were performed using needle gauze 14.

Standard mammographic views (Mediolateral oblique and Craniocaudal views) were performed in accordance with the international atomic energy agency (IAEA) human health series [18]. The imaging plates were then processed using the computed radiography system inorder to print CR mammograms. The mammograms were subsequently viewed systematically on a dedicated mammographic film viewer box by a team that consisted of the Consultant Radiologists and radiology residents. The mammographic breast density category was categorized according to the ACR BI-RADS atlas breast density categories recorded as 1,2,3 or 4. The final conclusion reached on consensus by the team on the breast density category and final mammographic diagnosis was documented on the questionnaire by the principle investigator. The BI-RADS atlas was available to the team and was helpful in sorting out interobserver disagreements that arose during interpretation.

Bilateral whole breast ultrasound scan was performed on all the study participants for atleast one of the following reasons;

Further evaluation of mammographically dense breast tissue inorder to complete breast image work up or ultrasound guided biopsy of the detected breast lesions when indicated.

The process of breast sonographic examination was explained to the patient before performing it. While observing privacy in the examination room all patients had to change to a clean examination gown with adequate exposure of chest wall. A chaperone was present during the procedure.

The patients were positioned lying supine oblique on a clean examination bed with the ipsilateral hand extended above the head to stabilize and flatten breast against the chest wall. This positioning was done for both breasts.

An acoustic gel was applied on the breast prior to scanning using the linear probe.

Both breasts were systematically scanned with overlapping scans in a radial and antiradial pattern from the nipple to the periphery. The retroareolar region including both axillae were scanned separately with angled probe views to ensure the complete coverage of all breast tissue. The images were saved as a soft copy in the US machine and copied to DVD blanks. A hard copy print on thermal paper was also made for some patients.

A report on breast sonographic findings was written down in accordance with the BI-RADS US lexicon adapted from the American college of radiology for standardization and given to the study participants.

Sonographs were blinded to the mammograph results.

A total of 45 US guided core biopsies were performed on breast mass lesions categorized as BI-RADS final assessment categories 4, 5 as well as some category 3 cases.

Biopsy procedure

An informed consent for biopsy was obtained after thorough explanation of the procedure to the study patients.

Both breasts including the axillae were systematically scanned with overlapping scans in a radial and antiradial pattern until a mass lesion was localized.

Under local anaesthesia and aseptic technique ultrasound guided core needle biopsy of solid breast masses were performed by a standard free hand technique using a disposable automated 14-gauge needle with a 22 mm throw. The breast tissue sampled was put in a biopsy bottle containing formalin and taken for histopathological analysis. At least 3 biopsy samples was taken from each lesion for diagnostic adequacy of the sample.

In case the lesions were sonographically similar then only one of the most prominent lesions was biopsied.

If the lesions are sonographically differing in appearance then at least two of the lesions were biopsied. Ultrasound guided fine-needle aspiration biopsy was done for complex cysts or masses, sample was air dried for 5 seconds prior to fixing it on the slide using ethanol 95% solution.

We took the biopsy samples to pathology laboratory for cytopathological analysis.

Data management

Questionnaires were checked for completeness. Data was entered into the computer using EPI DATA version 3.1. It was exported to STATA version 2013 for analysis. Statistical methods to analyze the data included univariate, bivariate analyses. Categorical and nominal variables were summarized using proportions, frequency tables, pie chart, and histograms.

Quality control

Quality control was ensured using the following measures:

The questionnaire was pre tested before commencement of the study to ascertain if the required information could be obtained using the specified questions.

Breast imaging interpretation was performed by a team, with BI-RADS atlas [12] available for reference to ensure correct interpretation was made.

Ethical consideration

Approval was obtained from Makerere University College of Health Sciences and IRB of Mulago Hospital.

Patient confidentiality was ensured.

Results

Out of the total 370 mammograms performed, 148 were categorized as BI-RADS density category 3 or 4 (mammographically dense breast tissues) and all underwent bilateral breast ultrasound scan. A total of 111 lesions were detected and described using the BI-RADS lexicon and final assessment categorization was made. US guided biopsy was done for 43 patients with BI-RADS final assessment category 4 or 5 lesions. 2 patients with breast masses categorized as BI-RADS 4 were not biopsied as they did not return for their biopsy appointment (see Figure 1).

The characteristics of lesions missed on mammography are indicated in Table 1.

Several BIRADS sonographic descriptors were used and included shape, orientation margins, boundaries, echo texture, posterior acoustic feature, surrounding tissues, calcification, lesion vascularity size and lymph nodes. Shape, orientation, margins, boarders and vascularity differentiated between benign and malignant, see Table 2.

In Figure 2 we show the presenting complaints; a lump being the most prevalent, followed by breast pain.

Figure 3A and B mammogram show a sample of a BIRADS 3 density. The mammogram shows BI-RADS density category 3 and no focal mass is demonstrable.

Figure 4 shows a sonogram of a solid mass with descriptors suggesting a malignancy is shown.

US guided biopsy revealed a poorly differentiated infiltrative lobular carcinoma.

Majority of the women were symptomatic with palpable breast lump. Only two women came for breast cancer screening.

Diagnostic performance of US scan and mammogram is described and shown in Table 3.

The most frequent histological type was ductal carcinoma 54% followed by lobular carcinoma. The most common benign lesions were fibroadenomas (see Table 4).

In all 22 breast cancer cases were correctly diagnosed using sonography and occurred in relatively young women averaging to 41 years in age (age range; 28-59 years), see Table 4.

Discussion

We set to investigate the incremental breast cancer detection rate of breast ultrasonography as a supplemental imaging tool in evaluation of symptomatic women with dense breasts (BIRADS 3 & 4). We found that US Scan detected 27% more malignant lesions than mammography did. The odds of mammography missing a malignant breast lesion in dense breasted women were 1 in 4.

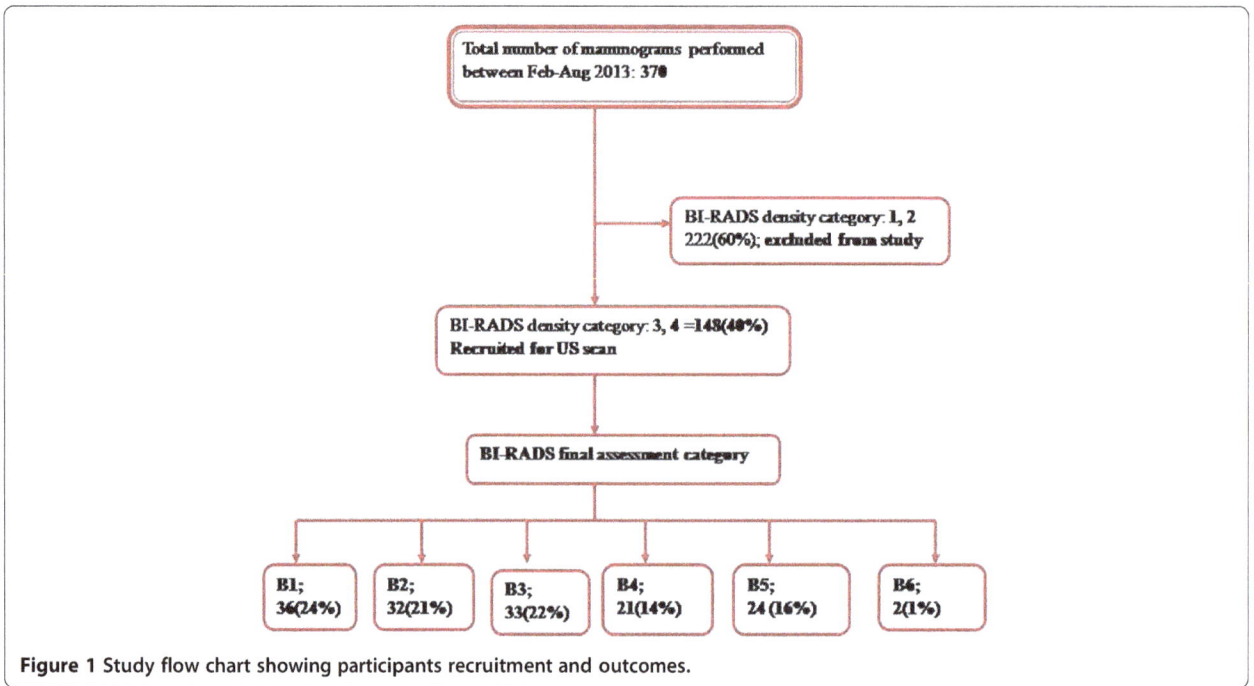

Figure 1 Study flow chart showing participants recruitment and outcomes.

The missed lesions were likely to be 10 mm or less in their widest diameter. Reasons for missing these malignant mass lesions could be the dense tissues obscuring visualization of those small sized tumors at mammography. However all the missed lesions were detected at US scan which is not limited by breast density. These findings are important because small lesions (less than 20 mm) are mostly early breast cancer lesions and are amenable to curative treatment. In addition ultrasound is more accessible than mammogram in our environment, therefore becomes an attractive supplement to mammography [3].

The BI-RADS sonographic lexicon was helpful in distinguishing benign from malignant solid breast masses with typical signs of malignancy being irregular shape, anti-parallel orientation, non circumscribed margin, echogenic halo, and increased lesion vascularity. Typical signs of benignity were oval shape and circumscribed margin (p < 0.005).

Mass echo texture, posterior acoustic features and surrounding tissues of a mass as well as presence or absence of lymph nodes were not reliable in differentiating between benign and malignant mass lesions (P > 0.005).

A total malignancy rate of 14.9% (22/148) is three fold higher compared to a previous study by Paulo et al. which showed a prevalence of 4.2% among symptomatic patients with dense mammograms [16].

Breast cancer occurred in relatively young women averaging to 41 years in age (age range; 28-59years). This finding is in keeping with literature which shows that more than half of women between 25 and 49 years of age have dense breasts with more cancer risks, as do approximately 29% of women older than 50 years [4,5].

Nearly all the women were symptomatic; 99% (n = 146) and only two women (1%) came in for breast cancer assessment.

Table 1 Characteristics of the mammographically missed cancer cases

Cases	Age	Complaint	BI-RADS density	Tumor size (mm)	US BI-RADS categorization
1	45	Pain	3	10	BI-RADS 4
2	31	Lump	4	12	BI-RADS 5
3	28	Lump	4	22	BI-RADS 4
4	35	Lump	4	15	BI-RADS 5
5	38	Discomfort	3	12	BI-RADS 4
6	29	Painful lump	4	9	BI-RADS 4

Table 2 Frequency of BI-RADS sonographic descriptors and its correlation with benign versus malignant outcome

BI-RADS sonographic descriptors	Frequency: n (%)	Malignant outcome: n (%)	Benign outcome: n (%)	P-Value
Shape				0.004
Oval	15 (13.9)	2 (13.3)	13 (86.7)	
Round	50 (46.3)	25 (50.0)	25 (50.0)	
Irregular	43 (39.8)	41 (95.4)	2 (4.6)	
Orientation				0.001
Parallel to skin	67 (62)	13 (19.4)	54 (80.6)	
Not parallel	41 (38)	40 (97.6)	1 (2.4)	
Margin				<0.001
Circumscribed	53 (49.1)	5 (9.4)	48 (90.6)	
Non circumscribed	55 (50.9)	52 (94.5)	3 (5.5)	
Lesion boundary				0.004
Abrupt interface	80 (74.1)	53 (66.3)	27 (33.7)	
Echogenic halo	28 (25.9)	26 (92.8)	2 (7.2)	
Echo texture				0.448
Anechoic	14 (13.0)	7 (50.0)	7 (50.0)	
Hypoechoic	74 (68.5)	53 (71.6)	21 (28.4)	
Complex	17 (15.7)	16 (94.1)	1 (5.9)	
Hyperechoic	3 (2.8)	0 (0.0)	3 (100)	
Posterior acoustic feature				0.458
No posterior feature	40 (37.0)	24 (60.0)	16 (40.0)	
Enhancement	32 (29.6)	21 (65.6)	11 (34.4)	
Shadowing	18 (16.7)	17 (94.4)	1 (5.6)	
Combined	18 (16.7)	16 (88.9)	2 (11.1)	
Surrounding tissues				0.448
Normal	65 (60.2)	15 (23.1)	50 (76.9)	
Architectural distortion	20 (18.5)	19 (95.0)	1 (5.0)	
Skin thickening	11 (10.2)	7 (63.6)	4 (36.4)	
Subcutaneous oedema	11 (10.2)	8 (72.7)	3 (27.3)	
Nipple retraction	1 (0.9)	1 (100.0)	0 (0.0)	
Calcification				0.406
Micro calcification	35 (32.4)	34 (97.1)	1 (2.9)	
Macro calcification	2 (1.9)	2 (100.0)	0 (0.0)	
No calcification	71 (65.7)	43 (60.6)	28 (39.4)	
Lesion vascularity				0.002
Increased vascularity in mass	41 (37.9)	37 (90.2)	4 (9.8)	
Avascular	56 (51.9)	29 (51.8)	27 (48.2)	
Increased surrounding vascularity	11 (10.2)	9 (81.8)	2 (18.2)	

Table 2 Frequency of BI-RADS sonographic descriptors and its correlation with benign versus malignant outcome *(Continued)*

Widest diameter of mass				NA
<1 cm	6 (5.6)	1 (16.7)	5 (83.3)	
1-2.5 cm	44 (40.7)	27 (61.4)	17 (38.6)	
>2.5 cm	58 (53.7)	52 (89.7)	6 (10.3)	
Abnormal lymph nodes				NA
Present	73 (67.6)	60 (82.2)	13 (17.8)	
Absent	35 (32.4)	19 (54.3)	16 (45.7)	

Note: Numbers in parentheses are percentages of each group.
Frequency: Number of times this US feature was reported to be present.
Malignant outcome = number of masses reported to have this feature that were considered malignant.
Benign outcome = number of masses reported to have this feature that were benign.
NA = Not applicable as the US feature is not a recognized BI-RADS descriptor according to ACR.

Tumors and glandular tissue have a similar dense appearance on mammography, making it difficult to distinguish metabolically active normal breast tissue from cancer. As a result, the performance of mammography in women with high breast density is poor [3,6-10]. The relative availability of ultrasound makes it an attractive imaging modality for evaluating women for breast cancer in resource-limited settings where other modalities like MRI are not readily available.

Correlation of sonographic features with benign versus malignant outcome

A standardized lexicon for sonography was developed in 2003 by the ACR in light of the increasing use of

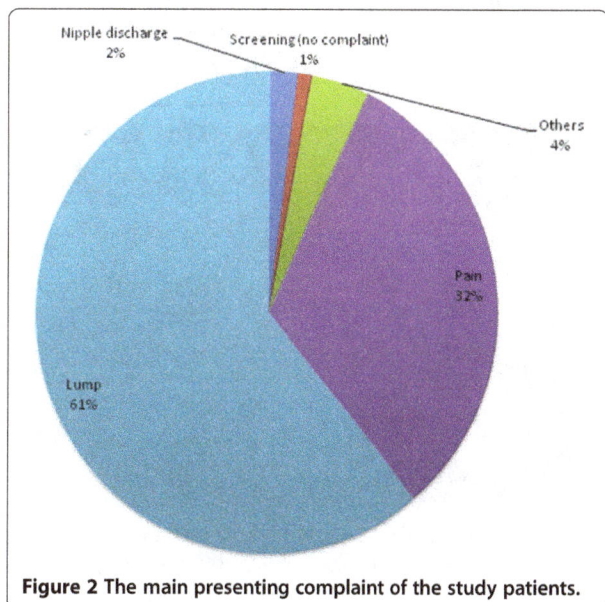

Figure 2 The main presenting complaint of the study patients.

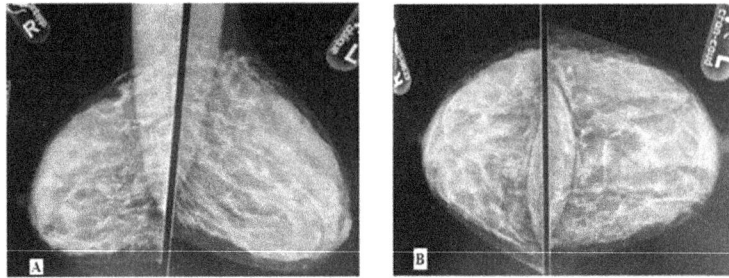

Figure 3 Mammographic films of a 31-year old woman who presented with a palpable left breast lump for 4 months, A: Oblique views B: craniocaudal views.

sonography in clinical practice. Like its mammographic counterpart, the sonographic BI-RADS lexicon was intended to provide a unified language for sonographic reporting and research and to avoid ambiguity in the communication and teaching of sonographic interpretation [12]. This lexicon helps the radiologist in describing sonographic features and defining the final assessment category that is associated with the most appropriate clinical management of the case.

Sonographic BI-RADS descriptors that most reliably characterized a mass as malignant study include an irregular shape, non circumscribed margin, non parallel orientation, echogenic halo around a mass, and increased vascularity within the mass.

In this study, Sonographic BI-RADS descriptors highly predictive of benignity of a mass were circumscribed margin; 90.6% (48/53), parallel orientation; 80.6% (54/67), and oval shape; 86.7 (13/15). Bi-variate analysis of these descriptors (margin, shape, orientation, lesion boundary and vascularity chosen were significantly reliable in differentiating malignant and benign ($p < 0.005$).

This is in conformity with prior study findings that, these BI-RADS descriptors represent an abnormal disease process in the breasts [11,13].

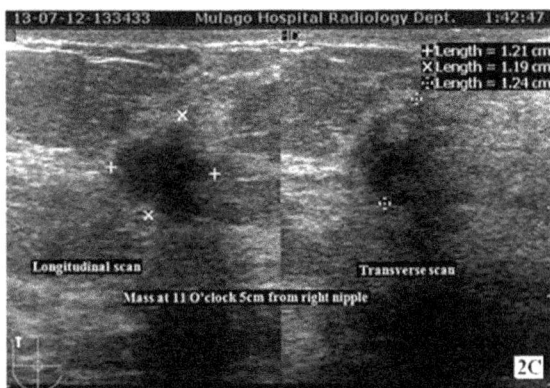

Figure 4 Sonogram shows a solid hypoechoic mass which is irregular in shape, has angular margin with surrounding echogenic halo at 11 O'clock 5 cm from right nipple.

A circumscribed margin is well defined or sharp, with an abrupt transition between the lesion and surrounding tissue usually predicts a benign outcome.

As in mammography, sonographic evidence of non circumscribed margins (which includes one of these options: spiculated, angular, microlobulated and indistinct margins) suggests infiltrating growth of the lesion into the surrounding tissue which is most times predictive of a malignant outcome.

Irregular shapes indicate inconsistent growth and advancement of the lesion edge which usually predicts a malignant outcome while for a benign mass usually takes on an oval or a round shape.

A parallel orientation is when the long axis of lesion parallels the skin line ("wider than tall" or horizontal) whereas a non-parallel orientation refers to a long axis, not oriented along the skin line ("taller than wide" or vertical, includes round masses).

Non-parallel orientation on sonography may suggest spread of the lesion through tissue-plane boundaries, a characteristic which is more likely to be associated with malignant lesions. In contrast, circumscribed margins and oval shapes represent smooth uniform growth without involvement of surrounding tissue and are associated more with a benign lesion. Similarly, parallel orientation suggesting containment in one tissue plane and indicative of a benign process.

Lesion boundary refers to the demarcation between the mass lesion and surrounding tissues. Identification of surrounding echogenic halo was a reliable BI-RADS descriptor in predicting a malignant outcome in this study. This agrees with previous studies which showed that identification of surrounding tissue effects had a high predictive value for malignancy, suggesting that recognition of such features could be helpful in the final assessment categorization at ultrasonography [12,13].

Increased vascularity within a mass lesion was a reliable BI-RADS descriptor of malignancy, a finding that agrees with literature.

Mass echo texture, posterior acoustic features and surrounding tissues of a mass as well as presence or absence

Table 3 Diagnostic performance of mammography versus ultrasound in visualizing mass lesion in women with mammographically dense breast tissue

Mass (lesion) seen	Mammogram	Ultrasound	Mammographic findings	Ultrasound plus Mammographic findings; (BI-RADS final assessment)
			Conclusive diagnosis	Conclusive diagnosis
	Frequency; N (%)	Frequency; N (%)	Frequency; N (%)	Frequency; N (%)
Yes	69 (62.2)	110 (99.1)	71 (64)	111 (100)
No	42 (37.8)	1 (0.9)	40 (36)	0 (0)
Total	111	100	111	100

of lymph nodes were not reliable in differentiating between benign and malignant mass lesions in this study.

The most common malignancy was invasive ductal carcinoma which accounted for 54.5% (n = 12) of histopathological examination results obtained. This histopathological finding confers with previous studies [14,15]. The cancer yield is comparable to the expected rate of malignancy in BI-RADS final assessment categories. Benign breast disease was also not uncommon with fibroadenoma being the most commonly encountered histological diagnosis.

Several factors limit the use of mammography in breast cancer detection in Uganda. First, breast cancer peaks in younger women who more frequently have denser breasts and, therefore the sensitivity of mammography is reduced. Second, younger women [17] are more sensitive to ionizing radiation. Several other benefits to using ultrasound include its relatively cheaper costs, its availability in resource-limited countries, no limitation by fibroglandular breast composition, its ability to be used for image guided-biopsies with relatively little additional training and equipment, and its portability [7-9]. For these reasons, ultrasound is an attractive imaging modality for evaluating women for breast cancer in a

resource-limited country such as Uganda. According to the latest BI-RADS atlas, it is mandatory that a mammographically dense breast tissue needs further additional imaging evaluation in order for the interpreting radiologist to make a conclusive radiological diagnosis. This further imaging evaluation is most times completed using high frequency breast ultrasound and rarely requiring MRI scan [10]. The are only five mammography machines which are inequitably distributed in Uganda compared to over 100 high frequency range ultrasound machines capable of breast sonography. This study was carried out with the aim of evaluating the use of bilateral whole breast ultrasound scan as an adjunctive imaging tool to detect cancer in women with dense breasts at Mulago hospital. Breast mass lesions detected were described according to the BI-RADS lexicon and final assessment categorization made.

Study limitations

This was a cross sectional descriptive study and so short term interval follow up of breast mass lesions categorized as benign and probably benign (BI-RADS 2 and BI-RADS 3 respectively) was not carried out to ascertain radiological and clinical stability of these mass lesions. Not all benign breast lesions were biopsied hence sensitivity and specificity of breast ultrasound could not be calculated.

Conclusion

Breast ultrasound scan resulted in significant incremental breast cancer detection rate (of 27%) among symptomatic women with mammographically dense breast tissue. We recommend that breast ultrasound scan should routinely be done in mammographically dense breasts (BI-RADS density category 3 and 4) in resource limited settings.

Table 4 Breast lump histological diagnoses

Breast cancer cases	
Histological type	Frequency; N (%)
Invasive ductal carcinoma	12 (54)
Infiltrating lobular carcinoma	2 (9)
Adeno carcinoma	6 (27)
Lymphoma	1 (5)
Alveolar rhabdomyosarcoma	1 (5)
Total	22 (100)
Benign breast conditions	
Fibro adenoma	7 (33)
Cystic mastopathy	4 (19)
Chronic inflammation	5 (24)
Sclerosis adenosis	1 (5)
Other benign conditions	4 (19)
Total (benign conditions)	21 (100)

Competing interest
The authors declare that they have no competing interest.

Authors' contributions
OJ conceived the concept. OJ and GM wrote the first draft. KH, BS and GM critically reviewed the manuscript for intellectual content. All authors approved content of the final manuscript.

Acknowledgement
We are grateful to the department of Radiology, Uganda Cancer Institute
and Breast Clinic staff at Mulago Hospital and St. Mary's hospital Lacor and
IAEA Uganda.

Author details
[1]Department of Radiology and Radiotherapy, Mulago National Referral and
University Teaching Hospital, Kampala, Uganda. [2]Department of Surgery,
College of Health Sciences, Makerere University, Kampala, Uganda.

References
1. Kelly KM, Dean J, Comulada WS, Lee SJ: Breast cancer detection using
    automated whole breast ultrasound and mammography in
    radiographically dense breasts. *Eur Radiol* 2010, **20:**734–742.
2. Boyd N, Guo H, Martin LJ, Sun L, Stone J, Fishell E, *et al:* Mammographic density
    and the risk and detection of breast cancer. *N Engl J Med* 2007, **356:**227–236.
3. Galukande M, Kiguli-Malwadde E: Rethinking breast cancer screening
    strategies in resource-limited Settings. *Afr Health Sci* 2010, **10**(1):89–92.
4. Stomper PC, D'Souza DJ, Di Nitto PA, Arredondo MA: Analysis of
    parenchymal density on mammograms in 1353 women 25–79 years old.
    AJR Am J Roentgenol 1996, **167:**1261–1265.
5. Kelemen LE, Pankratz VS, Sellers TA: Age-specific trends in mammographic
    density: the Minnesota breast cancer family study. *Am J Epidemiol* 2008,
    167:1027–1036.
6. Hersh MR: Imaging the dense breast. *Appl Radiol* 2004, **33:**22.
7. Buist DSM, Porter PL, Lehman C, Taplin SH, White E: Factors contributing to
    mammography failure in women aged 40–49 years. *J Natl Cancer Inst*
    2004, **96:**1432–1440.
8. Bevers TB, Anderson BO, Bonaccio E, Buys S, Daly MB, *et al:* National
    Comprehensive Cancer Network: Breast cancer screening and diagnosis.
    J Natl Compr Canc Netw 2009, **7:**1060–1096.
9. Berg WA, Blume JD, Cormack JB, Mendelson EB, Lehrer D, Böhm-Vélez M,
    Pisano ED, *et al:* Combined screening with ultrasound and
    mammography vs mammography alone in women at elevated risk of
    breast cancer. *JAMA* 2008, **299:**2151–2163.
10. Mandelson MT, Oestreicher N, Porter PL, White D, Finder CA, Taplin SH,
    et al: Breast density as a predictor of mammographic detection: comparison
    of interval- and screen-detected cancers. *J Natl Cancer Inst* 2000, **92:**1081–1087.
11. American College of Radiology. BI-RADS: *Mammography Atlas.* 4th edition.
    Reston, VA: American College of Radiology; 2003.
12. American College of Radiology BI-RADS: **Ultrasound, 1st Ed.** In *Breast
    imaging reporting and data system: BI-RADS atlas 4th ed.* Reston, VA:
    American College of Rad; 2003.
13. Zanello PA, Felipe A, Robim C, Mendes T, Oliveira G, et al. *Breast ultrasound
    diagnostic performance and outcomes for mass lesions using Breast Imaging
    Reporting and Data System category 0 mammogram,* http://www.ncbi.nlm.
    nih.gov/pmc/articles/PMC3072469/.
14. Hong AS, Rosen EL, Soo M, Jay A, *et al:* BI-RADS for Sonography: Positive and
    Negative Predictive Values of Sonographic Features. *AJR* 2005, **184:**1260–1265.
15. Sseggwanyi J, Galukande M, Fualal J, Jombwe J: Prevalence of HIV/AIDS
    among Breast Cancer Patients and the associated Clinico-pathological
    features. *Annals of African Surgery* 2011, **8:**22-27
16. Zanello P A, Andre Felipe Cica Robim, Tatiane Mendes Gonçalves Oliveira et al.
    *Breast ultrasound diagnostic performance and outcomes for mass lesions using
    Breast Imaging Reporting and Data System category 0 mammogram.*
    http://www.ncbi.nlm.nih.gov/pubmed/21552670 Accessed on line June 2014
17. Gakwaya A, Kigula-Mugambe JB, Kavuma A, Luwaga A, Fualal J, Jombwe J,
    Galukande M, Kanyike D: Cancer of the breast: 5-year survival in a tertiary
    hospital in Uganda. *Br J Cancer* 2008, **99:**63–67.
18. IAEA; *Quality assurance programme for screen film mammography.* Volume 2.
    Viena; ISSN 2075-3772; 2009.

3

Breast vibro-acoustography: initial experience in benign lesions

Azra Alizad[1,2]*, Mohammad Mehrmohammadi[1], Karthik Ghosh[2], Katrina N Glazebrook[3], Rickey E Carter[4], Leman Gunbery Karaberkmez[5], Dana H Whaley[3] and Mostafa Fatemi[1]

Abstract

Background: Vibro-acoustography (VA) is a newly developed imaging technology that is based on low-frequency vibrations induced in the object by the radiation force of ultrasound. VA is sensitive to the dynamic characteristics of tissue. Here, we evaluate the performance of VA in identifying benign lesions and compare the results to those of mammography.

Methods: An integrated mammography-VA system designed for in vivo breast imaging was tested on a group of female volunteers, age ≥ 18 years, with suspected breast lesions based on clinical examination. A set of VA scans was acquired after each corresponding mammography. Most lesions were classified as benign based on their histological results. However, in 4 cases, initial diagnosis based on clinical imaging determined that the lesions were cysts. These cysts were aspirated with needle aspiration and disappeared completely under direct ultrasound visualization. Therefore, no biopsies were performed on these cases and lesions were classified as benign based on clinical findings per clinical standards. To define the VA characteristics of benign breast masses, we adopted the features that are normally attributed to such masses in mammography. In a blinded assessment, three radiologists evaluated the VA images independently. The diagnostic accuracy of VA for detection of benign lesions was assessed by comparing the reviewers' evaluations with clinical data.

Results: Out of a total 29 benign lesions in the group, the reviewers were able to locate all lesions on VA images and mammography, 100% with (95% confidence interval (CI): 88% to 100%). Two reviewers were also able to correctly classify 83% (95% CI: 65% to 92%), and the third reviewer 86% (95% CI: 65% to 95%) of lesions, as benign on VA images and 86% (95% CI: 69% to 95%) on mammography.

Conclusions: The results suggest that the mammographic characteristics of benign lesion may also be used to identify such lesions in VA. Furthermore, the results show the ability of VA to detect benign breast abnormalities with a performance comparable to mammography. Therefore, the VA technology has the potential to be utilized as a complementary tool for breast imaging applications. Additional studies are needed to compare the capabilities of VA and traditional ultrasound imaging.

Keywords: Breast neoplasms, Breast ultrasonography, Mammography, Vibro-acoustography, Benign breast lesion

Background

There are several different medical imaging modalities for the screening and diagnosis of breast cancer [1-3]. However, benign breast lesions are much more common than malignant lesions, and accurate diagnosis of these lesions is important for optimal care of the patient [4].

Benign breast disease (BBD) is a well-known, significant risk factor for breast cancer [5]. BBD is diagnosed when a woman has a breast biopsy for a palpable or imaging abnormality in her breast that results in benign findings.

Any imaging evaluation of the breast with high sensitivity may also be associated with increased false positive results that may leads to unnecessary (i.e. benign) biopsies, resulting in high cost as well as significant trauma and anxiety for the patients due to this invasive procedure and in some instances, they may choose unnecessary extensive varieties of surgeries such as mastectomy [6,7]. Moreover,

* Correspondence: Alizad.azra@mayo.edu
[1]Department of Physiology and Biomedical Engineering, Mayo Clinic College of Medicine, 200 First Street SW, Rochester, MN 55905, USA
[2]Division of General Internal Medicine, Department of Medicine, Mayo Clinic College of Medicine, 200 First Street SW, Rochester, MN 55905, USA
Full list of author information is available at the end of the article

accurate identification of benign non-proliferative conditions such as cysts and fibroadenomas can reduce unwanted benign breast biopsies. It is, therefore, important to develop imaging tools with higher specificity to reduce false positive test results. Mammographic breast density (MBD), another known factor, reduces the sensitivity of mammograms [8]. Hence, there is an immense need for a noninvasive tool that can assess breast tissue characteristics while not influenced by MBD.

Conventional breast ultrasonography (US) is routinely used as an adjunct imaging tool to x-ray mammography for diagnosis of breast pathology; it improves sensitivity and has a considerable role in differentiation of cysts and solid nodules with higher specificity. US can also help to characterize solid breast masses [3,9-14]. US features such as lesion shape, orientation to the skin line, lesion boundary, margin characteristics, echo-pattern, posterior acoustic appearance, and effects on the surrounding breast tissue are employed to reach a Breast Imaging and Reporting Data System (BI-RADS) assessment [15]. In BI-RADS, the lesions are categorized into 7 categories numbered 0 to 6. Categories 1 to 3 indicate being negative, benign findings, or probably benign, respectively. Categories 4 and 5 are suspicious for malignancy, and 6 refers to having known biopsy proven malignancy [15]. Abnormalities on screening mammography that require further evaluation are assessed as category 0; similarly, calcifications found on breast US are also in category 0 assessment [16]. US is usually used for the subsequent evaluation of BI-RADS category 0 mammograms [17].

Benign breast lesions have a characteristic sonographic appearance; cysts appear as well-circumscribed, round or oval anechoic or hypoechoic masses with unnoticeable walls and posterior acoustic enhancement [18]. Fibroadenomas typically appear as oval, well-circumscribed masses with an abrupt interface and homogeneous iso- or hypoechoic echo texture. Benign papilloma masses appear as solid masses within a dilated duct with a vascular feeding pedicle seen on color Doppler imaging [2,9,14]. There is, however, an overlap between benign and malignant lesion US characteristics leading to a significant number of false-positive cases, which are recommended for US-guided percutaneous biopsy [14]. An additional sonographic tool to help decrease the number of unnecessary biopsies can play an important role to reduce such a large number of unnecessary biopsies. Imaging modalities, particularly those that provide palpation-like information, can help to better diagnose and identify breast lesions.

Elasticity imaging is an emerging field of medical imaging that provides such information. Elasticity imaging consists of magnetic resonance elastography (MRE) [23,24] which is expensive and not widely available [19,20], conventional quasi-static ultrasound elastography [21-23], Acoustic Radiation Force Impulse (ARFI) imaging [24-26]

and Shear Wave Elastography (SWE, also called SuperSonic Imaging (SSI)) [27-31]. ARFI and SWE use ultrasound radiation force to generate shear waves and quantify tissue elasticity from measured propagation speed of shear waves [32,33]. The results of studies using ARFI and SWE for breast have been very promising.

Vibro-acoustography (VA) is an imaging modality that also provides palpation-like information [34]. VA is introduced as a complementary technique to improve sensitivity and specificity in clinical breast imaging [35]. Principles of VA have been described extensively [34,36-39]. In VA, ultrasound is employed to produce a localized low-frequency force to vibrate the tissue. In technical terms, such a force is called "acoustic radiation force (ARF)". The low-frequency ARF is generated by two intersecting continuous wave (CW) focused ultrasound beams at slightly different frequencies. This force, which acts as a point force, vibrates the object at a frequency equal to the difference between two US frequencies (typically in kHz range). The resulting vibrations produce an acoustic emission field that is detected by a sensitive microphone (or hydrophone). Harder tissues normally produce a significantly different acoustic emission compared to normal soft tissues. Conceptually, VA resembles palpation; i.e., detects tissue response to an exerted force on tissue. [34,36]. However, VA benefits from a significant advantage of using a highly localized ARF, which leads to the possibility of assessing tissue properties on a small scale. As a result, VA can provide detailed information on tissue mechanics at high resolution [38,39].

Compared to conventional US imaging, VA images are speckle free, thus, the images have high-contrast that allows detection of small structures [4,40,41]. Thus VA can be a complementary tool to the existing breast imaging tools. Compared to elastography techniques, VA uses dynamic acoustic radiation force in the range of 10s of kHz, which is much higher than the frequency used in quasi-static elastography, ARFI, and shear wave imaging (normally in 10s to 100s Hz range). VA mages represent the acoustic response of tissue, which is a complex function of several parameters, including the elasticity and viscosity. However, elasticity cannot be directly and quantitatively measured from this acoustic response.

Our preliminary studies demonstrated the abilities of VA imaging in various tissues [40,42,43] including *in vivo* human breast [35,44]. In our previous studies [35,44], we used a confocal VA system combined with mammography to image various breast abnormalities, [35]. Since VA is a new modality, characteristic of different types of lesions (benign or malignant) in VA are not necessarily known. A goal of this paper is to determine and present VA characteristics of benign breast lesions. Another goal of this paper is to evaluate the performance of such characteristics in identifying benign lesions in VA and compare the results and compare the results to those of mammography. To define the VA characteristics of benign breast masses, we adopted the features that are normally attributed to such masses in mammography. Such features, which are often defined in contrast to those of malignant masses, include morphological attributes of the mass and information related to calcifications. We will test the validity and performance of these characteristics in a reader-based study.

Methods and materials

Study subjects

Under an approved protocol by the Mayo Clinic Institutional Review Board (IRB), female volunteers (18 and up) were chosen for the study and informed consent was obtained from all enrolled patients. Pregnant women were excluded from this study. We selected 36 patients with benign lesions based on pathology and clinical data. Five of the 36 patients examined were used for training and excluded from the study. Also, two participants were excluded from the study because of accidental hardware failure that occurred during the study. In the group of 29 women with benign lesions, 25 underwent ultrasound-guided core needle biopsy. The other 4 cases, based on radiologist impression of mammography and/or breast ultrasound, diagnosis of simple cyst was made and the cysts were aspirated and disappeared completely under direct ultrasound visualization, therefore, no histology was necessary for these 4 cystic lesions.

VA system

An experimental mammography-VA system, designed for *in vivo* breast imaging [35], was used to image patients with benign breast lesions. The VA system was integrated into a clinical stereotactic mammography machine (MammoTest system; Fischer Imaging, Inc, Denver, Colorado, USA) so that we could have matching VA and mammography images (from the same view angle) for comparison. Figure 1 represents the diagram of this system. It should be noted that VA is a noninvasive imaging tool, and it has been shown that VA can function at ultrasound intensities within the FDA limits. VA System parameters are: transducer frequency = 3 MHz, transverse resolution = 0.7 mm, scanning increments = 0.2mm, ultrasound intensity at the focal point = 700 mW/cm^2 in compliance with the FDA recommendation for *in vivo* diagnostic ultrasound [45]. The thermal safety of VA system is discussed in detail in [46].

The patient rested on an examination bed in a prone position. Through a hole in the bed, the breast was positioned between the back panel, including an x-ray detector, and a sliding panel that slightly compresses the breast. The compression was constant and at minimal level during VA acquisitions. A thin latex membrane covers the window of the compression panel that is transparent to the US beams, and the US transducer is

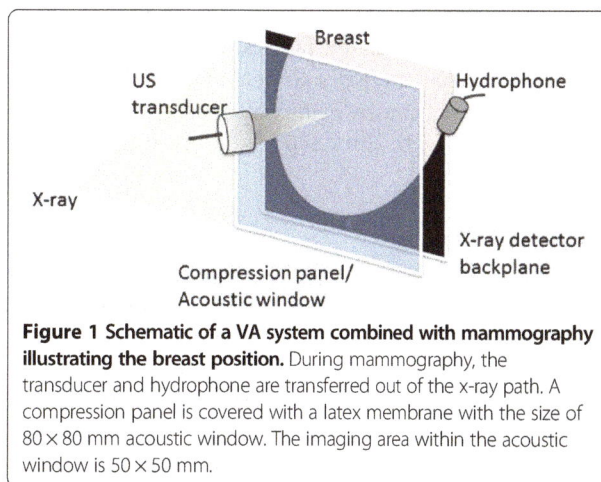

Figure 1 Schematic of a VA system combined with mammography illustrating the breast position. During mammography, the transducer and hydrophone are transferred out of the x-ray path. A compression panel is covered with a latex membrane with the size of 80 × 80 mm acoustic window. The imaging area within the acoustic window is 50 × 50 mm.

located behind the window. All VA images were acquired in the cranial-caudal view at various depths from the skin. The VA images were acquired by mechanically scanning the confocal VA probe, and each scan covered a 50 × 50 mm area with a scan step size of 200 μm in each direction. VA image resolution is determined by the spatial resolution of the mixed US beams (i.e. low frequency ARF) and was about 700 μm [34,47]. A hydrophone (Bruel & Kjaer model 8106) was placed on the side of the breast to receive the acoustic emission generated by the radiation force of US. Upon finishing a mammography scan, a set of VA scans at different depths was acquired by adjusting the distance between the confocal VA probe and breast tissue.

Reference standard documentation

After mammography, a set of VA scans was acquired by the experimental device. Then we selected the group of patients with benign lesions based on pathology, and in some cases, based on clinical findings and radiologist impression. To characterize the benign lesions' morphology, we reviewed all data including the corresponding X-ray mammograms acquired during the VA testing, other available clinical images such as clinical mammograms, US, and clinical data such as palpation information from the patient record. Based on these data, the shape and location of the benign lesion in the VA imaging window were determined.

Criteria for benign and malignant masses

Findings such as irregular or oval shaped; indistinct or ill-defined borders, presence of architectural distortion and or spiculations, presence of clustered pleomorphic microcalcifications are common characteristics of malignant breast masses. Round punctate calcifications are mostly benign unless appears as a segmental or linear distribution would be at least suspicious [48]. Other findings such as circumscribed and distinct borders, round shape and lobulated masses, or simple cysts with soft wall are characteristics of benign lesions. However, *intra cystic mass,* masses with eccentric cystic spaces or thick wall cysts with thick separation are usually malignant [18].

Reader interpretation

VA images were evaluated independently by three independent reviewers (radiology residents) who identified breast lesions and location. Because the reviewers did not have prior experience with VA imaging interpretation, they underwent a training session to learn about VA images and familiarize themselves with the general appearance of normal breast tissues. Masses and calcification in a typical VA image and five images used for training were excluded from the study. For training purposes, all the clinical data were given to the reviewers. However, for the remaining test set, we asked reviewers to locate and identify the benign lesion without having access to any clinical data. The reviewer evaluated each lesion based on the criteria for the benign masses including size, shape, margins, presence of microcalcifications, and presence of architectural distortion and/or spiculations, and determined if lesion was benign or not. In a separate session, the reviewers evaluated only the mammography images based on similar criteria.

Statistical considerations

Observer performance for detection of a breast lesion and correct classification of the lesion was measured using proportions and score confidence intervals.

Results

Women volunteers with abnormality in their clinical breast examination and/or mammography BI-RADS category 4 or less were included in this study. All patients underwent clinical mammography and breast US before participation in the study. VA imaging was done on all subjects. In total, 36 patients with benign lesions were evaluated; five were used for training and excluded from the evaluation. Also, two participants were excluded from the study because of accidental hardware failure that occurred during the study. A total of 29 patients, averaging 44 years old, with benign lesions were evaluated. The final diagnosis for 25 patients was based on histological results. In the remaining 4 patients, based on clinical imaging, the lesions were determined to be simple cysts. These cysts were aspirated with needle aspiration and disappeared completely under direct ultrasound visualization. Therefore, the final diagnosis includes six benign cysts, 15 fibroadenomas, three papillomas, and three of post-surgical scar tissue, and two focal atypical ductal hyperplasia with microcalcifications. The flow chart shown

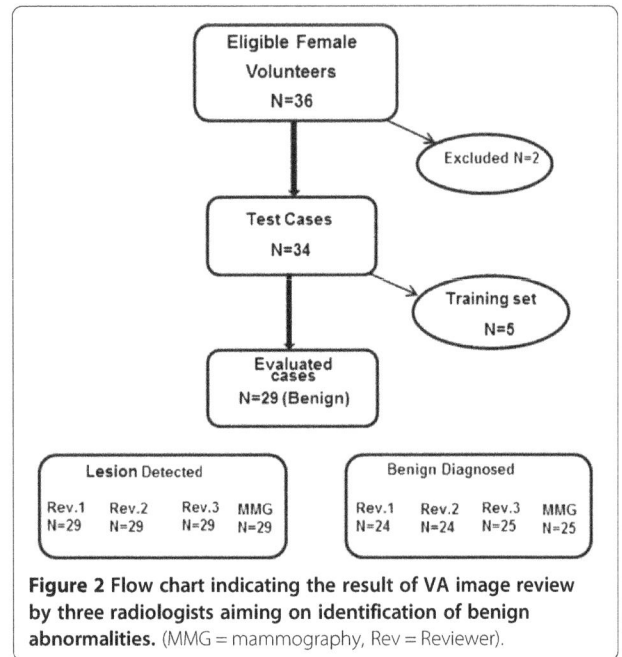

Figure 2 Flow chart indicating the result of VA image review by three radiologists aiming on identification of benign abnormalities. (MMG = mammography, Rev = Reviewer).

in Figure 2 demonstrates the results of VA image evaluation by three independent readers' reviews in 29 patients with benign lesions and their final diagnosis. The lesion detection rate for each radiologist was 100% with (95% confidence interval (CI): 88% to 100%). While all 29 lesions were confirmed to be benign (25 biopsy proven and 4 cysts with aspiration), the primary clinical imaging review of reference image (mammography) indicated that four lesions were suspicious for malignancy, therefore, the correct classification as benign was 86% (95% CI: 69% to 95%). This uncertainty was also observed using the new imaging modality. Correct classification as benign by the reviewers was either 83% (95% CI: 65% to 92%) or 86% (95% CI: 69% to 95%) as shown in Figure 2. Readers 1 and 2 misclassified three of the lesions as suspicious and two as malignant. Reader 3 misclassified three of the lesions as suspicious

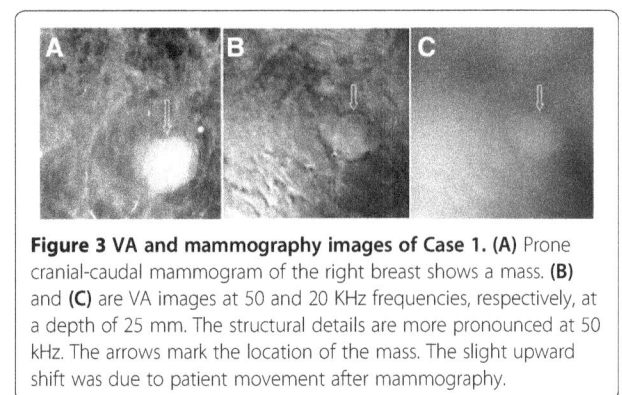

Figure 3 VA and mammography images of Case 1. (A) Prone cranial-caudal mammogram of the right breast shows a mass. **(B)** and **(C)** are VA images at 50 and 20 KHz frequencies, respectively, at a depth of 25 mm. The structural details are more pronounced at 50 kHz. The arrows mark the location of the mass. The slight upward shift was due to patient movement after mammography.

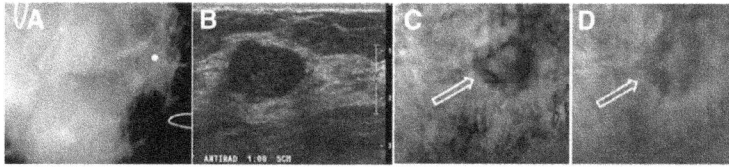

Figure 4 VA, US and mammography images of Case 2. (A) Prone cranial caudal mammogram image corresponding to the VA image showing only a marker placed in the vicinity of a palpable mass. **(B)** US of same breast shows a hypoechoic lobulated mass. **(C and D)** VA images of the same breast at 60 kHz and at 20 mm and 25 mm depths, respectively. Arrows mark the location of the breast mass.

and one as malignant. These misclassified cases are discussed in the following section.

Review of select cases

To further demonstrate the abilities of VA in detecting breast benign lesions, we present VA images of eight identified cases and compare VA results with that of conventional US and mammography. We also present three of the cases that were misclassified in mammography as well as VA images.

Cases of fibroadenomas identified by both mammography and VA

Case 1 The patient was a woman in her 70s. Her screening mammography showed scattered fibroglandular densities in both breasts and a mass lesion in her right breast (fibroadenoma). The prone cranial-caudal mammogram of the right breast showed a 2 cm, sharply marginated mass with coarse lobulations of a soft-tissue mass (Figure 3A). The fibroadenoma region was clearly seen in the VA images, taken at a depth of 25 mm below the skin (Figure 3B and C), denoted by arrows. The VA images could show the gentle coarse lobulation in the mass, a classic finding in fibroadenoma, and the margin very well. The mammogram additionally showed a well-circumscribed 3 mm calcification near the mass, but it was out of focus in the VA image, due to its different depth (Figure 3). This case demonstrates that VA can identify fibroadenomas.

Cases of fibroadenomas not seen on mammography but identified on VA

Case 2 The patient, a woman in her 40s, presented with a palpable mass in the right breast. Targeted US showed a $29 \times 19 \times 13$ mm well-defined lobulated and mildly hypoechoic mass. Her diagnostic mammography showed heterogeneous dense parenchyma in both breasts, but was not able to detect the palpable mass on right breast. A marker was placed on the skin to identify the approximate location of palpable mass as seen in the ultrasound (Figure 4A and B). The VA images indicated a round mass with a defined border and some lobulation inside denoted by arrows (Figure 4C and D). The pathology result revealed the mass to be a fibroadenoma. This case demonstrates that VA can identify mass lesions not seen on mammograms.

Case 3 The patient, in her 30s, presented with a palpable lesion in the left breast. Her mammography showed an extremely dense breast, and there is no discrete mammographic abnormality in the area of the palpable abnormality because of the highly dense tissue. The US image showed a benign appearing hypoechoic mass in the left breast. The VA image reveals a lobulated mass with a defined border (Figure 5). This case demonstrates that VA can identify mass lesions (in this case a biopsy proven fibroadenoma) not seen on mammograms.

Case 4 (Benign Papilloma) The patient was in her 50s. Her mammography demonstrated scattered fibroglandular

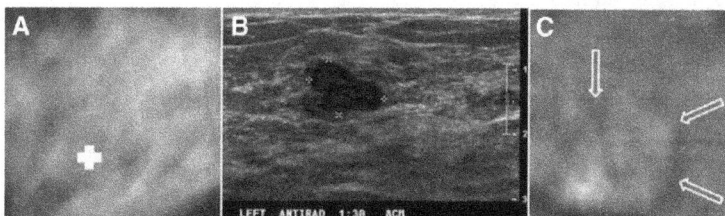

Figure 5 VA, US and mammography images of Case 3. (A) Mammography does not show any discrete abnormality, the lesion location marked by our radiologist. **(B)** US image of left breast shows a hypoechoic mass. **(C)** VA image shows a lobulated mass in an area of concern marked by our radiologist.

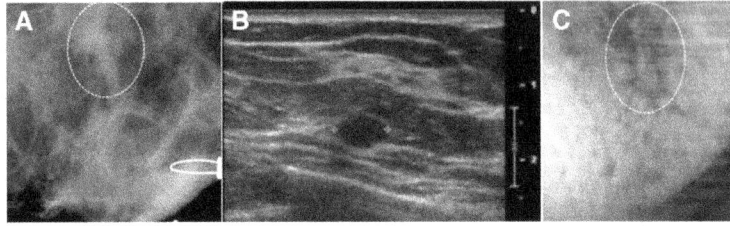

Figure 6 VA, US and mammography images of Case 4. (A) X-ray mammogram of the left breast, which corresponds to the same view as VA showing a small nodular density. **(B)** US of left breast shows 1 cm elongated solid circumscribed nodule. **(C)** VA image at a 30 mm depth shows the elongated solid nodule at the same location of X-ray.

density on both breasts and a small nodular density measuring about 10 mm in her left breast. Clinical US revealed a 10 mm elongated solid circumscribed nodule. VA images acquired at a 30 mm depth showed the same elongated nodule at the same location as that shown in X-ray (Figure 6). The result of pathology classified the lesion as a papilloma with stromal fibrosis. This case demonstrates the ability of VA in identifying a benign papilloma.

Cases of benign cysts
Case 5 The patient, in her 50s, presented with a palpable mass in the left breast. Her mammography demonstrated scattered fibroglandular densities (D2) in both breasts and a circumscribed lobulated mass measuring about 2 cm in the left breast. Targeted US indicated a benign cyst in the area comparable to mammography. VA images at a different depth (Figure 7) showed a well-defined mass about the same size and location seen in the mammogram (denoted by arrows). The patient was diagnosed with a benign cyst and the fluid was completely drained under guided US. This case demonstrates that VA can identify benign cystic lesions.

Case 6 The patient, in her 40s, presented with an oil cyst in the right breast near the nipple. Mammography demonstrated scattered fibroglandular tissue and a 20 mm radiolucent well-defined mass with soft border, which was consistent with an oil cyst, along with several calcifications near the larger cyst. Clinical US revealed the presence of the cyst as a hypoechoic mass. VA images acquired at 20, 25, and 30 mm depths (Figure 8) confirmed the presence of a well-defined circumscribed

mass with soft border. This case demonstrates that VA can identify a benign oil cyst.

Misidentified cases
Case 7 The patient, in her 50s, presented with a previous lumpectomy site above the left nipple. The patient was initially scheduled for a screening mammography, but a questionable new abnormality on the left breast necessitated additional imaging evaluation. Diagnostic mammogram demonstrated scattered fibroglandular densities in both breasts, and architectural distortion in a predominately radial pattern that could be due to resection of an invasive carcinoma approximately 5 years earlier or recurrence of cancer. VA images showed the area of concern as a spiculated or radial pattern architectural distortion (Figure 9). Final assessment was benign post-operative changes.

We had three cases of post-surgical scar tissue that imitated spiculation, the hallmark of a cancerous lesion; one shown in Figure 9. These cases were misidentified as malignant in both mammography and VA because of the misleading radial pattern distortion due to post-surgical scar tissue.

Case 8 The patient was in her early 50s. Her mammography shows extremely dense breasts. Diagnostic mammography demonstrated indeterminate calcifications, clustered and scattered, in the left breast. VA was also able to reveal this cluster of microcalcifications and ductal calcifications. Biopsy presented focal atypical ductal hyperplasia (ADH) with associated calcifications (Figure 10). This patient had an extremely dense breast and due to

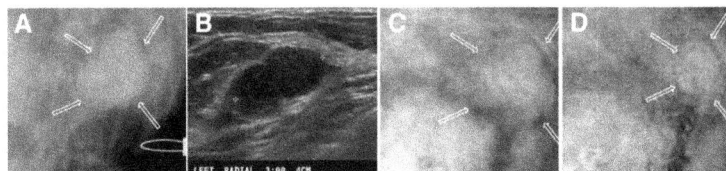

Figure 7 VA, US and mammography images of Case 5. (A) Mammogram showing a 20 mm circumscribed lobulated mass. **(B)** Targeted US showing a hypoechoic mass. **(C)** and **(D)** are VA images at depths of 30 mm and 35 mm, respectively. A mass with soft border is observed at the same location as the mammogram (denoted by arrows).

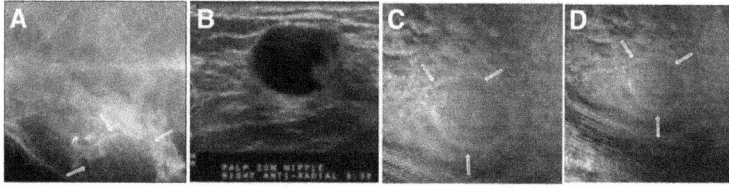

Figure 8 VA, US and mammography images of Case 6. (A) Mammogram taken corresponding to the VA view showing a 20 mm well-circumscribed lesion with soft border and several calcifications near the lesion. **(B)** Targeted US showing a hypoechoic mass confirmed as an oil cyst. **(C and D)** are VA images at 25 mm and 30 mm depths, respectively. The well-defined mass with soft border is seen in all VA images. Note: breast repositioned in **(D)** and cyst seen in center of the image.

indeterminate calcifications, both mammography and VA misidentified this case as malignant.

Discussion

The goal of this study was to primarily investigate the diagnostic accuracy of VA in detecting benign breast lesions. Various types of benign breast lesions including lipid cyst, benign cyst, benign fibroadenoma, and benign papilloma were studied with a laboratory-built VA system integrated with a mammography machine. The results of the study clearly show the efficacy of VA in detecting benign breast lesions. Also, the results show that the mammographic attributes of benign lesions can be adopted to identify such lesions in VA imaging.

We explored the VA characteristics of a wide range of benign lesions. Regular shape, well-defined lesion boundary, distinct or soft margin, and soft lobulation are the most benign characteristics we found on VA images. Cysts appeared on VA images as well-defined masses with a soft border as seen in Figures 7 and 8 and all reviewers could identify all cyst cases. Fibroadenomas, the most common solid breast masses that undergo breast biopsy, appeared on VA images as well-circumscribed ovoid or round masses

with gentle lobulation, and in some cases were calcified as seen in US and mammography, which happens in degenerating fibroadenomas [49,50].

Three cases of fibroadenomas and one case of papilloma that were unidentifiable by mammography were marked by our radiologist and detected by VA. Similarly seen in breast US [14], VA can help identify lesions that are obscured in mammography due to dense breast. VA also identified benign papilloma lesions as elongated nodules in a dilated duct; one papilloma was not identifiable on mammography but seen using VA. Diagnosis of papilloma is important and surgical excision should be considered for core needle biopsy proven benign papilloma - especially for lesions larger than 1.5 cm, regardless of imaging findings [41]. As expected, VA worked better than mammography in dense breast.

The cases that were misclassified by VA were also misidentified by mammography. Three of the misidentified cases were post-surgical scar tissue, as shown in Figure 9, presenting as a radial pattern distortion imitating spiculation, which is most seen in malignant tissue. It should be noted that mammographically only some of these changes can be differentiated based on morphological characteristics. Even though microcalcifications are often associated with breast carcinoma, not all spiculated lesions including microcalcifications are considered malignant. Mammography alone is often not a reliable imaging tool for making the definitive diagnosis in these cases. Additional mammographic views, breast US, clinical breast examination, and needle or surgical biopsy are often required [18].

Two other misclassifications occurred in focal atypical ductal hyperplasia (ADH) with associated calcifications as shown in Figure 10. The presence of a cluster of indeterminate microcalcifications is always suspicious of ADH or ductal carcinoma in situ (DCIS). ADH is a lesion with significant malignant potential. The diagnosis of ADH at needle core breast biopsy is normally considered as an indication for surgical excision [19,21,46]. In these two cases, VA and mammography were in agreement on suspicious lesions.

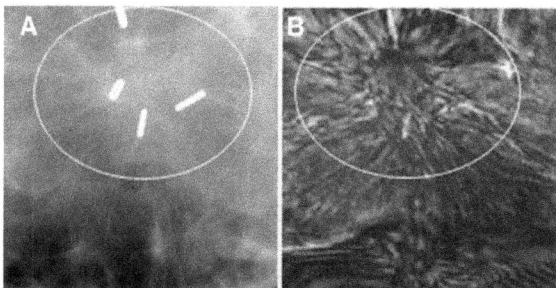

Figure 9 VA and mammography images of Case 7. (A) X-ray mammogram of left breast which corresponds to the same view as VA showing a radial pattern architectural distortion with surgical clips. **(B)** VA image at 20 mm depth showing the same speculated-like architectural distortion denoted by the circle. Parts of surgical clips can also be seen in the VA images.

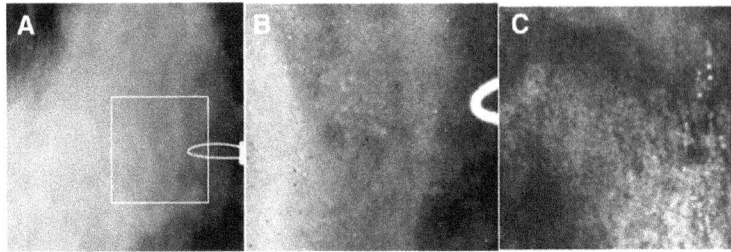

Figure 10 VA and mammography images of Case 8. (A) A cluster of calcifications and some scattered microcalcifications, which can be better seen in the magnified images of the square box part of x-ray shown in **(B)**. **(C)** VA image of the breast at 1 cm depth and normal sum of frequencies. The cluster of microcalcifications and ductal calcification are visible. Note: Due to patient's repositioning during the experiment, calcifications are seen on the far right of the VA image.

The VA images represented in the results section are simply reconstructed from the amplitude of the acoustic emission; additional signal and image processing algorithms were not required. The resolution of the VA images is determined by the spatial distribution of the ARF and is in the sub-millimeter range. Such resolution is generally sufficient for detecting the breast lesions. Since VA and US share common hardware (US scanner and transducer), we envision that in the future VA can be combined with conventional US imaging and become a hybrid imaging modality that can provide physicians with further clinically useful information.

We used mammography as the reference modality because the confocal VA system is integrated with a mammography machine that allowed acquiring matching mammography and VA images from the same view angle and through the same imaging window, which facilitated the comparison. We also note that traditional breast US and elastography images are obtained in the B-Plane, which is perpendicular to the C-plane images of VA. This difference in imaging plane makes it difficult to compare VA against US and elastography images to match the location of breast lesions. In contrast, we can obtain VA and mammography from an identical imaging window, thus one-to-one comparison becomes possible. We also emphasize that VA is introduced as a complementary technique to improve sensitivity and specificity in clinical breast imaging [35]. Compared to conventional US imaging, VA images are speckle free, thus, the images have high-contrast that allows detection of small structures such as microcalcifications. Thus VA can be a complementary tool to the existing breast imaging tools. Compared to elastography techniques such as ARFI [32] and SWI [33], VA uses dynamic acoustic radiation force in the range of 10s of kHz [34], which is much higher than the frequency used in quasi-static elastography, ARFI, and shear wave imaging (normally in 10s to 100s Hz range). VA images represent the acoustic response of tissue, which is a complex function of several

parameters, including the elasticity and viscosity. However, elasticity cannot be directly and quantitatively measured from this acoustic response.

VA imaging of the breast with a confocal VA system in the prone position has certain limitations. One of the drawbacks of this system is limited access to parts of the breast near the chest wall. This was due to mechanical limitations caused by the patient position (prone position) which put a part of the breast close to the chest wall outside the imaging window and thus not accessible. Also, the need for two-dimensional raster scanning of the transducer resulted in slow image acquisition. To overcome such limitations of confocal VA, we recently developed a new VA system with a handheld array transducer that is implemented on a clinical ultrasound scanner. This system is now being tested in an ongoing study on patients in supine position [51].

We understand that malignant lesions are clinically more important. We decided to focus this study on benign breast lesions, because benign lesions are also clinically important as they are much more common than malignant breast lesions. Benign breast lesions cover a wide range of abnormalities with different VA characteristic, thus warranting a separate a study.

Furthermore, the case selection did not represent a typical screening process. Nonetheless, this study represented an important first step in studying the utility of VA for detection and characterization of breast masses. Despite the mentioned limitations, the results of this study show the ability of the technique to identify the benign lesions with high clarity and present VA characteristics of a wide range of benign lesions.

Although the sample size in the present study was rather small, we believe that our results can be reproduced and validated in future clinical studies. We anticipate that by implementing VA on a clinical US scanner and by using a 2D US transducer [52], VA will become a more suitable tool for clinical usage. Additional studies are needed to compare the capabilities of VA and traditional ultrasound imaging.

Consent

Written informed consent was obtained from the patient(s) for publication of this manuscript and accompanying images.

Abbreviations

BBD: Benign breast diseases; ARF: Acoustic radiation force; VA: Vibro-acoustography; US: Ultrasonographic, ultrasonography, ultrasound; SWE: Shear wave elastography; SWI: Shear wave imaging; SSI: Supersonic imaging; ARFI: Acoustic radiation force impulse.

Competing interests

Disclosure: Drs. Fatemi and Alizad disclose Mayo Clinic's patents on the vibro-acoustography technology (discussed in this manuscript) as a potential financial conflict of interest.

Authors' contributions

AA: Leading the project and conducting human study, writing most of the manuscript; MM: writing a part of method section; KG: writing a part of introduction and manuscript editing; KNG: writing a part of introduction, image interpretation, operating the vibro-acoustography system, some of methods section; REC: statistical analysis; LGK: image processing and selection; DHW: patient selection and image interpretation; and MF: technique development, vibro-acoustography system design, writing the technical section of the paper, supervising data acquisition and signal processing. All authors read and approved the final manuscript.

Acknowledgements

This study was supported by BCTR0504550 from Susan G. Komen for the Cure, grants R21CA121579, R01CA148994, and R01CA127235 from the National Institute of Health. The content is solely the responsibility of the authors and does not necessarily represent the official views of the National Cancer Institute or the National Institutes of Health or Susan G Komen for the Cure. The authors are grateful to Dr. Matthew Urban and Dr. James Greenleaf for their helpful scientific discussions, to Mr. Randall Kinnick for technical support, to Mr. Thomas Kinter for computer support, and to Ms. Jennifer Milliken for administrative support.

Disclosure of conflict of interest: Mayo Clinic and some of authors have financial interests associated with the technology used in this research; the technology has been licensed in part to industry.

Author details

[1]Department of Physiology and Biomedical Engineering, Mayo Clinic College of Medicine, 200 First Street SW, Rochester, MN 55905, USA. [2]Division of General Internal Medicine, Department of Medicine, Mayo Clinic College of Medicine, 200 First Street SW, Rochester, MN 55905, USA. [3]Department of Radiology, Mayo Clinic College of Medicine, 200 First Street SW, Rochester, MN 55905, USA. [4]Division of Biomedical Statistics and Informatics, Department of Health Sciences Research Mayo Clinic College of Medicine, 200 First Street SW, Rochester, MN 55905, USA. [5]Bolu IBD Hospital, Radiology, Sanayi Sitesi 32. Blok Demirciler Ve Nalburcular Odasi Hiz. Binasi Alti, No:1, 14100 Bolu, Turkey.

References

1. Byrne C, Schairer C, Brinton LA, Wolfe J, Parekh N, Salane M, Carter C, Hoover R: Effects of mammographic density and benign breast disease on breast cancer risk (United States). *Cancer Causes Control* 2001, 12(2):103–110.
2. Sickles EA, Filly R, Callen P: Benign breast lesions: ultrasound detection and diagnosis. *Radiology* 1984, 151(2):467–470.
3. Berg WA, Blume JD, Cormack JB, Mendelson EB, Lehrer D, Böhm-Vélez M, Pisano ED, Jong RA, Evans WP, Morton MJ: Combined screening with ultrasound and mammography vs mammography alone in women at elevated risk of breast cancer. *JAMA* 2008, 299(18):2151–2163.
4. Fatemi M, Wold LE, Alizad A, Greenleaf JF: Vibro-acoustic tissue mammography. *Med Imaging IEEE Trans* 2002, 21(1):1–8.
5. Hartmann LC, Sellers TA, Frost MH, Lingle WL, Degnim AC, Ghosh K, Vierkant RA, Maloney SD, Pankratz VS, Hillman DW: Benign breast disease and the risk of breast cancer. *N Engl J Med* 2005, 353(3):229–237.
6. Burke Beckjord E: Diagnostic breast magnetic resonance imaging and contralateral prophylactic mastectomy. *Ann Surg Oncol* 2009, 16(6):1597–1605.
7. Katipamula R, Degnim AC, Hoskin T, Boughey JC, Loprinzi C, Grant CS, Brandt KR, Pruthi S, Chute CG, Olson JE: Trends in mastectomy rates at the Mayo Clinic Rochester: effect of surgical year and preoperative magnetic resonance imaging. *J Clin Oncol* 2009, 27(25):4082–4088.
8. Vachon CM, Brandt KR, Ghosh K, Scott CG, Maloney SD, Carston MJ, Pankratz VS, Sellers TA: Mammographic breast density as a general marker of breast cancer risk. *Cancer Epidemiol Biomark Prev* 2007, 16(1):43–49.
9. Stavros AT, Thickman D, Rapp CL, Dennis MA, Parker SH, Sisney GA: Solid breast nodules: use of sonography to distinguish between benign and malignant lesions. *Radiology* 1995, 196(1):123–134.
10. Corsetti V, Houssami N, Ghirardi M, Ferrari A, Speziani M, Bellarosa S, Remida G, Gasparotti C, Galligioni E, Ciatto S: Evidence of the effect of adjunct ultrasound screening in women with mammography-negative dense breasts: Interval breast cancers at 1year follow-up. *Eur J Cancer* 2011, 47(7):1021–1026.
11. Gordon PB, Goldenberg SL: Malignant breast masses detected only by ultrasound. A retrospective review. *Cancer* 1995, 76(4):626–630.
12. Kolb TM, Lichy J, Newhouse JH: Comparison of the performance of screening mammography, physical examination, and breast us and evaluation of factors that influence them: an analysis of 27,825 patient evaluations1. *Radiology* 2002, 225(1):165–175.
13. Berg WA, Zhang Z, Lehrer D, Jong RA, Pisano ED, Barr RG, Böhm-Vélez M, Mahoney MC, Evans WP III, Larsen LH: Detection of breast cancer with addition of annual screening ultrasound or a single screening MRI to mammography in women with elevated breast cancer risk. *JAMA* 2012, 307(13):1394–1404.
14. Sehgal CM, Weinstein SP, Arger PH, Conant EF: A review of breast ultrasound. *J Mammary Gland Biol Neoplasia* 2006, 11(2):113–123.
15. Mendelson E, Baum J, Berg W, Merritt C, Rubin E: *Breast imaging reporting and data system, BI-RADS: ultrasound.* Reston: American College of Radiology; 2003.
16. Berg W, Mendelson E, Merritt C, Blume J, Schleinitz M: ACRIN 6666: screening breast ultrasound in high-risk women. *American College of Radiology Imaging Network* 2007.
17. Zanello PA, Robim AFC, Oliveira TMG, Elias-Junior J, Andrade JM, Monteiro CR, Sarmento-Filho JM, Carrara HHA, Muglia VF: Breast ultrasound diagnostic performance and outcomes for mass lesions using Breast Imaging Reporting and Data System category 0 mammogram. *Clinics* 2011, 66(3):443–448.
18. Berg WA, Campassi CI, Ioffe OB: Cystic lesions of the breast: sonographic-pathologic correlation 1. *Radiology* 2003, 227(1):183–191.
19. Mariappan YK, Glaser KJ, Ehman RL: Magnetic resonance elastography: a review. *Clin Anat* 2010, 23(5):497–511.
20. Sinkus R, Siegmann K, Xydeas T, Tanter M, Claussen C, Fink M: MR elastography of breast lesions: understanding the solid/liquid duality can improve the specificity of contrast-enhanced MR mammography. *Magn Reson Med* 2007, 58(6):1135–1144.
21. Garra BS, Cespedes EI, Ophir J, Spratt SR, Zuurbier RA, Magnant CM, Pennanen MF: Elastography of breast lesions: initial clinical results. *Radiology* 1997, 202(1):79–86.
22. Barr RG: Real-time ultrasound elasticity of the breast: initial clinical results. *Ultrasound Q* 2010, 26(2):61–66.
23. Cho N, Moon WK, Kim HY, Chang JM, Park SH, Lyou CY: Sonoelastographic strain index for differentiation of benign and malignant nonpalpable breast masses. *J Ultrasound Med* 2010, 29(1):1–7.
24. Meng W, Zhang G, Wu C, Wu G, Song Y, Lu Z: Preliminary results of acoustic radiation force impulse imaging of breast lesions. *Ultrasound Med Biol* 2011, 37(9):1436–1443.
25. Yao M, Wu J, Zou L, Xu G, Xie J, Wu R, Xu H: Diagnostic Value of Virtual Touch Tissue Quantification for Breast Lesions with Different Size. *BioMed Research International* Vol. 2014, Article ID 142504, 7 pages pp.1-7. Hindawi Publishing Corporation http://dx.doi.org/10.1155/2014/142504.
26. Bai M, Du L, Gu J, Li F, Jia X: Virtual touch tissue quantification using acoustic radiation force impulse technology initial clinical experience with solid breast masses. *J Ultrasound Med* 2012, 31(2):289–294.

27. Plecha DM, Pham RM, Klein N, Coffey A, Sattar A, Marshall H: **Addition of shear-wave elastography during second-look mr imaging–directed breast US: effect on lesion detection and biopsy targeting.** *Radiology* 2014.

28. Lee SH, Cho N, Chang JM, Koo HR, Kim JY, Kim WH, Bae MS, Yi A, Moon WK: **Two-view versus single-view shear-wave elastography: comparison of observer performance in differentiating benign from malignant breast masses.** *Radiology* 2014, **270**(2):344–353.

29. Chang JM, Moon WK, Cho N, Yi A, Koo HR, Han W, Noh D-Y, Moon H-G, Kim SJ: **Clinical application of shear wave elastography (SWE) in the diagnosis of benign and malignant breast diseases.** *Breast Cancer Res Treat* 2011, **129**(1):89–97.

30. Cosgrove DO, Berg WA, Doré CJ, Skyba DM, Henry J-P, Gay J, Cohen-Bacrie C: **Shear wave elastography for breast masses is highly reproducible.** *Eur Radiol* 2012, **22**(5):1023–1032.

31. Barr RG, Zhang Z: **Effects of precompression on elasticity imaging of the breast development of a clinically useful semiquantitative method of precompression assessment.** *J Ultrasound Med* 2012, **31**(6):895–902.

32. Nightingale K, McAleavey S, Trahey G: **Shear-wave generation using acoustic radiation force:** *in vivo* **and** *ex vivo* **results.** *Ultrasound Med Biol* 2003, **29**(12):1715–1723.

33. Bercoff J, Tanter M, Fink M: **Supersonic shear imaging: a new technique for soft tissue elasticity mapping.** *Ultrason Ferroelectr Freq Control IEEE Trans* 2004, **51**(4):396–409.

34. Fatemi M, Greenleaf JF: **Vibro-acoustography: an imaging modality based on ultrasound-stimulated acoustic emission.** *Proc Natl Acad Sci* 1999, **96**(12):6603–6608.

35. Alizad A, Whaley DH, Urban MW, Carter RE, Kinnick RR, Greenleaf JF, Fatemi M: **Breast vibro-acoustography: initial results show promise.** *Breast Cancer Res* 2012, **14**(5):R128.

36. Fatemi M, Greenleaf JF: **Ultrasound-stimulated vibro-acoustic spectrography.** *Science* 1998, **280**(5360):82–85.

37. Fatemi M, Greenleaf JF: **Probing the dynamics of tissue at low frequencies with the radiation force of ultrasound.** *Phys Med Biol* 2000, **45**(6):1449.

38. Fatemi M, Manduca A, Greenleaf JF: **Imaging elastic properties of biological tissues by low-frequency harmonic vibration.** *Proc IEEE* 2003, **91**(10):1503–1519.

39. Fatemi MGJ: **Imaging and evaluating the elastic properties of biological tissues.** *BMUS* 2000, **8**:16–18.

40. Alizad A, Fatemi M, Wold LE, Greenleaf JF: **Performance of vibro-acoustography in detecting microcalcifications in excised human breast tissue: a study of 74 tissue samples.** *Med Imaging IEEE Trans* 2004, **23**(3):307–312.

41. Urban MW, Alizad A, Aquino W, Greenleaf JF, Fatemi M: **A review of vibro-acoustography and its applications in medicine.** *Curr Med Imaging Rev* 2011, **7**(4):350.

42. Alizad A, Wold LE, Greenleaf JF, Fatemi M: **Imaging mass lesions by vibro-acoustography: modeling and experiments.** *Med Imaging IEEE Trans* 2004, **23**(9):1087–1093.

43. Alizad A, Fatemi M, Whaley DH, Greenleaf JF: **Application of vibro-acoustography for detection of calcified arteries in breast tissue.** *J Ultrasound Med* 2004, **23**(2):267–273.

44. Alizad A, Whaley D, Greenleaf J, Fatemi M: **Potential applications of vibro-acoustography in breast imaging.** *Technol Cancer Res Treat* 2005, **4**(2):151–158.

45. Alizad A, Whaley DH, Greenleaf JF, Fatemi M: **Critical issues in breast imaging by vibro-acoustography.** *Ultrasonics* 2006, **44**:e217–e220.

46. Chen S, Aquino W, Alizad A, Urban MW, Kinnick R, Greenleaf JF, Fatemi M: **Thermal safety of vibro-acoustography using a confocal transducer.** *Ultrasound Med Biol* 2010, **36**(2):343–349.

47. Fatemi, M and Greenleaf, JF: **Imaging the Viscoelastic Properties of Tissue.** In Fink et al. (Eds.): Imaging of Complex Media with Acoustic and Seismic Waves. Topics Appl. Phys. 84. 257-275 (2002). Springer-Verlag berlin Heidelberg.

48. Berg WA, Campassi C, Langenberg P, Sexton MJ: **Breast Imaging Reporting and Data System: inter-and intraobserver variability in feature analysis and final assessment.** *Am J Roentgenol* 2000, **174**(6):1769–1777.

49. Weinstein SP, Conant EF, Mies C, Acs G, Lee S, Sehgal C: **Posterior acoustic shadowing in benign breast lesions sonographic-pathologic correlation.** *J Ultrasound Med* 2004, **23**(1):73–83.

50. Moon HJ, Kim MJ, Kwak JY, Kim E-K: **Probably benign breast lesions on ultrasonography: a retrospective review of ultrasonographic features and clinical factors affecting the BI-RADS categorization.** *Acta Radiol* 2010, **51**(4):375–382.

51. Mehrmohammadi M, Fazzio RT, Whaley DH, Pruthi S, Kinnick RR, Fatemi M, Alizad A: **Preliminary** *in vivo* **breast vibro-acoustography results with a quasi-2-D array transducer: a step forward toward clinical applications.** *Ultrasound in Medicine & Biology* 2014.

52. Urban MW, Chalek C, Kinnick RR, Kinter TM, Haider B, Greenleaf JF, Thomenius KE, Fatemi M: **Implementation of vibro-acoustography on a clinical ultrasound system.** *Ultrason Ferroelectr Freq Control IEEE Trans* 2011, **58**(6):1169–1181.

4

Fuzzy technique for microcalcifications clustering in digital mammograms

Letizia Vivona, Donato Cascio*, Francesco Fauci and Giuseppe Raso

Abstract

Background: Mammography has established itself as the most efficient technique for the identification of the pathological breast lesions. Among the various types of lesions, microcalcifications are the most difficult to identify since they are quite small (0.1-1.0 mm) and often poorly contrasted against an images background. Within this context, the Computer Aided Detection (CAD) systems could turn out to be very useful in breast cancer control.

Methods: In this paper we present a potentially powerful microcalcifications cluster enhancement method applicable to digital mammograms. The segmentation phase employs a form filter, obtained from LoG filter, to overcome the dependence from target dimensions and to optimize the recognition efficiency. A clustering method, based on a Fuzzy C-means (FCM), has been developed. The described method, Fuzzy C-means with Features (FCM-WF), was tested on simulated clusters of microcalcifications, implying that the location of the cluster within the breast and the exact number of microcalcifications are known.
The proposed method has been also tested on a set of images from the mini-Mammographic database provided by Mammographic Image Analysis Society (MIAS) publicly available.

Results: The comparison between FCM-WF and standard FCM algorithms, applied on both databases, shows that the former produces better microcalcifications associations for clustering than the latter: with respect to the private and the public database we had a performance improvement of 10% and 5% with regard to the *Merit Figure* and a 22% and a 10% of reduction of false positives potentially identified in the images, both to the benefit of the FCM-WF. The method was also evaluated in terms of Sensitivity (93% and 82%), Accuracy (95% and 94%), FP/image (4% for both database) and Precision (62% and 65%).

Conclusions: Thanks to the private database and to the informations contained in it regarding every single microcalcification, we tested the developed clustering method with great accuracy. In particular we verified that 70% of the injected clusters of the private database remained unaffected if the reconstruction is performed with the FCM-WF. Testing the method on the MIAS databases allowed also to verify the segmentation properties of the algorithm, showing that 80% of pathological clusters remained unaffected.

Keywords: Breast cancer, Microcalcifications, Spatial filters, Clustering, Fuzzy logic, C-means, Mammography, Segmentation

Background

Breast cancer is the most common cancer affecting women worldwide. It is visible in two forms: microcalcifications (small calcium deposits appearing as small bright dots on the mammogram) and massive lesions. These forms exhibit different typical characteristics, such as density, size, shape and number. For this reason,

the algorithms implemented to detect both types of lesions have to be different.

The main difficulties for radiologists to detect microcalcifications are due to their small size (0.1–1 mm, mean diameter ~ 0.3 mm) and low contrast compared to the background of the images. In this context, a CAD system may help physicians to improve their performance [1-3]: a good CAD system must be able to suppress the noise in the image in order to improve the contrast between the Region Of Interest (ROI hereafter) and the

* Correspondence: donato.cascio@unipa.it
Dipartimento di Fisica e Chimica, Università Degli Studi di Palermo, Palermo, Italy

background, and extract/select the lesions for a correct classification process.

In a CAD system, an unidentified microcalcification at the initial phase of image processing is considered completely lost, with severe limitations for later stages; for this reason several filtering techniques are applied to reduce the signal to noise ratio (SNR) [4]. But an equally important role is carried out by the classification phase, where training based procedures such as artificial neural networks are used, and a feature reference pattern set is required in order to correctly assign an unknown pattern, related to a lesion or to a particular membership class [5-9].

The clusters of microcalcifications are an important warning sign for breast cancer and they are present in 30 - 50% of screening mammography cases [10], therefore, their identification plays an important role in the phase image processing. The clustering is a type of classification imposed on a finite set of objects, characterized as points in a d-dimensional metric space in which every dimension corresponds to a feature (e.g. color, size, shape, position) [11].

Many techniques may be used for microcalcifications clustering: some are based on the simple Euclidean distance evaluation, others are related to the most significant features.

The procedure described by Nishikawa et al. [12] was applied to signals defined by a single pixel: signals with several pixels in area are reduced to single pixel by means of a recursive transformation. The number of signals within a small region, typically 3.2 mm × 3.2 mm, are counted: only if three or more signals are present within such a region, they are preserved in the output image. 78 mammograms were examined containing 41 clusters and a reduction in the false positives rate detection from 4.2 to 2.5 per image was found, while maintaining a sensitivity of approximately 85%.

Estevez et al. [13] proposed an algorithm (interactive selective and adaptive clustering, ISAAC) for assisting the radiologist in looking for small clusters of microcalcifications. This algorithm can be divided into two successive steps: selective clustering and interactive adaptation. The first step reduces the false positives number by identifying the microcalcifications subspace in the feature space; the second step allows the radiologist to improve results by identifying interactively additional false positive or true negative samples. The algorithm was tested on a 15 mammograms database. Performance of the method have been evaluated not by numerical parameter but by asking to three radiologists to determine, on a scale of 1 to 10 how helpful the method was in locating suspicious microcalcifications cluster areas, and by valuing capability of two other radiologists of identifying clusters observing the mammograms before and after the ISAAC application.

Mao et al. [14] proposed a distance-based and dense-to-sparse grouping method: the basic idea is to group the microcalcifications close enough to each other by examining the distance among them. The most closely distributed regions can be grouped into clusters first and relatively more widely distributed regions can be gradually grouped from evident cluster centers if they are still near enough to the centers. Several experiments were performed on a set of 30 mammograms containing 40 microcalcification clusters. The method yields a result independent of the distribution orientation of clusters.

Arodz et al. [15] performed a sequence of morphological operations on the filtered image with the goal of eliminating small or isolated objects: an area opening operation (removal of objects smaller than threshold), followed by dilation (for removing isolated objects). The technique was applied to 50 mammograms, each of them showing a region of the breast with an area of 25 cm2 containing a suspicious lesion, and displayed higher efficiency levels for those clusters with a probability of 40% to be malignant. Performance of the method was evaluated by valuing the average number of clusters detected on mammograms processed by the system but not detected on original mammograms and by valuing the average estimate of detection improvement resulting from using the system.

Cihan et al. [16] used the subtractive clustering; this subtractive clustering is a fast one-pass algorithm for estimating the number of clusters and the cluster centers in a dataset, if no prior knowledge of number of clusters is available. The point with the highest number of neighbours may be a center point and is selected as the first cluster. The method has been applied to 34 mammograms with a total of 72 micro-calcification clusters. The results show a success rate of 93% for the proposed algorithm.

Riyahi-Alam et al. [17] proposed an automated segmentation of suspicious clustered microcalcifications on digital mammograms. The algorithm consists of three main processing steps for this purpose. In the first step, the improvement of the microcalcifications appearance by using the "a trous wavelet" transform which could enhance the high frequency content of breast images were performed. In the second step, individual microcalcifications were segmented using wavelet histogram analysis on overlapping subplanes. Then, the extracted histogram features for each subplane used as an input to a fuzzy rule-based classifier to identify subimages containing microcalcifications. In the third step, subtractive clustering was applied to assign individual microcalcifications to the closest cluster. Finally, features of each cluster were used as input to another fuzzy rule-based classifier to identify suspicious clusters. The results of the applied algorithm for 47 images containing 16 benign and 31 malignant biopsy cases showed a sensitivity of 87% and the average of 0.5 false positive clusters per image.

Cordella *et al.* [18] proposed a method based on a graph-theoretical cluster analysis for automatically finding clusters on mammographic images. The proposed method starts by describing with a graph all the microcalcifications detected by an automatic algorithm: the graph nodes correspond to microcalcifications, while the edges of the graph encode the spatial relationships between microcalcifications. Each micro-calcification is linked, by an edge, to all the other ones. The weight of each edge is the Euclidean distance in the 2D space between the nodes connected by that edge. After such a graph is obtained, the GTC analysis is employed to remove all the tree edges with weights greater than a threshold value: in this way, the GTC method automatically groups vertices (microcalcifications) into clusters. Successively, clusters with less than three nodes are eliminated. The approach has been tested on a standard database of 40 mammographic images and turned out to be very effective even when the detection phase gives rise to several false positives. Performance of the method were measured in terms of Precision and Recall giving rise to a Precision value of 1 and a Recall value of 0.94.

Wang *et al.* [19] presented an approach based on fuzzy clustering to detect small lesions, such as microcalcifications and other masses, that are hard to recognize in breast cancer screening. A total of 180 mammograms were analyzed and classified by radiologists into three groups (n = 60 per group): those with microcalcifications; those with tumors; and those with no lesions. Analysis by fuzzy clustering achieved a mean accuracy of 99.7% compared with the radiologists' findings.

Quintanilla-Dominguez *et al.* [20] presented a method for the automatic detection of microcalcifications implemented by feature extraction and sub-segmentation steps. The feature extraction step is improved using a top-hat transform such that microcalcifications can be highlighted. In a second step a sub-segmentation method based on the possibilistic fuzzy c-means clustering (PFCM) algorithm is applied in order to segment the images and as a way to identify the atypical pixels inside the regions of interest as the pixels representing microcalcifications. Once the pixels representing these objects have been identified, an ANN model is used to learn the relations between atypical pixels and microcalcifications, such that the model can be used for aid diagnosis, and a medical could determine if these regions of interest are benign or malignant. The classifier presented in this work has been tested on four different combination of features, obtained the following results: Sensitivity: 98.21%, 98.70%, 88.93%, 88.73%; Accuracy: 99.54%, 99.56%, 98.22%, 98.18%.

Malar *et al.* [21] proposed an approach for detection and classification of mammographic microcalcifications

using wavelet analysis and Extreme Learning Machine (ELM). A total of 55 mammograms, including normal and microcalcifications images have been used, producing an Accuracy of 94%.

Cheng *et al.* [22] presented an approach to microcalcification detection based on fuzzy logic and scale space techniques (FLSS). First, they employ fuzzy entropy principal and fuzzy set theory to fuzzify the images. Then, they enhance the fuzzified image. Finally, scale-space and Laplacian-of-Gaussian filter techniques are used to detect the sizes and locations of microcalcifications. A dataset of 40 mammograms containing 105 clusters of microcalcifications is studied. Experimental results demonstrate that the proposed method can archive an accuracy greater than 97% with the FP rate of three clusters per image.

In the following paragraphs we will explain the algorithm and its application to a set of digital images. The findings will be subsequently presented.

Materials and methods

According to the report of the radiologist, a cluster of microcalcifications must have precise geometrical and morphological requirements: a cluster is a set of localized microcalcifications, therefore a potential microcalcification cannot be associated with a cluster that is spatially "distant".

As a further observation, the spatial association of microcalcifications is a necessary but not sufficient condition for proper clustering: a good microcalcifications clustering must be able to gather objects not only spatially "near", but also "near" from a point of view of the form and the visual information contained in them.

Moreover, another frequently encountered difficulty in developing clustering algorithms is the lack of knowledge of the number of clusters present in an image with microcalcifications. Within this context, this paper describes a method that aims to achieve two objectives: the first is to use a more powerful clustering process (FCM-WF) based on the standard FCM algorithm appropriately modified with the addition of some features; the second objective is to determine the optimal number of microcalcifications clusters that may be present in an image.

In order to better evaluate the efficiency of the method, i.e. the correct identification of the cluster and the number of micro belonging to it, testing the algorithm on pathological images reported by the radiologists could not be sufficient because we need to know exactly both the correct position of the cluster and the number of microcalcifications belonging to the cluster. For this reason in this paper we have chosen to test the algorithm on images obtained by healthy images with an artificial injection of microcalcifications. The microcalcifications clusters used for simulation are extracted from real pathological images reported by several radiologists.

The procedure followed in this preliminary phase is shown in Figure 1.

The first step of the procedure is the segmentation (Section Microcalcifications Segmentation), which is preliminary to other phases of the process as in all CAD system. Each cluster, with a number of micro variables depending on the lesions structure, is stored to build a database of real clusters (gold database). The mode of creating this "gold database" makes it possible to maintain in the cluster all relevant information present in the original image, with the consequent possibility to use them at a later stage (Section Databases). Afterwards, some clusters, or part of these, are injected on healthy images by creating a sample of pathological images "artificial" that will become our new "gold database artificial". Finally, with a new segmentation process performed on sample images, we obtain N objects used as a starting point to test the FCM-WF algorithm and to determine the number of clusters, as described in Section The Fuzzy C-MEANS Implemented With Features (FCM-WF) and Section K Clusters Best Value. The procedure was tested on images belonging to a private anonymous database collected in the Policlinic Hospital of Palermo. Policlinic Hospital is a hospital firm of University of Palermo in which formation, scientific research and health service are well integrated. Policlinic Hospital assess that every research involving human being is carried out in compliance with the Helsinki Declaration

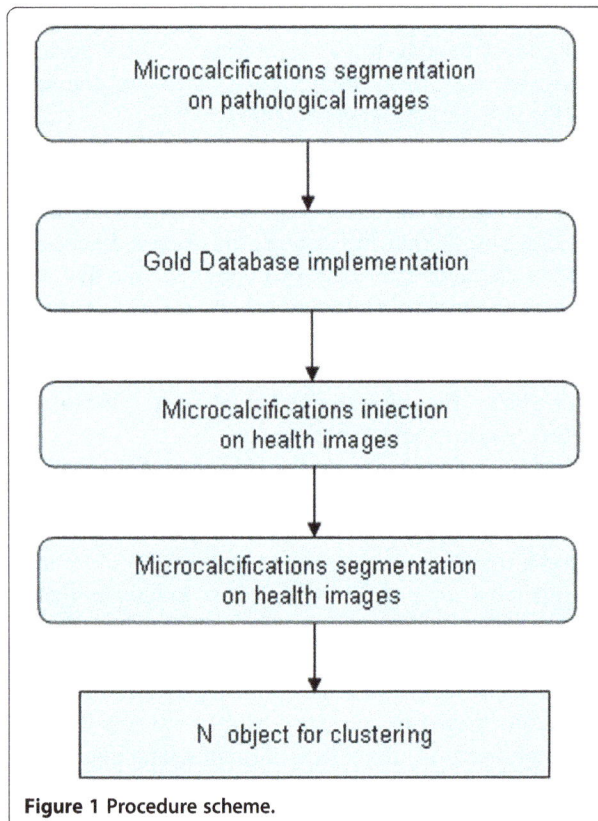

Figure 1 Procedure scheme.

and correctly informing the patients previously. Policlinic Hospital of Palermo, in the person of Dr. Raffaele Ienzi who provided us the images, assessed that every precaution has been taken to protect the privacy of the patients and the confidentiality of their personal information. Only the images belonging to patients who given a free informed consent in writing have been used to create the database.

Anyway, since each paper described in the state-of-the-art is tested on different image databases and as such does not provide a perfectly fair comparison, in order to provide strong justification for the effectiveness of our work, we applied the FCM-WF algorithm even on the publicly available MIAS database (/http://peipa.essex.ac.uk/info/mias.html). The characteristics of this database will be described in Section The MIAS database.

Microcalcifications Segmentation

In a CAD system, an important role is performed by the ROI extraction phase [23], because at this level a missed microcalcifications is definitely lost. The algorithms designed to enhance the contrast of microcalcifications may improve the ROI extraction performance [24].

It is possible to recognize microcalcifications within an image using mammography features edge detection [25]. The enhancement stage must be sensitive enough to emphasize low contrast objects while, at the same time, it must have the required specificity to suppress the background [26]. Usually the background corresponds to some smoothed regions of the image which don't give relevant information about pathologies in many cases. Background suppression can be implemented by using high pass filtering. In order to detect contours, the Laplacian of Gaussian (LoG) is often used in practice; it combines the Gaussian filter with the search properties of the edges of the Laplacian. The filter equation is represented by:

$$-\nabla^2 H_\sigma(x, y) = -\frac{1}{\pi\sigma^2}\left(\frac{x^2 + y^2 - 2\sigma^2}{2\sigma^4}\right)e^{-\frac{x^2+y^2}{2\sigma^2}} \qquad (1)$$

The parameter σ of Gaussian controls the effect of the LoG: the rise of its value increases the smoothing effect but with the lost of the ability to discriminate the details; therefore it is closely correlated to the size of the objects to identify. In equation 1), standard deviation σ is related to the target of size [27]. The relationship between the parameter σ and the dimensions of the target to identify has as effect, for microcalcifications recognition, a variability in the ability of individualization of the filter inside the range of dimensions of microcalcifications. This dependence implies that, if the size of the object to identify varies as in our case, we must use a method of analysis that uses several forms of convolution, with different values of σ. Conversely, in a multiscale approach, the final result can derive from mean or from maximum value among different obtained results (different values of σ) but in both cases the same problems occur: in the first case the scales different from that with the best coupling between the value of σ and the size of the object have as a result the reduction of detection power; in the second case we have a high sensitivity to noise.

To overcome the dependence from target dimensions and to optimize the recognition efficiency, it has been necessary to study and implement a spatial filter with a form that allows the detection of small and large microcalcifications. This form-filter, designed with the sum of the weights equal to zero in order to get the effect on the derivative, is characterized by three regions:

1. a first central region, circular (of radius equal to R_1), whose pixels have positive intensity, and area equal to the smallest size of a single micro, with the shape of the positive part of the Laplacian of Gaussian (LoG);
2. a second region, also circular, adjacent to the first region and outer, whose pixels have zero intensity, which extends up an area equal to the maximum size of a micro detectable (distance R_2);
3. a third region, the most external and quite narrow, with negative values obtained from the same LoG function and renormalized so that the sum of the intensities of its pixels, negative, is equal to the sum of the intensity of the first region, positive.

By assuming $\Delta R = R_2 - R_1$, mathematically the three regions of developed filter F(x, y) may be defined as follows:

$$F(x,y) = \begin{cases} Log(x,y) & \text{where}: \quad x^2 + y^2 < R_{1^2} \\ 0 & \text{where}: \quad R_{1^2} \leq x^2 + y^2 \leq R_{2^2} \\ \alpha Log[(x-\Delta R), \ (x-\Delta R)] & \text{where}: \quad x^2 + y^2 \geq R_{2^2} \end{cases}$$

where α is a normalization factor chosen such that the volumetric integral I_{S1}, within the circle of radius R_1, is equal to the volumetric integral I_{S2} of the surface outer to the circle of radius R_2.

From an analytic perspective, the filter function here realized is a LoG translated function: the negative LoG tail (that is: the third region of the developed filter) has been translated with ΔR, and the subsequent emptied region (the filter's second region, a circular crown of width ΔR) has been assigned a null value. Actually, the second region of the filter has the objective to make negligible the convolution contribution of the pixels characterized by distances between R1 and R2 and thus to obtain a constant detection performance on the pathology interval [R1, R2]; in fact, all the pixels of a ROI falling in the interval [R1, R2] and geometrically lying on a circular crown, will give no contribution in the computing of the convolution. So we can strongly reduce the dependence of the

recognition process from the variability of the dimensions of microcalcifications. Since the aforementioned translation occurs in the plane and quadratically increases the number of interested pixels, a renormalization (performed by acting on the parameter α from the third region) becomes compulsory in order to fulfill the null sum condition (as required by the derivative filter definition). If one analyzes the LoG filter and the result of its application on a generic (x,y) position of an image, one notes that for obtaining a positive value in (x,y) the ROI must correspond to the positive part of the filter, while the background must overlap with the negative part. The filter developed here allows also partial overlaps of the ROI and the positive part of the filter. In fact, for ROI characterized by linear dimensions between R1 and R2, the positive part which will overlap with the filter still remains the part of linear dimensions R1.

Figure 2 shows the 3-D representation of the filter, Figure 3 shows the 2-D projection and its renormalization due to the effect of placing the region with null values. In our case, application to a discrete image, the 3-D integrals are equivalent to the sum of the pixels intensities of the two affected areas, positive and negative, respectively.

Figures 4 and 5 show how the filter implemented can emphasize the presence of microcalcifications: Figure 4 shows original mammograms in which microcalcifications clusters are hidden by breast tissues; Figure 5 shows the microcalcifications that remain after the segmentation process: in this figure it is possible to recognize the five clusters hidden in Figure 4. The image colours are inverted for better visualization.

Databases
Gold Database Implementation and Injection Process

A medical image data set is the starting point for important epidemiological and statistical studies. Usually, such a set is used to develop and test algorithms for computer aided detection (CAD) systems but it is used also for teaching and training medical students or as an archive of cases. The development of a CAD system is intimately linked to collection of a dataset of selected images [28]. The purpose of this step was the creation of a gold database of mammographic images [29] containing microcalcification clusters to be used for the evaluation of the clustering process. We used a private database because we need to know all the truth and the details of microcalcifications clusters, i.e. not only the healthy or pathological nature of microcalcifications, but even all the useful properties like the mean intensity over the background, the number and the position inside a cluster, the geometrical and spatial distribution of clusters on breast tissue and so on.

Two expert radiologists took place to the segmentation process: after the comparison, they segmented

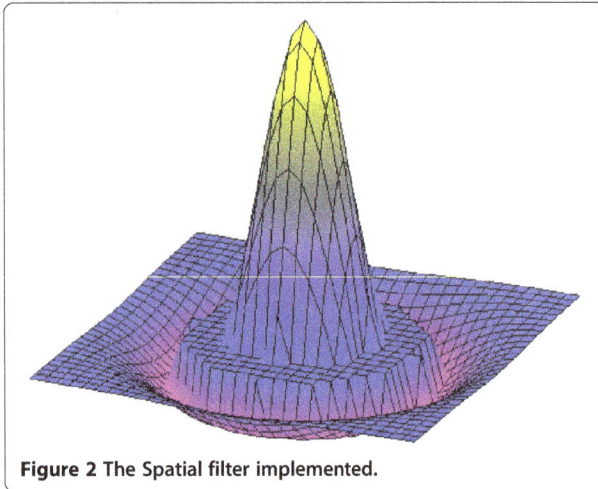

Figure 2 The Spatial filter implemented.

semi-automatically the ROI they though being microcalcifications. The health microcalcifications have been confirmed by a 2 years follow up and the pathological ones with histological exam.

Among all the ROI extracted by segmentation process, only those "cluster of ROI" identified by the physician as pathological cluster are kept to constitute the gold database of microcalcifications, while all other ROI are discarded. For all the microcalcification of each cluster we have recorded: mean intensity, number and coordinates of pixels, and membership cluster.

Since the properties that make possible to classify a group of microcalcifications as a cluster certainly take into account the parameters of size, intensity over the

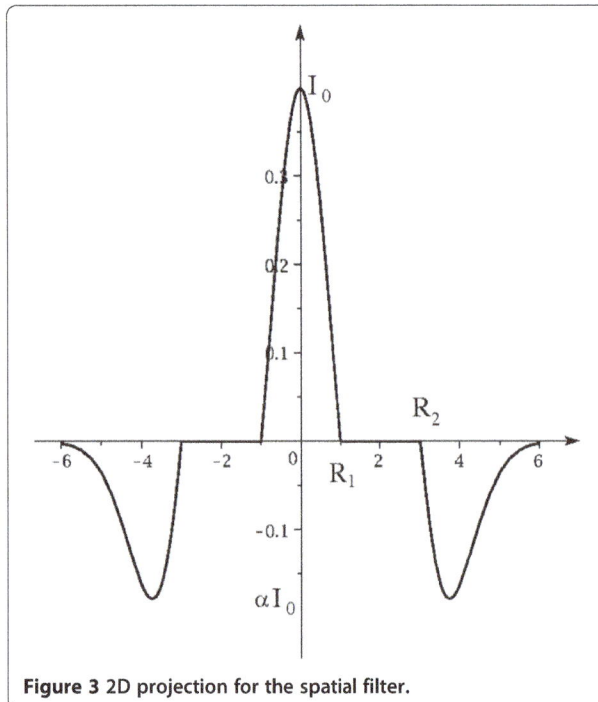

Figure 4 Digital mammography.

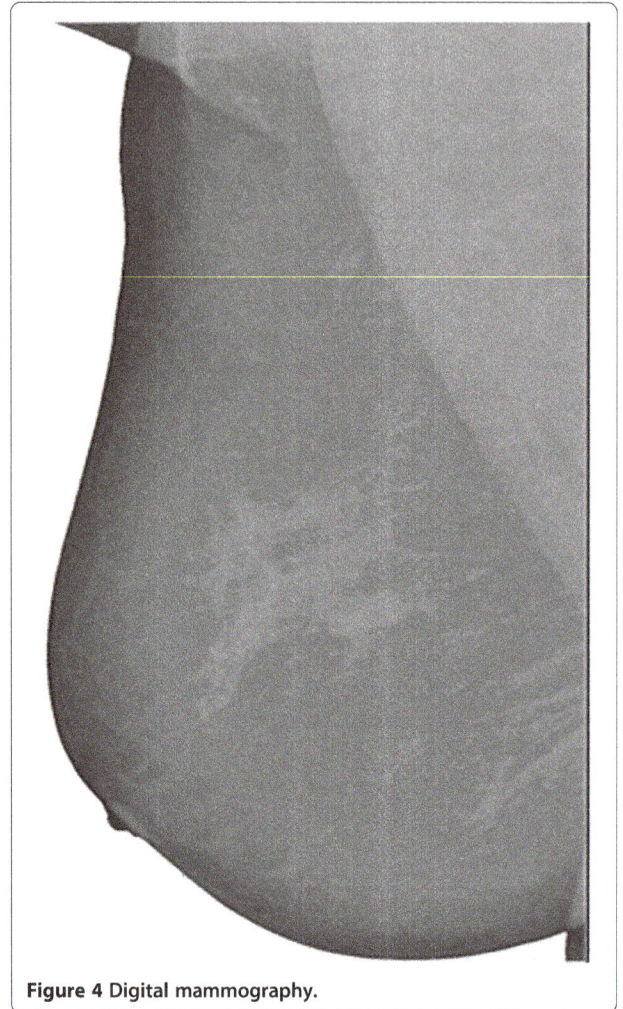

Figure 3 2D projection for the spatial filter.

background, relative distances of the microcalcifications and cluster geometry itself, each simulated cluster must retain all informations of original cluster. From these data, we injected the cluster of microcalcifications in healthy images according to the following steps:

1. random extraction of one microcalcification from a cluster (mother cluster);
2. random selection of a position within the breast and injection of the extracted microcalcification;
3. random extraction of a new microcalcification from the same "mother cluster" and its injection on the breast retaining angles and distance with the previous microcalcification.

Step 3 is repeated until injection of a microcalcification number n in the range [P,M], where M is the micro number within the mother cluster and P is the nearest integer to M*0.8 (20% less), with condition $M \geq 4$.

To not interfere with the healthy breast tissue, this injection method takes into account the average intensity

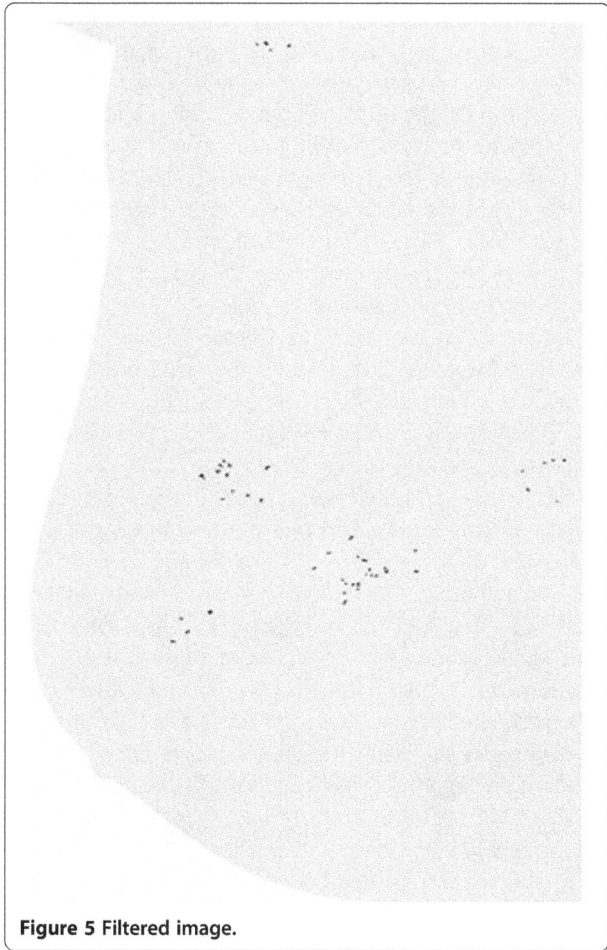

Figure 5 Filtered image.

of each cluster related to the intensity of the parenchyma where the cluster is injected.

At the end of the injection process of microcalcification, the healthy image is segmented with the same method used for the pathological images. The number N of objects segmented will be used for the following step, that is the clustering algorithm.

The MIAS database

The images collected from the Mammographic Image Analysis Society (MIAS), an organization of research groups in UK, are available via the Pilot European Image Processing Archive (PEIPA) at the University of Essex. The database contains 322 digitized films of 161 subjects with both right and left breast images and it also includes the so called ground truth on the locations of any abnormalities that may be present [21].

To test the method we have to know position and number of microcalcifications belonging to the clusters, so among all the images contained in this database only the 20 images in which centre locations and radii of clusters are known have been used. Particularly, since the database provide only the centre locations and radii

of clusters, and we need to know even position and number of every microcalcification belonging to it, we considered as "truth" about pathological microcalcifications the objects found inside the indicated circle after the segmentation process. An example is shown in Figure 6 and in Figure 7: Figure 6 shows the original mammogram (image mdb209), Figure 7 shows the same mammogram after the segmentation process, in which the centroids of all the segmented objects are indicated. In both figures the circle of cluster is present. We considered as microcalcifications belonging to the cluster only the objects found in the circle.

The images of MIAS database used contain one cluster, except images mdb223, mdb239, mdb249 (two clusters) and image mdb227 (three clusters), for a total of 25 clusters.

The Fuzzy C-MEANS Implemented With Features (FCM-WF)

As already explained in Paragraph 1, clusters of microcalcifications are an important warning sign for breast cancer so their identification plays an important role in developing a CAD system. Anyway, detecting all microcalcifications clusters is not an easy task, as there is often poor contrast on mammograms between microcalcifications and the surrounding tissue. Since microcalcifications belonging to the same cluster have similar properties

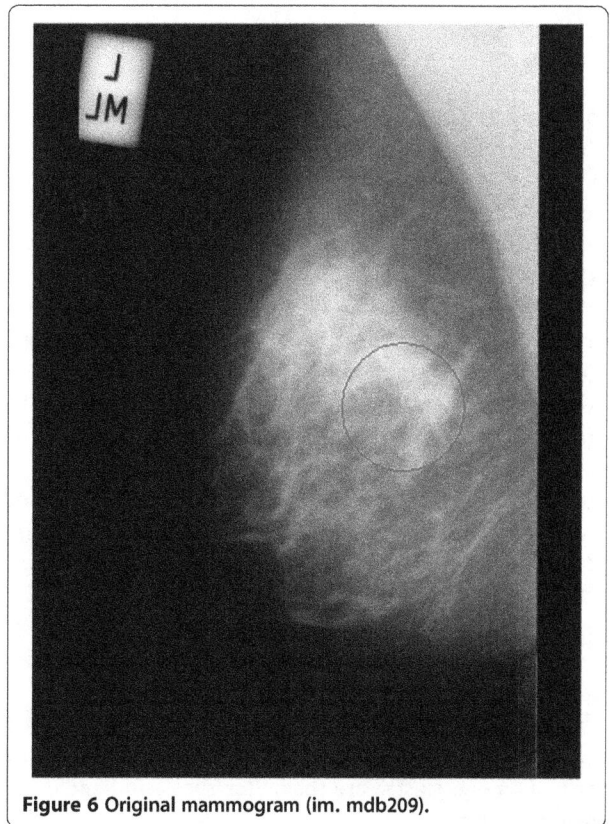

Figure 6 Original mammogram (im. mdb209).

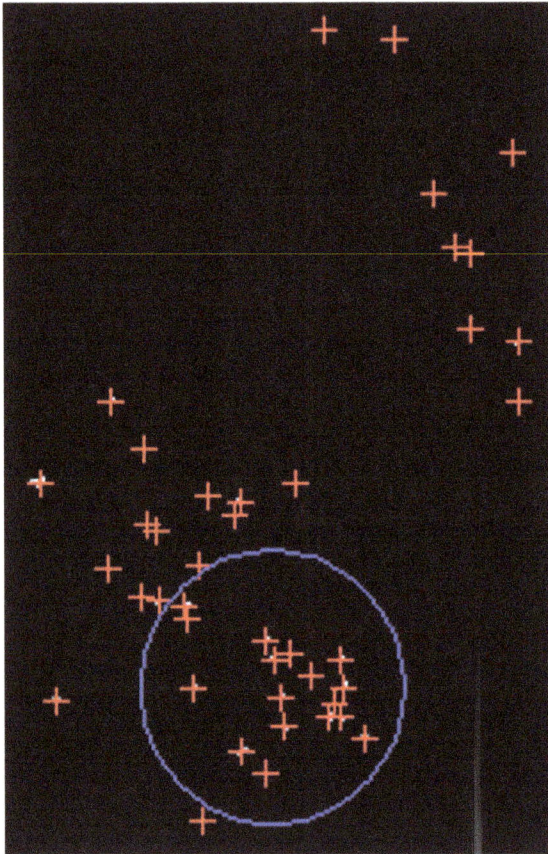

Figure 7 Mammogram after segmentation process.

In the fuzzy clustering methods an object can belong to more than one cluster with a degree of membership continuously variable between 0 and 1. For ordinary clusters, the degree of membership for an object x is 1 if it belongs to the cluster and 0 if it does not; for the fuzzy clusters, larger is the membership degree to the clusters, greater will be the confidence level that the object belongs to that cluster [30-33]. The output of a fuzzy algorithm not only includes a partition but also additional information in the form of membership value.

The most known fuzzy clustering algorithm is the Fuzzy C- Means (FCM), fuzzy version of the K-means algorithm, which usually takes into account as feature only the position of microcalcification for the clustering process.

The method proposed here, instead, in addition to the spatial information used in the standard Fuzzy C-Means makes use of seven other features (in the following we refer to our method as Fuzzy C-Mean – With Features, FCM-WF) that add information about the structure of each single micro [34-36]. Three of these features take into account the geometric shape of an individual micro: area, perimeter, eccentricity. The other four take into account the pixels intensity variability of each micro: average, standard deviation, skewness and kurtosis of the intensity. In FCM-WF algorithm, clustering is performed not in Euclidean space but in multidimensional features space *F*.

Given a set of N object, fuzzy partitioning in K clusters is carried out through an iterative optimization process that minimizes the following objective function

$$J_m = \sum_{i=1}^{N} \sum_{j=1}^{K} u_{ij}^m \left\| X_i - C_j \right\|^2 \qquad (2)$$

where X_i is the i-th object of the set $X = \{X_1, X_2, ...X_N\}$ used to perform the clustering, with $X_i \in R^F$, i = 1 ..... N; similarly C_j is the j-th centroid of the set $C = \{C_1, C_2, ... C_K\}$ with $C_j \in R^F$, j = 1 ..... K. Finally u_{ij}, is equal to the degrees of membership of the X_i object to the cluster C_j. In Figure 8 we report the flow chart of the process. The initial values of the matrix U elements u_{ij} are randomly assigned; correspondently the objective function assumes the initial value J_0. The iteration continues until reaching the absolute minimum of the objective function. The corresponding configuration of the clusters is considered as the best final result of the procedure used.

It has been necessary to normalize all the features [37] because they are not dimensionless quantities, variable in a predetermined range; so, if x is a generic feature, its normalization in the range (0–1) can be carried out with the formula (3):

(or *features*) such as grey level intensity, the main objective of a clustering process is to evaluate this similarity according to a distance measure between the microcalcifications and the prototypes of groups, and each microcalcification is assigned to the group with the nearest or most similar prototype [20].

Several algorithms should be proposed to solve the problem of microcalcifications clustering. Among them, partitional clustering methods are useful in this contest because they generate a single partition of the data in an attempt to recover the natural groups present in the data. Partitional methods are especially appropriate for the efficient representation and compression of large databases, as in the case of microcalcifications clustering [11].

If the clusters are compact and well separated, there is no uncertainty in assigning the objects to one cluster, but if the clusters are touching or overlapping, as is the case with microcalcifications clusters, the assignment of objects to clusters is difficult. So clustering methods based on fuzzy logic, according to which an object can belong to more than one cluster, are the better choice to handle the mammograms [22].

$$x_{norm} = \frac{x - \min}{\max - \min} \qquad (3)$$

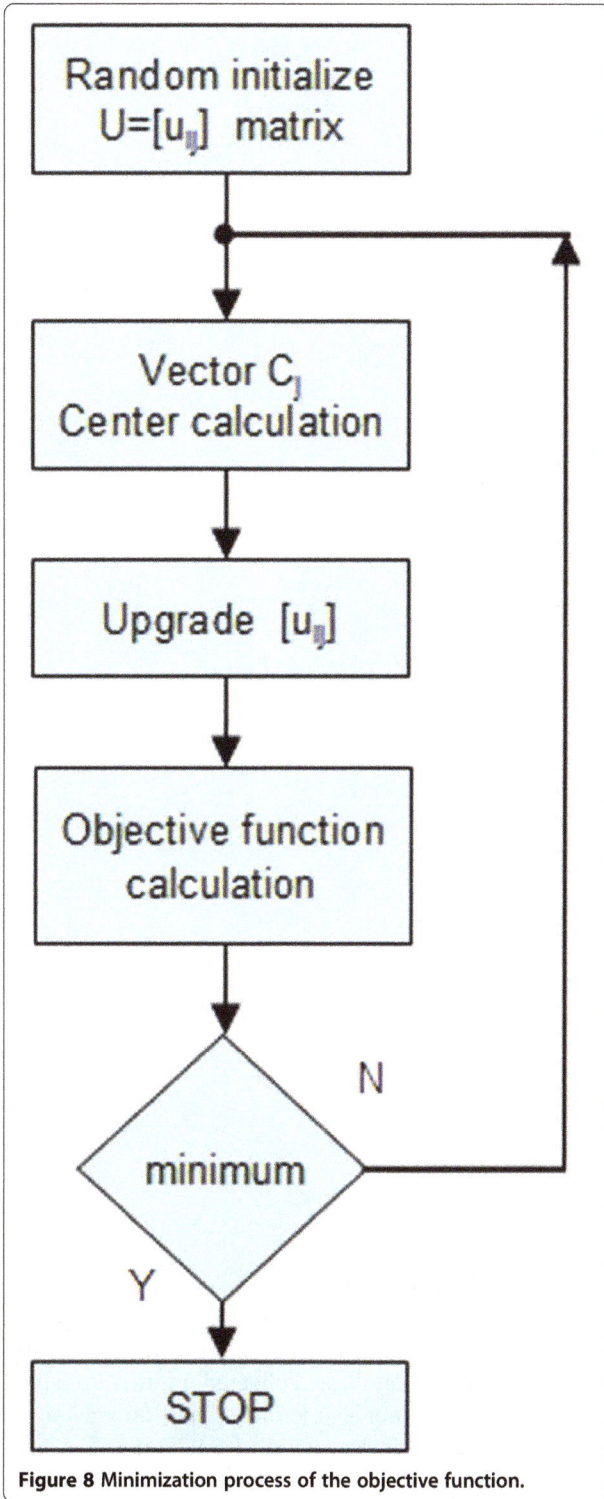

Figure 8 Minimization process of the objective function.

where, min = (*mean* - 4 *σ) and max = (*mean* + 4 *σ) and *mean* and σ are the mean value and the *standard deviation* of the feature x respectively. In Figure 9 the distributions of values for pathological and non-pathological segmented objects are compared for each feature.

K Clusters Best Value

One of the problems in developing clustering algorithms is the *a priori* lack of knowledge of the number of clusters present in images. In Paragraph 5 we described the FCM-WF method, but we must remember that the number of clusters we are looking for is an input parameter to the clustering algorithm [34], K_{ini}; it follows that it will be found always a number of clusters equal to the imposed value. For this reason we proposed a method to automatically determine the number of clusters present in an image based on the result of segmentation process: if the number of objects after the segmentation process is equal to N, since a disease cluster cannot have less than 3 micro, we can safely assume that the maximum number of clusters present in an image cannot exceed N/3. Moreover, we have a limit on cluster size because a pathological cluster has a maximum size of about 250 pixel (1 px = 0.07 mm).

If we start the clustering process on an image with the limit value $K_{ini} = N/3$ on the number of clusters, the minimization of the objective function will lead to a final configuration with N/3 clusters, some of which may have less than 3 micro (and they will be removed since they are not pathological) and other clusters with sizes that exceed the maximum size.

For this reason, at the end of the clustering process, the input value K_{ini} is reduced by N_{down} (number of clusters with less than 3 micro) and increased by N_{up} (number of clusters with spatial dimensions greater than the maximum), finding, at last, according to the equation 4, a final number W of residual clusters that may be less than K_{ini}.

$$W = K_{ini} - N_{down} + N_{up} \tag{4}$$

Furthermore, since the clustering process starts with a random position of the centroids and with random values of the U matrix, the final number W of residues clusters could be dependent from the initial conditions. To get a more reliable estimate of W, we repeat the FCM-WF process several times starting with the same value of K_{ini} (for every image there is a different value of K_{ini}, dependent from the number of segmented object present in the image), and calculate the average value $\bar{W}$ and the corresponding standard deviation σ_W. Finally, to improve the significance of the average value $\bar{W}$, we introduce a rejection criterion: the elimination of the W_i values at a distance greater than 3* σ_W from $\bar{W}$. After this rejection, we recalculate the new $\bar{W}$ and σ_W values starting from a new value of K_{ini}, according to the equation 5:

$$K_{ini} = \bar{W} + 3 * \sigma_W \tag{5}$$

If the average value of W differs from K_{ini} for less than 3* σ_W, the iterative process stops and a final run start with $K_{ini} = \bar{W}$.

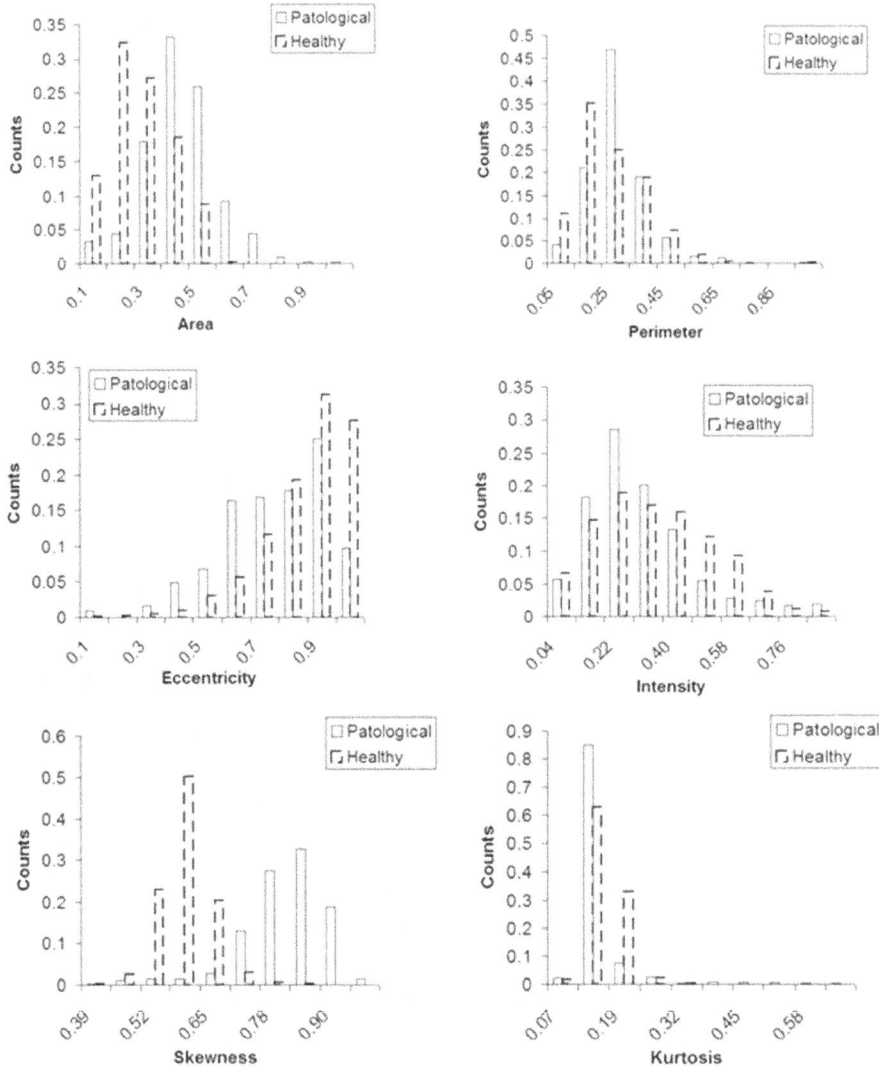

Figure 9 Features comparison: pathological/healthy.

The iterative process just described in the flow chart in Figure 10 that starts with $K_{ini} = N/3$ and repeat the process N_{Loop} times (in the example $N_{Loop} = 50$).

Figure 11 shows the histogram of the values $W(L_p)$, with $L_p = 1,...N_{Loop}$, obtained using an image with 261 segmented object and K_{ini} equal to 87. Figure 12 shows the histogram of the value $W(L_p)$ for the same image and positioned in the same range of variability as before but with a K_{ini} value equal to 72. This makes the process independent from the initial value of K_{ini}, provided that this is greater than the number of residual final clusters.

Figure 13 shows the histogram of the value $W(L_p)$ obtained starting from an initial condition (value of K_{ini}) closest to the final expected (stability condition).

Results and discussions

The procedure described in the previous paragraphs was tested on 39 images of healthy patients belonging to a private database collected in the Policlinic Hospital of Palermo; every image has dimension of 4096×3328 and pixel spacing of 0.07 mm. The procedure was tested also on 20 images of the MIAS database; the size of all the images is 1024×1024 pixels.

Since in all the images the FCM-WF algorithm was able to recognize the clusters but the reconstruction turned out to be characterized by the lack of a few micros and the presence of some more objects (noise), we defined a *Merit Figure* as follows:

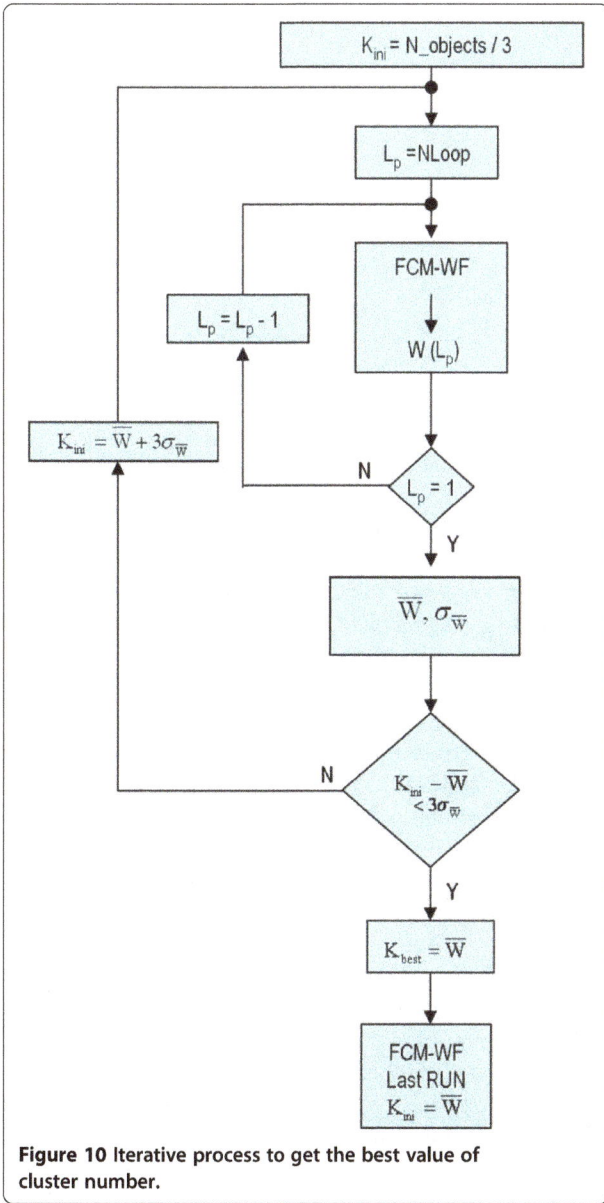

Figure 10 Iterative process to get the best value of cluster number.

$$F_M = \frac{N_{ini} - N_{miss}}{N_{ini} + N_{noise}} \quad (6)$$

In which is the number of micros belonging to the clusters, is the number of micros missing and is the number of noise objects added to the reconstructed cluster.

The performance of FCM-WF algorithm were compared with that of standard FCM. Indeed, to compare the results obtained by our proposed method with the existing ones, we used the following parameters:

TP = number of pathological micro correctly associated to the injected cluster;
FP = number of healthy segmented object erroneously associated to the injected cluster;
FN = number of pathological micro lost;
TN = number of healthy segmented object correctly associated to healthy clusters.

And evaluated also the following merit figures:

- Sensitivity = $\frac{TP}{(TP+FN)}$
- Accuracy = $\frac{TP+TN}{TP+TN+FP+FN}$
- FP/Image = FP/tot. of segmented objects
- Precision = $\frac{TP}{TP+FP}$

We reported in Table 1 the comparison between the performance of our method and that of the method already described with more details in paragraph 1, while the obtained results are presented in Section Results on private database and Section Results on MIAS database.

Results on private database
Every image of the private database was injected with a pathological cluster with the mechanism described in Paragraph 4.1. The performance of the FCM-WF method has been evaluated by examining its capability of correctly recognize the injected clusters, i.e. by counting the number of microcalcifications correctly associated to

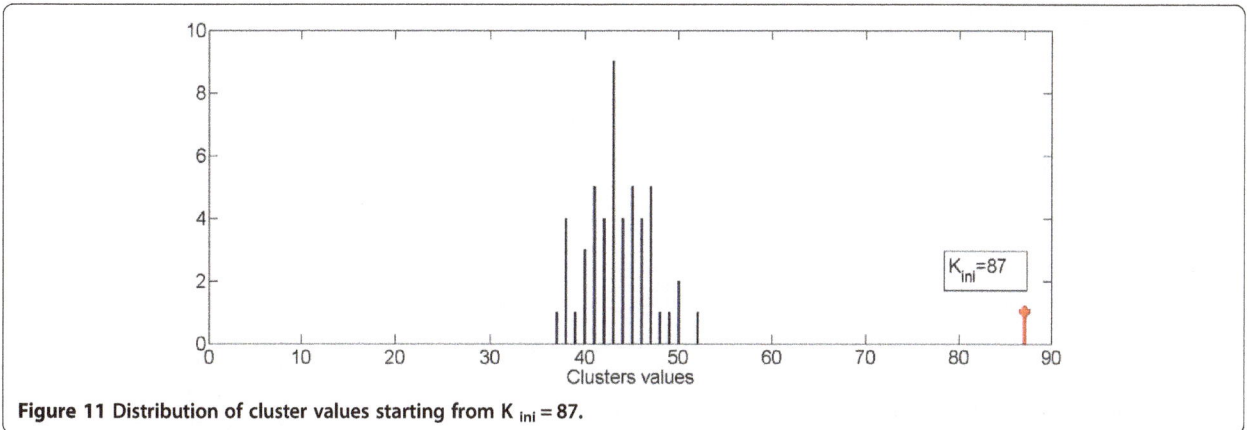

Figure 11 Distribution of cluster values starting from K $_{ini}$ = 87.

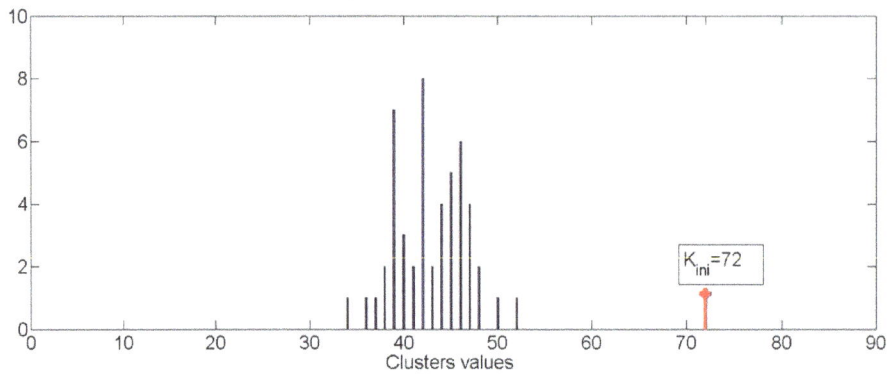

Figure 12 Distribution of cluster values starting from K $_{ini}$ = 72.

the clusters. For this reason, as explained in Paragraph 4.1, it has been necessary to create a gold database in order to know all the truth and the details of microcalcifications clusters.

In Figure 14 each point's coordinates represent the values of the *Merit Figure* obtained with the two methods: FCM (abscissa) and FCM-WF (ordinate); it is visible the improvement of the cases corresponding to the points above the diagonal line; the solid line corresponds to the cases that do not benefit in any way from the implemented method. Figure 15 highlights the relative performance (ratio) improvement as a function of the number of segmented objects in an image. If we denote by F_{M1} and F_{M2} the *Merit Figures* for the two methods FCM and FCM-WF respectively, the mean value of the two *Merit Figures* are 0.61 and 0.67 respectively, with an increase of about 10% in favor of the FCM-WF.

For an expert system, such as a CAD, the clustering process is a preliminary step done before the classification stage. Therefore, while the presence of injected disease clusters is definitely positive for both methods FCM and FCM-WF because it does not alter the efficiency of disease

detection, the presence of a large number of clusters in an image may have a negative effect by increasing the risk to accept an excessive number of false positives after the classification stage. Practically, with the method FCM-WF there has been a steady reduction in the number of residual clusters.

In Figure 16 a histogram is displayed which illustrates the capacity of the FCM-WF method to reduce the number of residual clusters compared to the standard method FCM; in only one case there is a consistent increase in the number of residual clusters. In Figure 17 the reduction of the number of clusters is displayed as a function of the number of segmented objects present in the image before the clustering processes. It is easy to see from this graph that the reduction of the residual clusters does not depend on the number of objects initially present in the image. If we calculate the false positives number in the two methods FCM and FCM-WF for each of the 39 images used, we obtain a false positives average number reduction equal to about 22%.

The histogram in Figure 18 illustrates the ability of the two methods to maintain the pathological cluster:

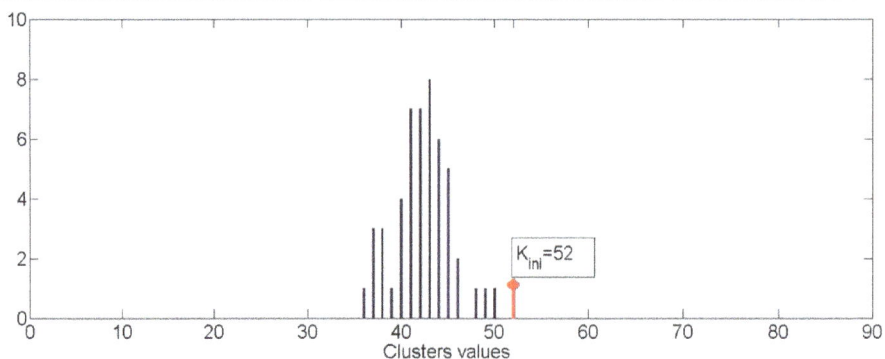

Figure 13 Distribution of cluster values starting from K $_{ini}$ = 52.

Table 1 Performance comparison of clustering methods for breast cancer detection

Author	Clustering method	N. of mammograms (clusters)	Sensitivity	Accuracy	FP/Im	Precision
Nishikawa [12]	Spatial clustering	78 (41)	85%	-	-	-
Cihan [16]	Subtractive clustering	34 (72)	93%	-	-	-
Riyahi [17]	Wavelet transform and Fuzzy clustering	47 (47)	87%	-	0.5%	-
Cordella [18]	Graph-theoretical cluster analysis	40 (102)	94%	-	-	100%
Wang [19]	EFCM	180	-	99.7%	-	-
Quintanilla [20]	PFCM and ANN	-	98.2%	99.5%	-	-
Malar [21]	Wavelet and ELM	55	-	94%		-
Cheng [22]	FLSS	40 (105)	-	> 97%	14%	-
Our method (Private database)	FCM-WF	39 (39)	93%	95%	4%	62%
Our method (MIAS database)	FCM-WF	20(25)	82%	94%	4%	65%

the results point out that FCM-WF achieves a better performance with respect to the conventional method. In particular, among the injected clusters, 70% remain unaffected if the reconstruction is performed with the FCM-WF.

The method was also evaluated in terms of Sensitivity, Accuracy, FP/image and Precision obtaining the following results:

- Sensitivity = $\frac{TP}{(TP+FN)} = 93\%$
- Accuracy = $\frac{TP+TN}{TP+TN+FP+FN} = 95\%$
- FP/Image = FP/tot. of segmented objects = 4%
- Precision = $\frac{TP}{TP+FP} = 62\%$

Results on MIAS database

The FCM-WF method has been tested also on 20 images belonging to the mini-MIAS database. As explained in Section The MIAS database, the database provide only the centre locations and radii of clusters, and since we need to know even position and number of every microcalcification belonging to it, we considered as "truth" about pathological microcalcifications the objects found inside the indicated circle after the segmentation process.

For this database we defined also a "segmentation efficiency" as the number of cluster found in the images after the segmentation process, which is equal to 80%.

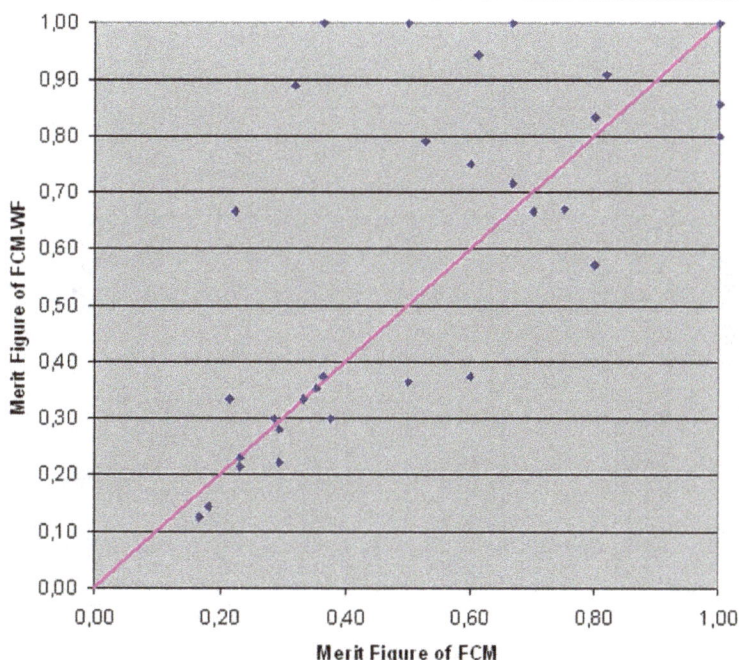

Figure 14 Comparison between the *Merit Figures*.

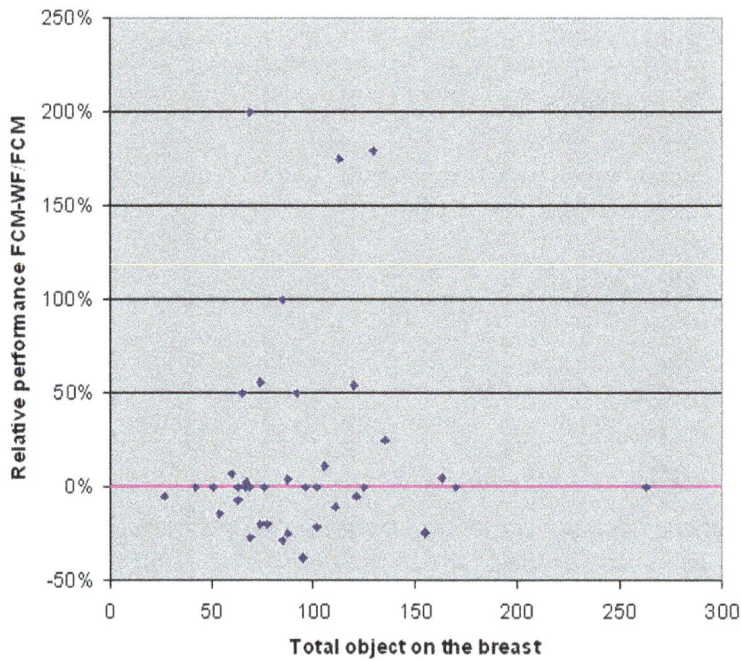

Figure 15 Relative performance improvement vs. total injected object.

In Figure 19 each point's coordinates represent the values of the *Merit Figure* obtained with the two methods: FCM (abscissa) and FCM-WF (ordinate); even for this database it is visible the improvement of the cases corresponding to the points above the diagonal line. Figure 20 highlights the relative performance (ratio) improvement as a function of the number of segmented objects in an image. If we denote by F_{M1} and F_{M2} the *Merit Figures* for the two methods FCM and FCM-WF respectively, the mean

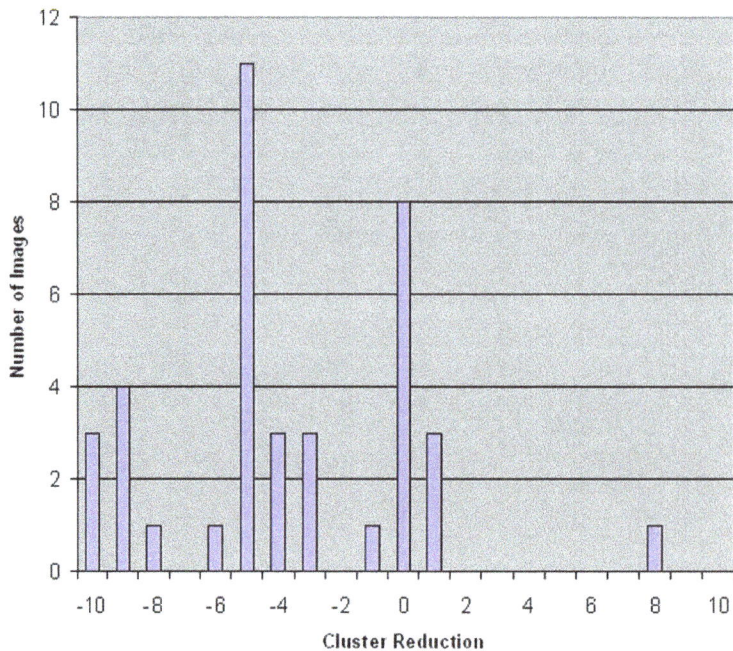

Figure 16 Residual clusters number reduction histogram.

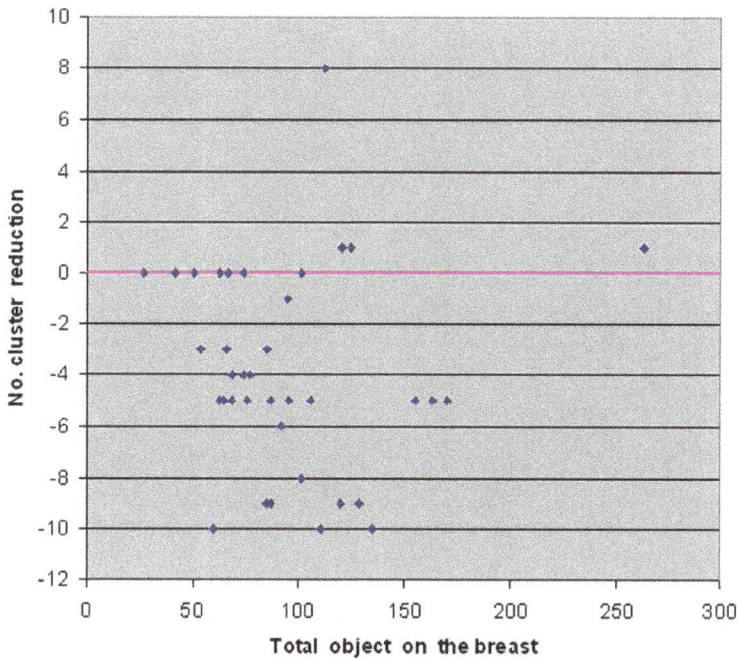

Figure 17 Residual clusters number reduction vs. total object on the breast image.

value of the two *Merit Figures* are 0.45 and 0.50 respectively, with an increase of 5% in favor of the FCM-WF.

If we calculate the false positives number in the two methods FCM and FCM-WF for every image of the MIAS database used, we obtain a false positives average number reduction equal to about 10%.

The method was also evaluated in terms of Sensitivity, Accuracy, FP/image and Precision obtaining the following results:

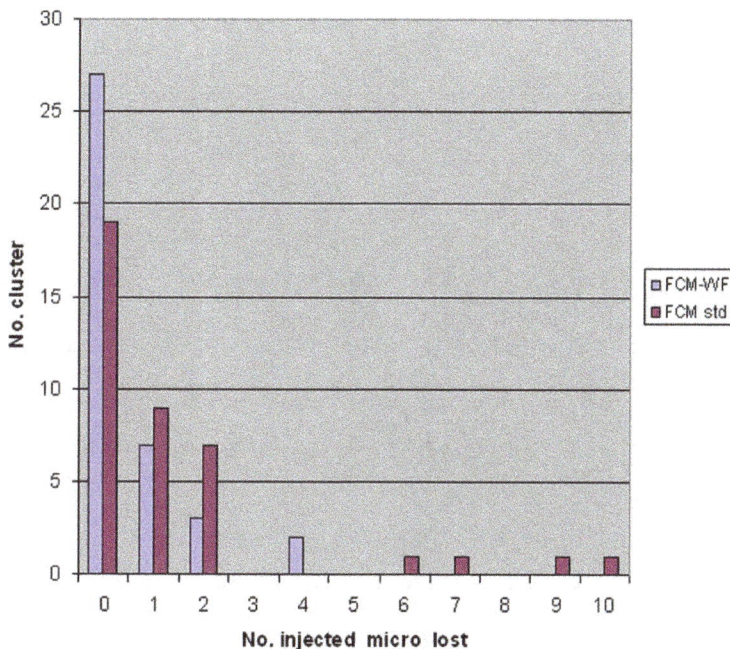

Figure 18 Number of lost injected micros.

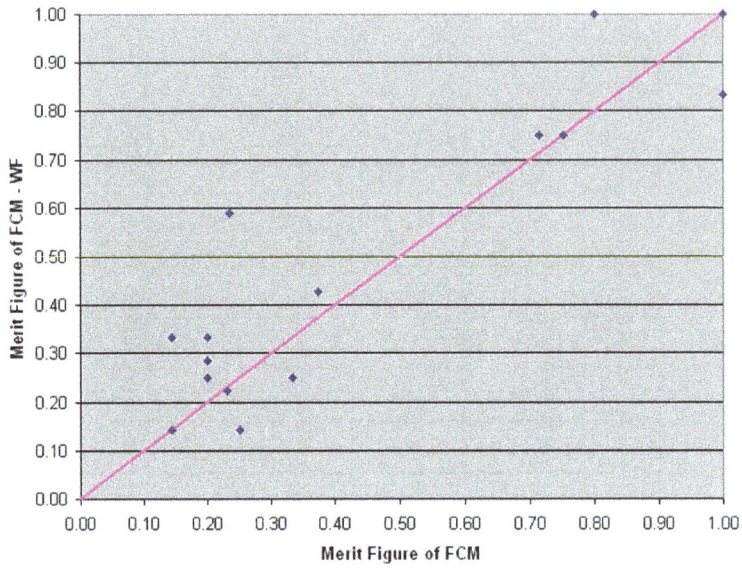

Figure 19 Comparison between the *Merit Figures.*

- Sensitivity = $\frac{TP}{(TP+FN)}$ = 82%
- Accuracy = $\frac{TP+TN}{TP+TN+FP+FN}$ = 94%
- FP/tot. of segmented objects = 4 %
- Precision = $\frac{TP}{TP+FP}$ = 65%

Conclusions

In this paper we presented a clustering method for microcalcifications based on fuzzy logic. This method, called Fuzzy C-Mean With Features (FCM-WF) allows microcalcifications clustering not only according to their distance but also to their relevant features.

The method was tested on a database of simulated images obtained by injecting a pathological cluster on healthy images: in this way we know the "truth" about the exact position of a cluster and the number of microcalcifications belonging to it.

Thanks to this database and to the informations contained in it regarding every single microcalcification, we tested the developed clustering method with great accuracy: actually, for every cluster, we verified the difference between the desired and obtained result with the *Merit Figure* of equation 6. In particular, we verified that 70% of the injected clusters remained

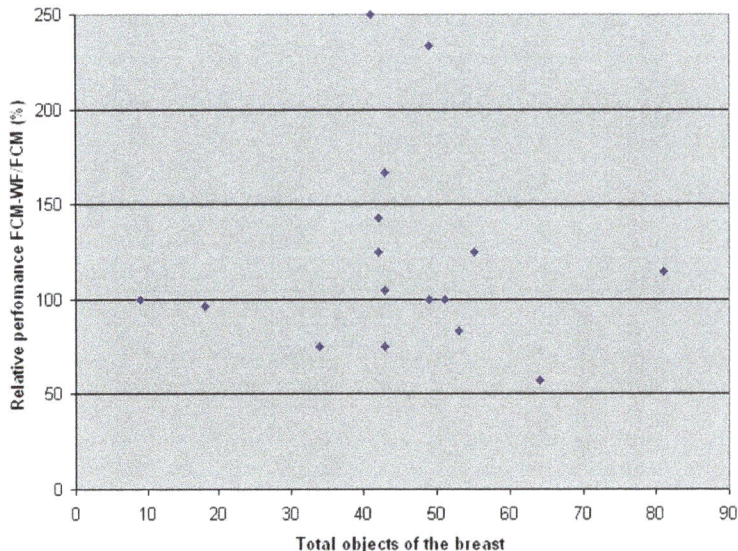

Figure 20 Relative performance improvement vs. total injected object.

unaffected if the reconstruction is performed with the FCM-WF.

Moreover, the automatic determination of the number of clusters in an image result in further improvements of the overall performance of the FCM-WF method over the standard FCM.

Finally, we want to put in evidence in this paper that the technique of placing the micro image in a healthy described here is not equivalent to a classic simulation process by injection of small spots of pixels of variable amplitude and positions randomly, but consists in the placing of real pathological cluster that retain and transfer the original information through the features used here, allowing us to consider the database simulated as a real database of reported image (Gold Standard Database).

In order to provide strong justification for the effectiveness of our work, we applied the FCM-WF algorithm even on the publicly available MIAS database. However, since to test the method we have to know position and number of microcalcifications belonging to the clusters, we didn't use all images of the database but only the images in which centre locations and radii of clusters are known. We considered as "truth" about pathological microcalcifications the objects found inside the indicated circle after the segmentation process, so we defined a "segmentation efficiency" as the number of cluster found in the images after the segmentation process, which is equal to 80%. For this database we obtained an increase of 5% of the Merit Figure of the FCM-WF compared to that of FCM and a false positives average number reduction equal to about 10%.

Competing interests

We haven't received in the past five years reimbursements, fees, funding, or salary from an organization that may in any way gain or lose financially from the publication of this manuscript, either now or in the future. We don't hold any stocks or shares in an organization that may in any way gain or lose financially from the publication of this manuscript, either now or in the future. We don't hold or we aren't currently applying for any patents relating to the content of the manuscript. We haven't received reimbursements, fees, funding, or salary from an organization that holds or has applied for patents relating to the content of the manuscript. We haven't any other financial competing interests. There aren't any non-financial competing interests (political, personal, religious, ideological, academic, intellectual, commercial or any other) to declare in relation to this manuscript.

Authors' contributions

LV conceived of the study, carried out the Clustering algorithm implementation and determination of K best value, performed the statistical analysis and drafted the manuscript. DC carried out the microcalcifications segmentation, the gold database creation and injection process. FF and GR conceived of the study, participated in the design and coordination of the manuscript, and helped to its draft. All authors read and approved the final manuscript.

Acknowledgements

Authors thanks Policlinic Hospital of Palermo and in particular Dr. Raffaele Ienzi for providing the images.

References

1. Ciatto S, Cascio D, Fauci F, Magro R, Raso G, Ienzi R, Martinelli F, Simone MV: Computer-Assisted Diagnosis (CAD) in Mammography: Comparison of Diagnostic Accuracy of a New Algorithm (Cyclopus®, Medicad) with Two Commercial Systems. Radiol Med 2009, 114:626–635. 10.1007/s11547-009-0396-4.
2. Cascio D, Fauci F, Iacomi M, Raso G, Magro R, Castrogiovanni D, Filosto G, Ienzi R, Vasile MS: Computer-aided diagnosis in digital mammography: comparison of two commercial systems. Imaging in Medicine 2014, 6(1):13–20.
3. Karssemeijer N, Hendriks JHCL: Computer-assisted reading of mammograms. Eur Radiol 1997, 7:743–748.
4. McLoughlin KJ, Bones PJ, Karssemeijer N: Noise equalization for detection of microcalcification clusters in direct digital mammogram images. IEEE Trans Med Imag 2004, 23(3):313–320.
5. Fu JC, Lee SK, Wong STC, Yeh JY, Wang AH, Wu HK: Image segmentation feature selection and pattern classification for mammographic microcalcifications. Comput Med Imaging Graph 2005, 29:419–429.
6. Halkiotis S, Botsis T, Rangoussi M: Automatic detection of clustered microcalcifications in digital mammograms using mathematical morphology and neural networks. Signal Process 2007, 87:1559–1568.
7. Vedkamp WJH, Karssemeijer N: Automated classification of clustered microcalcifications into malignant and benign types. Med Phys 2000, 27(11):2600–2608.
8. Cascio D, Magro R, Fauci F, Iacomi M, Raso G: Automatic detection of lung nodules in CT datasets based on stable 3D mass-spring models. Comput Biol Med 2012, 42(11):1098–1109.
9. Cascio D, Magro R, Fauci F, Iacomi M, Raso G: Automatic detection of lung nodules in low-dose computed tomography. Comput Assist Radiol Surg 2007, 2(supplement 1):357–360.
10. Wei L, Yang Y, Nishikawa RN, Jiang Y: A study on several machine-learning methods for classification of malignant and benign clustered microcalcifications. IEEE Trans Med Imag 2005, 24(3):371–380.
11. Jain AK, Dubes RC: Algorithms for clustering data. Upper Saddle River, NJ, USA: Prentice Hall; 1988:55–143.
12. Nishikawa RM, Giger ML, Doi K, Vyborny CJ, Schmidt RA: Computer-aided detection of clustered microcalcifications: an improved method for grouping detected signals. Med Phys 1993, 20(6):1661–1666.
13. Estevez L, Kehtarnavaz N, Wendt R: Interactive selective and adaptive clustering for detection of microcalcifications in mammograms. Digit Signal Process 1996, 6:224–232.
14. Mao F, Zhang Y, Song D, Qian W, Clarke LP: An improved method of region grouping for microcalcification detection in digital mammograms". Proc of IEEE 1998, 20(2):740–743.
15. Arodz T, Kurdziel M, Popiela TJ, Sevre E, Yuen D: Detection of clustered microcalcifications in small field digital mammography". Comput Methods Prog Biomed 2006, 81:56–65.
16. Cihan IK, Senel HG: An application of topological median filter on detection and clustering of microcalcifications in digital mammograms. IEEE 2006, 10:1136–1139.
17. Riyahi-Alam N, Ahmadian A, Nasehi Tehrani J, Guiti M, Oghabian MA: Segmentation of suspicious clustered microcalcifications on digital mammograms: using fuzzy logic and wavelet. 7th International Conference on Signal Processing Proceedings, ICSP 2004, 3:2228–2230.
18. Cordella LP, Percannella G, Sansone C, Vento M: A graph-theoretical clustering method for detecting clusters of microcalcifications in mammographic images. Proceedings of the IEEE CBMS 2005, 15:20.
19. Wang Y, Shi H, Ma S: A new approach to the detection of lesions in mammography using fuzzy clustering. J Int Med Res 2011, 39:2256–2263.
20. Quintanilla-Dominguez J, Ojeda-Magana B, Marcano-Cedeno A, Barròn-Adame JM, Vega-Corona A, Andina D: Automatic detection of microcalcifications in ROI images based on PCFM And ANN. Int J Intell Comput Med Sci Image Process 2013, 5(2):161–174.
21. Malar E, Kandaswamy A, Chakravarthy D, Giri DA: A novel approach for detection and classification of mammographic microcalcifications using wavelet analysis and extreme learning machine. Comput Biol Med 2012, 42:898–905.
22. Cheng HD, Wang J, Shi X: Microcalcification detection using fuzzy logic and scale space approaches. Pattern Recogn 2004, 37:363–375.
23. Fauci F, Bagnasco S, Bellotti R, Cascio D, Cheran SC, De Carlo F, De Nunzio G, Fantacci ME, Forni G, Lauria A, Lopez Torres E, Magro R, Masala GL, Oliva P, Quarta M, Raso G, Retico A, Tangaro S: Mammogram segmentation by

contour searching and massive lesion classification with neural network. *IEEE Nucl Sci Symp Conf R* 2004, **5**:2695–2699.

24. Fauci F, Cascio D, La Manna A, Magro R, Raso G, Vasile M, Iacomi M: **A fourier-based algorithm for micro-calcification enhancement in mammographic images.** *IEEE Nuclear Science Symposium Conference Record, article number 4774254* 2008:4388–4391.

25. Liu J, Chen J, Liu X, Chun L, Tang J, Deng Y: **Mass segmentation using a combined method for cancer detection.** *BMC Syst Biol* 2011, **5**(SUPPL. 3): art. no. S6.

26. Iacomi M, Cascio D, Fauci F, Raso G: **Mammographic images segmentation based on chaotic map clustering algorithm.** *BMC Med Imaging* 2014, **14**(1):12.

27. Marr D: *Vision: A computational investigation into the human representation and processing of visual information: San Francisco. ; 1982.*

28. Tangaro S, Bellotti R, De Carlo F, Gargano G, Lattanzio E, Monno P, Massacra R, Delogu P, Fantacci ME, Retico A, Mazzocchi M, Bagnasco S, Cerello P, Cheran SC, Lopez Torres E, Zanon E, Lauria A, Sodano A, Cascio D, Fauci F, Magro R, Raso G, Ienzi R, Bottigli U, Masala GL, Oliva P, Meloni G, Caricato AP, Cataldo R: **MAGIC-5: an Italian mammographic database of digitized images for research.** *La Radiologia Medica* 2008, **113**(4):477–485.

29. Youn H, Han Jong C, Cho Min K, Jang SY, Kim HK, Kim JH, Tanguay J, Cunningham IA: **Numerical generation of digital mammograms considering imaging characteristics of an imager.** *Nucl Instrum Meth A* 2011, **652**:810–814.

30. Berthold M, Hand DJ: *Intelligent data analysis.*: Book: Springer; 1999:321–351.

31. Vivona L, Cascio D, Magro R, Fauci F, Raso G: **A fuzzy logic C-means clustering algorithm to enhance microcalcifications clusters in digital mammograms.** *IEEE Nucl Sci Symp Med Imaging Conf* 2012:3048–3050. art. No. 6152551.

32. Bellotti R, De Carlo F, Gargano G, Tangaro S, Cascio D, Catanzariti E, Cerello P, Cheran SC, Delogu P, De Mitri I, Fulcheri C, Grosso D, Retico A, Squarcia S, Tommasi E, Golosio B: **A CAD system for nodule detection in low-dose lung CTs based on region growing and a new active contour model.** *Med Phys* 2007, **34**(12):4901–4910.

33. Rusina R, Kukal J, Bělíček T, Buncová M, Matěj R: **Use of fuzzy edge single-photon emission computed tomography analysis in definite Alzheimer's disease - a retrospective study.** *BMC Med Imaging* 2010, 10 , art. no. 20.

34. Masala GL, Golosio B, Oliva P, Cascio D, Fauci F, Tangaro S, Quarta M, Cheran SC, Lopez Torres E: **Classifiers trained on dissimilarity representation of medical pattern: a comparative study".** *Nuovo Cimento della Società Italiana di Fisica C* 2005, **28**(6):905–912.

35. Masala GL, Tangaro S, Golosio B, Oliva P, Stumbo S, Bellotti R, De Carlo F, Gargano G, Cascio D, Fauci F, Magro R, Raso G, Bottigli U, Cgincarini A, De Mitri I, De Nunzio G, Gori I, Retico A, Cerello P, Cheran SC, Fulcheri C, Lopez Torres E: **Comparative study of feature classification methods for mass lesion recognition in digiteized mammograms".** *Nuovo Cimento C, Geophysics and Space Physics* 2007, **30**(3):305–316.

36. McKeen-Polizzotti L, Henderson KM, Oztan B, Bilgin CC, Yener B, Plopper GE: **Quantitative metric profiles capture three-dimensional temporospatial architecture to discriminate cellular functional states".** *BMC Med Imaging* 2011, 11, art. no. 11.

37. Kim SY, Lee JW, Bae JS: **Effect of data normalization on fuzzy clustering of DNA microarray data.** *BMC Bioinformatics* 2006, 7, art. no. 134.

5

Automatic detection of anomalies in screening mammograms

Edward J Kendall[1*], Michael G Barnett[2] and Krista Chytyk-Praznik[3]

Abstract

Background: Diagnostic performance in breast screening programs may be influenced by the prior probability of disease. Since breast cancer incidence is roughly half a percent in the general population there is a large probability that the screening exam will be normal. That factor may contribute to false negatives. Screening programs typically exhibit about 83% sensitivity and 91% specificity. This investigation was undertaken to determine if a system could be developed to pre-sort screening-images into normal and suspicious bins based on their likelihood to contain disease. Wavelets were investigated as a method to parse the image data, potentially removing confounding information. The development of a classification system based on features extracted from wavelet transformed mammograms is reported.

Methods: In the multi-step procedure images were processed using 2D discrete wavelet transforms to create a set of maps at different size scales. Next, statistical features were computed from each map, and a subset of these features was the input for a concerted-effort set of naïve Bayesian classifiers. The classifier network was constructed to calculate the probability that the parent mammography image contained an abnormality. The abnormalities were not identified, nor were they regionalized.

The algorithm was tested on two publicly available databases: the Digital Database for Screening Mammography (DDSM) and the Mammographic Images Analysis Society's database (MIAS). These databases contain radiologist-verified images and feature common abnormalities including: spiculations, masses, geometric deformations and fibroid tissues.

Results: The classifier-network designs tested achieved sensitivities and specificities sufficient to be potentially useful in a clinical setting. This first series of tests identified networks with 100% sensitivity and up to 79% specificity for abnormalities. This performance significantly exceeds the mean sensitivity reported in literature for the unaided human expert.

Conclusions: Classifiers based on wavelet-derived features proved to be highly sensitive to a range of pathologies, as a result Type II errors were nearly eliminated. Pre-sorting the images changed the prior probability in the sorted database from 37% to 74%.

Background

Breast cancer is the most common form of cancer among Canadian women, and is second only to lung cancer in mortality [1-3]. Women in higher risk groups, are encouraged receive a screening x-ray mammogram every two years, with further screening for very high risk patients, such as those with familial history or genetic predisposition.

Treatment efficacy is linked to early detection of tumors. The challenge in x-ray mammography is that features associated with pathology may be patent or subtly represented in the image. For example, micro-calcifications sometimes signal the presence of cancer. Due to calcium's relatively high absorption of x-ray photons they appear as small bright regions in the mammogram and readily detected by CAD and human reviewers [4-8]. On the other hand, masses are evident in an x-ray if their density differs from that of the surrounding tissue, and this is often not the case. Masses may have almost any size, shape or structure [4,7,9-17]. Occasionally, masses are evident only by

* Correspondence: edward.kendall@mun.ca
[1]Discipline of Radiology, Janeway Child Health Centre, Memorial University of Newfoundland, Newfoundland A1B 3V6, Canada
Full list of author information is available at the end of the article

inducing deformation of adjacent tissue. These architectural distortions are difficult to detect thereby limiting the sensitivity of the screening procedure [18].

In response to these challenges, a range of software tools have been developed to help radiologists recognize subtle abnormalities in mammograms [7,19-23]. These tools typically use a common second reader model: the radiologist first examines the raw image and notes suspicious regions [24]. The tool then processes the image marking potentially suspicious regions and the results are compared.

Such systems have a significant drawback: they tend to have low specificity and so require nearly every image to be examined twice: once unaided, and then again to compare to the regions marked as suspicious by the software [25]. This is impractical for screening mammography where fewer than 1% of the images will have tumors. In that setting, the unintended consequence of CAD search routines is an increase the time required to report normal findings. In addition, increasing the number of prompts for review apparently does not guarantee an increase in accuracy [25].

Here we report the performance of a wavelet-map feature classifier (WFC), designed as a pre-sorting tool. The WFC identifies and removes normal images from the radiologists review queue, leaving those images with a higher probability of showing abnormalities. For this technique to be optimally safe, the algorithm is designed to perform at high sensitivity, detecting all or nearly all abnormalities; for it to be effective, it has sufficient specificity to remove enough normal images to usefully increase the relative frequency of suspicious images in the product queue.

The pre-screening algorithm was developed using the Digital Database for Screening Mammography (DDSM) database (http://marathon.csee.usf.edu/Mammography/Database.html) [26-28], a publicly available resource. A smaller unrelated Mammographic Images Analysis Society's database (MIAS) database (http://peipa.essex.ac.uk/info/mias.html) [29] provided a confidence check that the algorithm was not over-specified. These data provided a useful proving ground for testing various incarnations of the algorithm.

The DDSM data set consisted of 1714 images, 1065 of which were classified as normal, in that they showed no abnormalities. The other 649 images showed some type of abnormality that would merit further study. These included: 119 benign calcifications, 120 cancerous calcifications, 213 benign masses and 197 cancerous masses. There was a range of tissue composition and breast size in the DDSM data set, making it representative of the variety of images that may be seen in a clinical setting.

The MIAS data set contained 303 images. There were 205 normal images and 98 images that showed some type of abnormality that included: 11 benign calcifications, 12 cancer-associated calcifications, 38 benign masses, 18 cancerous masses, and 19 architectural distortions (9 from benign masses and 10 from cancerous masses that were not directly visible). Again, the images were from a wide variety of patients, such that the tissues imaged varied widely in terms of breast size and tissue composition.

The wavelet filter classifier process

The Wavelet Filter Classifier (WFC) proceeds in several discrete stages: regularizing the raw digital x-ray image, transforming it to produce scale maps, extracting features from the maps, classifying the features and generating the probability that the image contains some abnormality as an output.

Regularizing the images

Digital mammograms were pre-processed [30] to reduce non-pathological variations between images, such as background noise, artifacts, and tissue orientation. All images were rescaled to 200 micron pixel resolution, and were padded or cropped to be 1024 × 1024 pixels, or 20.48 × 20.48 cm. The analysis presented here was restricted to medial-lateral views and the presentation of both breasts was adjusted to a single orientation.

The DDSM (and MIAS) mammograms were scanned from film images. As a result they contained label, noise and other artifacts that are not present in direct digital images. These artifacts were removed using a threshold and segmentation procedure. Otsu's method [30] was used to determine the optimal pixel intensity threshold for distinguishing background and foreground (tissue) pixels. The segmented non-tissue regions were set to zero without changing pixel values within the tissue region. The processed images were rescaled to maximum pixel intensity.

Wavelet decomposition

The normalized mammograms were decomposed using 2D discrete wavelet transformation. This filtering process created four outputs: horizontal, vertical and diagonal detail maps from the high pass component and an approximation map using the low pass component applied vertically and horizontally. After each filter pass every second output pixel was kept. Figure 1 provides an example image and its feature maps generated at the second scale level using the Daubechies 2 wavelet. The high pass component produces scale maps at half the resolution of the parent image. They further emphasize features based upon how the image is sampled (horizontal, diagonal, vertical). The approximation image is the low-pass component and forms the input for the next scale transformation.

Eight decomposition levels were created in a serial process, applying the transformation to the approximation

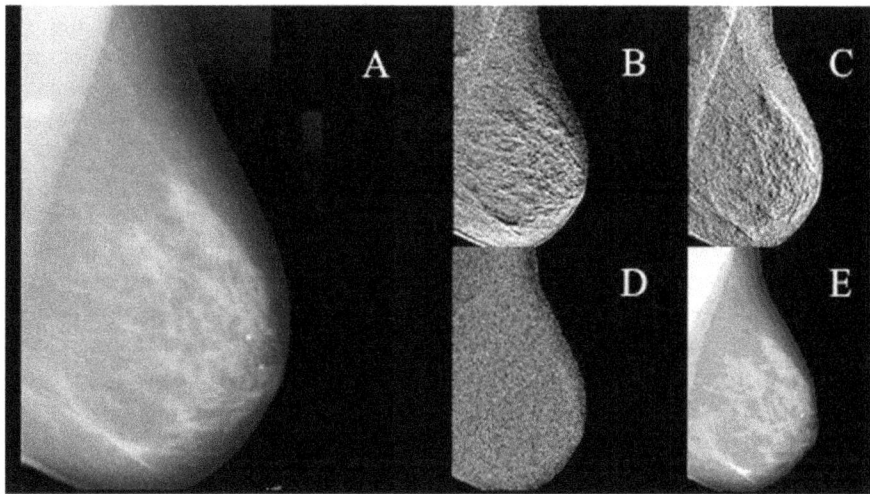

Figure 1 Panel A. Digitized film image masked to tissue. **Panels B - E** are Db2 wavelet coefficient maps at 2nd level of decomposition. **B**. horizontal detail, **C**. vertical detail, **D**. diagonal detail, **E**. approximation. Features were calculated from the tissue area.

map to create four more maps. Since the approximation map had half the resolution of the input image, the wavelet sampled structures that were twice as large as in the original image. The set of all maps derived from a single original image formed a decomposition tree. The highest levels of the tree had the highest resolution and were most sensitive to structures with small spatial extent, while the lowest levels of the tree had the lowest resolution and were most sensitive to structures with large spatial extent.

Many wavelet bases are available, each with unique sampling characteristics. Several, including the Biorthogonal, Debuchies and Haar appeared promising for detecting subsets of the broad range of shapes and intensity gradients potentially associated with pathology [4,31-33]. Eleven wavelets were selected from these families, Haar, Db2, Db4, Db8, Bior1.5, Bior2.2, Bior2.8, Bior3.7 Bior4.4, Bior5.5, Bior6.8. The Haar wavelet is a square function that usefully interrogates sharp discontinuities. The other wavelets are more complex. The notation used suggests some of the features. For example, Db2 (Daubechies 2) is an orthogonal function that samples polynomials that have constant and linear scaling regions. The Bior1.5 describes a bi-orthogonal fifth order sampling function that requires a first order reconstruction algorithm.

The decompositions were initially performed in Matlab using the wavelet toolbox and later ported to C++ to improve computational efficiency. Moments of the mean generated from the output maps formed the input features for classification.

Feature extraction

Four whole-image statistical features, mean, standard deviation, skewness and kurtosis of pixel intensity, were computed for each of the four wavelet-maps at each of the eight decomposition levels. This produced 132 scalar features for each of the eleven wavelet-bases applied to an x-ray image. The classification trials were restricted to using a combination of one, two or three features to avoid over-specifying the final classifier to the training set. Every combination of one, two or three features from the 132 member set were tested for every wavelet basis. The feature sets with the highest sensitivity for finding the images with known abnormalities were selected.

Mean and standard deviation are familiar metrics, skewness and kurtosis less so. The skewness value provides a measure of the asymmetry of a data distribution. Thus, the presence of a small number of unusually dark or bright pixels may alter skewness even when the mean and standard deviation values are not significantly affected. Here the skewness value may be sensitive to the representation of microcalcifications in an image. While these are only a few pixels in size they are unusually bright. Similarly, skewness may report the presence of bright (dense) masses. Since skewness measures the imbalance between the parts of the distribution above and below the mean, the presence of a dense mass will raise the skewness value relative to that found for a normal image.

Kurtosis reports the sharpness of the central peak of a distribution. Since it depends on the fourth power of the difference from the mean, it is highly sensitive to the addition of distant-valued points. Here, increasing numbers of bright microcalcification-containing pixels may be expected to raise kurtosis values. Interestingly, in some cases the kurtosis measure also detected masses. The post hoc rationale developed was based on the observation that when masses appear brighter than normal stromal tissue, they produced additional structure in wavelet maps at several scales. Adding intensity to normally dark pixels altered the kurtosis value sufficiently to distinguish it from the normal range. Of course for any feature, selection of wavelet bases and scale levels that correlate well with the shape of the anomaly was expected to provide the best differential. This was examined using eleven wavelet bases.

Selecting a subset of the candidate features added flexibility to the design of each individual classifier: for example, one classifier could use a feature subset sensitive to micro-calcifications while another could use a feature subset sensitive to masses.

Each classifier was limited to one wavelet basis and two of the four types of parameters generated from the maps. This reduced the feature pool size to 64. Combinations of these features were searched exhaustively to select the most effective combination.

The performance metric used to select the most effective feature subset was a weighted sum of the number of true positive classifications, NTP, and the number of true negative classifications, NTN. This score S was calculated as:

$$s = w(NTP) + (1-w)(NTN)$$

where w is a weighting factor that varies between zero and one. A high weighting factor favors a more sensitive classifier while a low weighting factor favors a more specific classifier. Since in this work, normal images were not subject to further analysis, the true positive fraction was maximized with a 0.995 weighting factor. When two feature subsets produced the same number of true positives the feature subset with the higher true negative fraction was selected.

The individual classifiers could also be designed to maximize detection of a specific abnormality (e.g. masses). To search for a single abnormality, NTP was replaced with the number of correctly classified images containing the specified abnormality, and NTN was replaced with the number correctly classified images of all other types. To ensure that other abnormalities were not missed by the complete system, the outputs of the individual classifiers were combined.

Classification using feature subset and naïve Bayesian classifiers

The goal was to assist a reviewing physician make an informed decision in selecting images for further study. To do this, the classification scheme must provide a measure of the confidence that an image contains an abnormality. Since single naïve Bayesian classifiers do not generate confidence measures, a naïve Bayesian classifier network was constructed. The network's performance classifying known images was used to calculate a classification confidence statistic. Training and

testing was achieved using the leave-one-out cross-validation approach. Here, all but one of the samples were used to train the classifier, and the classifier is tested on the lone remaining sample. The overall performance of the classifier was measured by averaging the classification results when each sample in the data set was used as the test sample.

In all cases the selected scalar features calculated from an image's wavelet maps formed the inputs. The network of classifiers was constructed by passing the normal and suspicious output images from one classifier into additional classifiers for further analysis; several network configurations were evaluated.

Determining classification confidence from classifier network

The predicted confidence levels for a realistic distribution of normal and suspicious images were inferred from the results from a small data set after correcting for its inherent bias. In the DDSM data set [26-28], for example, 649 of the 1714 images were abnormal, this was a higher relative frequency than typically found in a screening clinic (1 in 20) [34]. To correct for this, the relative probability that a given input image was normal or suspicious, $P_i(N)$ and $P_i(S)$, respectively was rescaled.

In the following discussion, lower case n and s refer to images classified as normal or suspicious, while upper case N and S refer to actual number of normal or suspicious images. If the number of normal images counted in a normal bin experimentally is $\eta_{exp}(n,N)$, then the expected fraction of all images from a realistic distribution that are normal and are in the same bin, $F_{real}(n,N)$ was calculated as:

$$F_{real}(n,N) = \eta_{\exp}(n,N)\frac{P_{real}(N)}{T_{\exp}(N)}$$

where $P_{real}(N)$ was the probability of an image from the realistic distribution being normal and $T_{exp}(N)$ was the total number of normal images used in the experimental data set.

The realistic fraction of suspicious images in a normal bin, $F_{real}(n,S)$, was similarly found from the experimentally counted number of suspicious images in the bin, $\eta_{exp}(n,S)$.

The predicted confidence level for an image from a realistic distribution to be correctly placed into a certain normal bin, $C_{real}(N)$, was calculated for each bin using the results measured from a small data set:

$$C_{real}(N) = \frac{F_{real}(n,N)}{F_{real}(n,N) + F_{real}(n,S)} = \frac{1}{1 + \frac{1}{\alpha}\frac{\eta_{\exp}(n,S)}{\eta_{\exp}(n,N)}}$$

where α is a constant defined by:

Table 1 Mean performance of statistical features across all 11 wavelet bases tested

Feature[§]	DDSM			MIAS		
	Sensitivity* (%)	Specificity[†] (%)	Classification rate[‡] (%)	Sensitivity (%)	Specificity (%)	Classification rate (%)
M	89.2	26.6	50.3	86.8	24.1	44.4
σ	94	27.6	52.8	87	27.7	46.9
S	90.8	29.4	52.7	91.9	20.6	43.6
K	92.8	23.7	49.8	93.5	16.8	41.6
M + σ	97.4	33.9	57.9	89.7	23.7	45
M + S	97.2	38.1	60.5	91.9	25.1	46.8
M + K	96.1	35.6	58.5	94	19.6	43.6
σ + S	95.6	29.1	54.3	93.2	23.1	45.8
σ + K	96.3	28.5	54.1	94.3	18	42.6
S + K	94.2	32.2	55.7	93.9	19.5	43.6

§M - mean, σ- standard deviation, S - skewness, K - kurtosis.
*Sensitivity is defined as TP/(TP + FN).
†Specificity is defined as TN/(TN + FP).
‡Classification rate is defined as (TP + TN)/(TP + TN + FP + FN).

$$\alpha = \frac{P_{real}(N)\,T_{exp}(S)}{P_{real}(S)\,T_{exp}(N)}$$

α characterizes the relative frequencies of normal and suspicious images in the experimental data set and in a realistic data set. For the DDSM data set [26-29] with 649 suspicious and 1065 normal images and for a clinic where 1 in 20 images are suspicious, $\alpha = 11.57$. For the MIAS data set with 98 suspicious and 205 normal images and for a clinic where 1 in 20 images are suspicious, $\alpha = 9.08$. A similar argument was used to calculate the confidence level ($C_{real}(S)$) for an image from a realistic distribution to be correctly placed into a certain suspicious bin.

Confidence levels were calculated for the various classifier networks by counting the number of normal and suspicious images assigned to each output bin of the classifier network and using the value of α appropriate for the data set in question.

The relatively low number of suspicious images that occur in practice dominates the realistic confidence levels and makes all bins have a large confidence for containing normal images. To facilitate feature comparisons the theoretical case for an equal chance for an image to be normal or suspicious was also calculated. Thus, $C_{real}(N)$ gave the realistic likelihood that an image in a bin was normal, while $C_{even}(N)$ was useful for comparing the relative confidence levels of different bins

Table 2 Comparison of the performance of wavelet bases on the DDSM dataset

Wavelet basis[§]	Best feature combination			Sensitivity* (%)	Specificity[†] (%)	Classification rate[‡] (%)
Haar	M-h1	M-d1	S-h3	99.2	36.6	60.3
Db 2	M-h3	M-d8	S-h5	97.4	42.7	63.4
Db 4	M-h8	M-d1	S-h5	95.2	20.8	49
Db 8	M-h6	S-v8	S-d3	97.5	40.4	62
Bior 1.5	M-d4	S-h6	—	96.9	38.8	60.8
Bior 2.2	M-h5	M-v2	S-d2	98.8	44.8	65.2
Bior 2.8	M-d4	S-d2	S-a5	92.9	46.9	64.4
Bior 3.7	M-d4	S-h4	S-d4	98.9	28.1	54.9
Bior 4.4	M-h1	M-d4	S-d2	96.1	43	63.1
Bior 5.5	M-h6	M-d5	S-d2	98.5	38.1	61
Bior 6.8	M-v3	M-d4	S-d2	98	39	61.3

§Wavelet basis notation: Dbn where n describes the number of coefficients used in the wavelet. Db2 encodes polynomials with two coefficients, i.e. constant and linear components. Biorm.n where n describes the order for decomposition and m is the order used for reconstruction.
*Sensitivity is defined as TP/(TP + FN).
†Specificity is defined as TN/(TN + FP).
‡Classification rate is defined as (TP + TN)/(TP + TN + FP + FN).
The best triplet feature was selected for each wavelet.

Table 3 Comparison of the performance of wavelet bases on the MIAS dataset

Wavelet basis[§]	Best feature combination			Sensitivity[*] (%)	Specificity[†] (%)	Overall[‡] classification rate (%)
Haar	S-h1	K-a2	K-a8	90.8	32.7	51.5
Db2	K-a3			93.9	14.1	39.9
Db4	K-h5			94.9	9.3	37.0
Db8	S-h3	S-a4	K-d4	91.8	27.3	48.2
Bior 1.5	K-h3	K-a1	K-a8	94.9	13.7	39.9
Bior 2.2	K-a2			94.9	14.1	40.3
Bior 2.8	S-d5	K-a4		94.9	27.3	49.2
Bior 3.7	S-d6	K-d8	K-a7	93.9	23.9	46.5
Bior 4.4	K-h6	K-a2	K-a5	93.9	16.1	41.3
Bior 5.5	K-a1			93.9	14.1	39.9
Bior 6.8	S-h3	K-h7	K-a3	94.9	22.0	45.5

§Wavelet basis notation: Dbn where n describes the number of coefficients used in the wavelet. Db2 encodes polynomials with two coefficients, i.e. constant and linear components. Bior$m.n$ where n describes the order for decompositiona and m is the order used for reconstruction.
*Sensitivity is defined as TP/(TP + FN).
†Specificity is defined as TN/(TN + FP).
‡Classification rate is defined as (TP + TN)/(TP + TN + FP + FN).
The best triplet feature was selected for each wavelet.

when deciding which images are most likely normal. The mapping is monotonic, so bin ranking is the same using either a realistic or equal chance measure.

In summary, images were subjected to wavelet decomposition using a variety of bases and producing 32 scale maps per basis per image. Moments of the mean were calculated for each of the maps resulting in a total of 132 features per image per basis. A Bayesian classifier using leave-one-out cross validation was used to segregate the images into two groups: normal or suspicious. To enhance classification accuracy combinations of up to three features were evaluated. Where classifier networks were employed, a confidence level for the final classification was calculated.

Results and discussion
Feature selection
The moments of the mean features were evaluated on both the DDSM and MIAS databases to identify those features that best detected abnormal images. Single features provided sensitivity and specificity ranging from 89 to 94% and 17 to 38% respectively (Table 1). Better performance was observed using the DDSM than the MIAS

database. The mean classification rate achieved on the DDSM database ranged from 50–60%. Whereas, the best performance on the smaller MIAS database did not exceed 47%. As a single feature, mean values provided the lowest sensitivity using either dataset. Standard deviation for DDSM and kurtosis for MIAS demonstrated the highest sensitivity. The best classification rate and sensitivity were obtained using a combination of features (Table 1). For example, using mean intensity and skewness together gave a sensitivity of 97%, and overall classification rate of 61%. Thus it appears that the sensitivity performance of the features, at least for some, was additive. These results were generally confirmed on the MIAS database, here the combination of mean and skewness achieved a sensitivity and classification rate of 92% and 47% respectively. In the case of this smaller database the individual components achieved sensitivities of 87% 92% respectively with classification rates near 44%.

The best single features obtained from the DDSM database were exhaustively tested for each wavelet over all scales and maps to identify the best combination of one, two or three features (Table 2). Sensitivities ranged from 93 to 99% with overall classification rates of 49 to 65%. The Bior 2.2 triplet combination of mean values

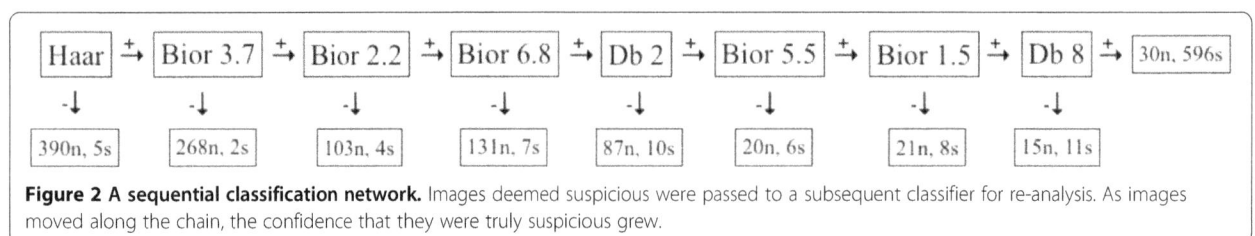

Figure 2 A sequential classification network. Images deemed suspicious were passed to a subsequent classifier for re-analysis. As images moved along the chain, the confidence that they were truly suspicious grew.

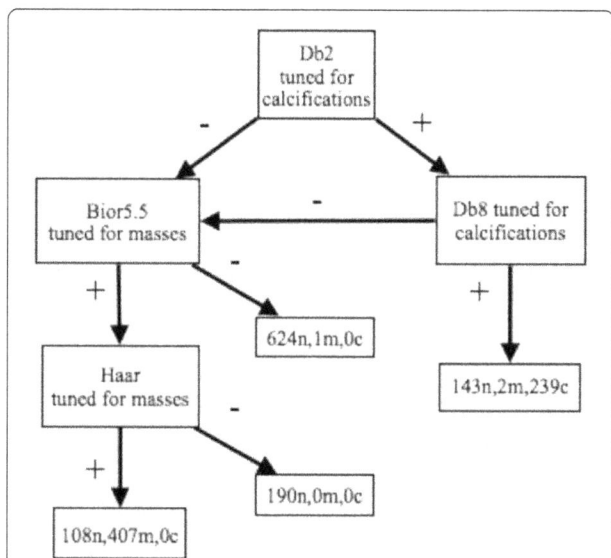

Figure 3 A four-tap branched network. Classifiers were tuned to preferentially detect calcifications or masses. Tuning refers to selecting the feature set to optimize sensitivity for the anomaly.

horizontal map combined with the kurtosis features from the approximation maps at levels 2 and 8, produced the best classification rate at 51%, but did so at the expense of sensitivity. All of the other wavelet bases tested provided higher sensitivity. The Bior2.8 basis using the doublet combination of the skewness value from the diagonal map at level 5 and the kurtosis value from the approximation map at level 4 provided the best combination of sensitivity (95%) and specificity (27%) and an overall classification rate of 49.2%. For this smaller dataset, four single and one double feature achieved the best performance for some wavelet bases. It may be noted in Table 3 that when single features exhibited good sensitivity they did so with a large specificity penalty.

The data had been normalized to 1024^2 leaving open the possibility that the interpolation process may have influenced classifications rates. However, this was found not to be the case. A subset of the data was re-sampled to 256^2 and to 512^2 and classified using mean features from the Haar wavelet. The lower resolution images provided classification rates indistinguishable from the 1024^2 resolution (not shown, see also [35]).

The results obtained (Tables 1, 2 and 3) suggested that no single combination of wavelet basis and feature would correctly classify all the images. Therefore, a network of classifiers was conceived in an attempt to achieve an acceptable classification rate.

Two general network designs were developed and tested: 1) A sequential series of classifiers that passed images along a line of classifiers, removing them from the queue once found to be normal (Figure 2); 2) A branched network of classifiers initially tuned to just masses or just

from the horizontal detail map at scale 5 and the vertical detail map at scale 2, combined with the skewness value for the diagonal detail map at scale 2 achieved a sensitivity of 99% and an overall classification rate of 65%. In only one case, Bior 1.5, did a combination of just two features provide the best performance.

A similar procedure was performed on the MIAS database (Table 3). Here the best features were found to be skewness and kurtosis. The Haar wavelet, using the triplet combination of skewness feature from the level 1

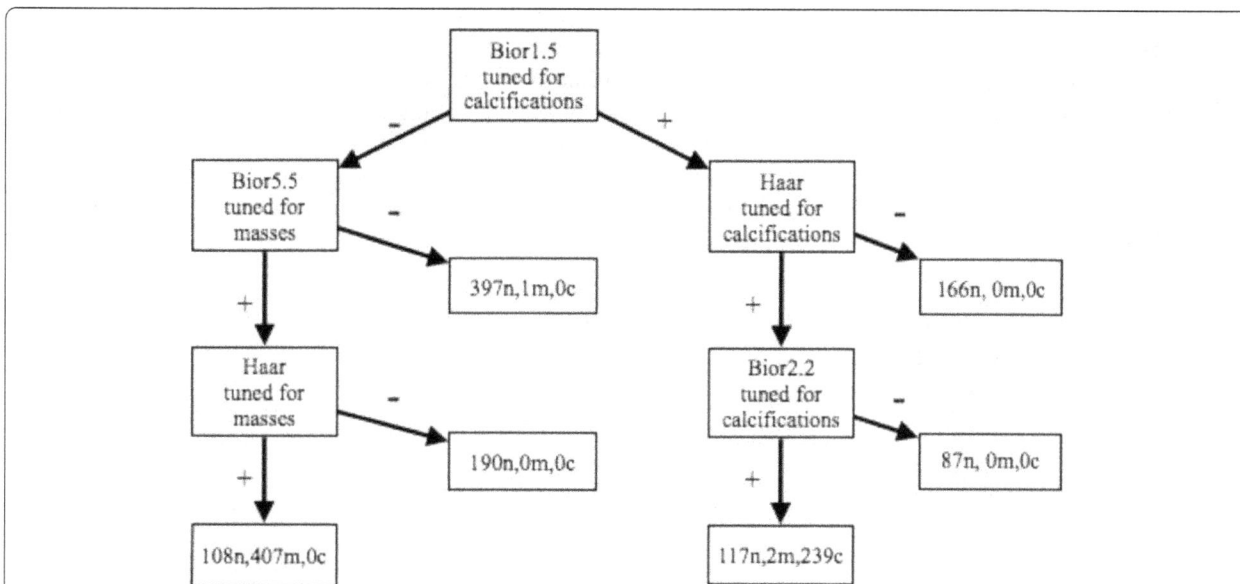

Figure 4 A six-tap branched network. Classifiers were tuned to preferentially detect calcifications or masses. Tuning refers to selecting the feature set to optimize sensitivity for the anomaly.

Table 4 Performance of sequential classifiers using the DDSM database

Wavelet basis[§]	Classified normal		Classified suspicious		Confidence level (%)	
	Actually normal	Actually suspicious	Actually normal	Actually suspicious	$C_{even}(N)$	$C_{even}(S)$
Haar	390	5	675	644	97.9	61
Bior 3.7	268	2	407	642	98.8	72.1
Bior 2.2	103	4	304	638	94	77.5
Bior 6.8	131	7	173	631	91.9	85.7
Db 2	87	10	86	621	84.1	92.2
Bior 5.5	20	6	67	615	67	93.8
Bior 1.5	21	8	45	607	61.5	95.7
Db 8	15	11	30	596	45.5	97

[§]Wavelet basis notation: Dbn where n describes the number of coefficients used in the wavelet. Db2 encodes polynomials with two coefficients, i.e. constant and linear components. Bior$m.n$ where n describes the order for decompositiona and m is the order used for reconstruction.
Suspicious images were passed to the next classifier in the chain.

calcifications (Figures 3 and 4). The classifier features selected for the networks were those that had proven superior when tested alone. The findings from these approaches are presented below.

Sequential network classifier

In the sequential configuration (Figure 2), an image's wavelet map features (best set) were passed to the first classifier, images deemed normal were removed from the queue, while images classified as suspicious were passed on to the next classifier for re-analysis. Thus, the further an image passed along the chain before being found normal, the higher was its "suspicious" probability.

Classifiers selected for maximal sensitivity to any abnormality were organized in a sequential series. To increase the independence of the component classifiers, no wavelet basis was used more than once in a series. This criterion left eleven possible classifiers to choose among for the sequential design, one for each wavelet basis tested. An eight-member sequential series (Figure 2) was developed and the leave-one-out methodology was used for training and testing. Each individual classifier was the most sensitive for that wavelet basis. Tables 4 and 5 show the performance of the classifiers in the

sequence that they were used on the DDSM and MIAS data respectively.

For the DDSM data, the Haar based classifier correctly identified 390 of the 1065 normal images in the set and misidentified 5 of the 649 suspicious images as normal. This provided a confidence level, using an equal prior probability of normal or suspicious, of 97.9% for normal and 61% for suspicious. Images classified as suspicious were passed down the chain configured with Biorthogonal and Daubechies based classifiers. After stage five in the chain, the confidence that an image classified as normal, was normal, declined sharply. This implied that the incidence of type II error (false negative) rose at this stage and beyond. Considering the emphasis placed on detection in this study, the data suggested that this eight member sequential network might be terminated at stage 5 to maintain high sensitivity. Overall, the DDSM-trained sequential network achieved 91.8% sensitivity for abnormal images with a specificity of 97.2%. Eight percent of the positive images escaped detection.

Re-evaluation on the MIAS-trained network (using different features) achieved 88.8% sensitivity to abnormal images with a specificity of 67.3% at stage 5. These results were very encouraging and led to the second network approach.

Table 5 Performance of sequential classifiers on the MIAS database

Wavelet basis[§]	Classified normal		Classified suspicious		Confidence level (%)	
	Actually normal	Actually suspicious	Actually normal	Actually suspicious	$C_{even}(N)$	$C_{even}(S)$
Bior 2.8	56	5	149	93	84.3	56.6
Bior 6.8	23	0	126	93	100.0	60.7
Bior 3.7	9	1	117	92	81.1	62.2
Haar	50	5	67	87	82.7	73.1
Db 8	5	3	62	84	44.3	73.9

[§]Wavelet basis notation: Dbn where n describes the number of coefficients used in the wavelet. Db2 encodes polynomials with two coefficients, i.e. constant and linear components. Bior$m.n$ where n describes the order for decompositiona and m is the order used for reconstruction.
Suspicious images were passed to the next classifier in the chain.

Table 6 Performance of branched network classification

Dataset	TP	TN	FP	FN	Sensitivity	Specificity	Class. rate	$C_{real}(N)$	$C_{real}(S)$
DDSM									
four-tap	748	814	251	1	1.0	0.764	0.861	0.975	1
six-tap	648	840	225	1	1.0	0.789	0.868	0.979	1
MIAS									
4 tap	98	95	110	0	1.0	0.463	0.637	0.975	1
6 tap	98	134	71	0	1.0	0.654	0.766	0.979	1

Network tuned for particular abnormalities

The alternative embodiment used classifiers that were tuned to detect specific types of abnormalities, either masses or calcifications. The goal was to determine if performance might be improved by deploying specialized classifiers. Images were first passed through several classifiers looking for one type of abnormality; if they were not suspicious for it, they were passed on to several classifiers looking for the other type of abnormality. These classifiers, with more specific targets, had potentially higher sensitivities. Figures 3 and 4. show two networks designed in this way. The number of images that are normal (n), show calcifications (c), or show masses (m) are listed at each stage of the network with the appropriate letter label. The wavelet features selected were those that had best identified the anomaly as a single feature classifier.

The tuned classifier networks were configured with four or six output taps. This offered the additional potential to distinguish among normal, calcifications and masses. The network selected calcifications first. The four-tap network (Figure 3) used the Db2 wavelet feature tuned for calcifications. Suspicious images were passed to a Db8 classifier also tuned for calcifications. Normal images from the Db8 classifier went to the queue with normal images from the Db2 classifier, to be reexamined using Bior5.5 and Haar classifiers tuned for masses. The Db8 classifier output on the calcifications leg, was a bin with all the images containing calcifications, a few masses and some normal images. On the masses leg of this network the suspicious tap contained most of the masses (all but one), no calcifications and some normal images. The normal output bins on this leg contained 814 of the 1065 normal images, one mass and no calcifications. This configuration achieved 99.8% sensitivity, a specificity of 76.4% and a classification rate of 86.1%.

For the six-tap network, classification began with the Bior1.5 (Figure 4). Suspicious images from this were passed successively to Haar and Bior2.2 classifiers both tuned for calcifications. The suspicious output on this leg was a bin containing all the calcifications, 2 masses and 117 normal images. There were two normal output bins on this leg, these bins contained only normal images. The normal output from the Bior1.5 was passed to Bior5.5 and Haar classifiers tuned for masses. On this leg the classifiers identified all but one of the masses. The two normal bins contained no calcifications and a single mass. This configuration provided a sensitivity of 99.8%, a specificity of 78.9% and an overall classification rate of 86.8%. This configuration successfully removed 840 of the 1065 images from the suspicious bin. To achieve this result, the penalty was one incorrectly classified mass-containing image.

When similar networks were evaluated on the MIAS data set equivalent results were obtained (not shown). Here again, in the four-tap configuration calcifications were identified first, then masses. The six-tap configuration searched for masses first, then calcifications. Using this smaller dataset the four-tap configuration achieved 100% sensitivity and 46.3% specificity with an overall classification rate of 63.7%. The six-tap network also achieved 100%

Table 7 Segmentation of mammograms containing masses from those containing calcifications

Dataset	T-Norm	F-Norm	T-Mass	F-Mass	T-Calc	F-Calc	C_{even} (Norm)	C_{even} (Mass)	C_{even} (Calc)
DDSM									
four- tap	814	1	407	108	239	145	0.764	0.993	1.000
six- tap	840	1	407	1078	239	119	0.770	0.993	1.000
MIAS									
4 tap	95	0	71	86	23	28	0.463	0.947	1.000
6 tap	134	0	75	66	23	5	0.654	1.000	1.000

sensitivity, and 65% specificity. Here the overall classification rate achieved was 76.6%.

Table 6 collects the results for each of the network configurations and provides the realistic confidence for the classification. The sensitivity of the systems was such that even in a realistic data set, when the incidence of abnormality was 5%, it is likely that all abnormalities will be detected.

The networks also achieved a strong segmentation between images with calcifications and images with masses. The data is collected in Table 7 where it is evident that the networks were perfectly sensitive for calcifications although perhaps less efficient with the smaller MIAS data set. It is tempting to speculate that this is due to under-representation of the range of normal mammogram types in MIAS.

The networks were designed conservatively; each wavelet classifier was configured for maximum sensitivity. A more aggressive design could have removed more normal images, but may have sacrificed overall sensitivity; that was not considered an acceptable tradeoff.

The classifiers developed in this paper offer a useful approach for binary classification of mammographic x-ray images. In practice, an analyst could use the WFC, tuned to a confidence threshold of their choosing, to remove or re-prioritize normal images. This pre-screening technique should improve subsequent detection of those few images showing abnormalities that merit further analysis [5,36].

For an algorithm to be effective and optimally safe as a preliminary screening tool, it must be able to correctly identify a significant number of normal images while minimizing the number of suspicious images that are incorrectly identified as normal. That is, the algorithm must offer sensitivity higher than current clinical levels, which have been estimated to be between 75% and 90% [2,3,5,34,36-38], while offering a non-negligible specificity. Both branched networks tested in this study achieved sensitivity superior to current clinical performance.

Conclusion

An x-ray mammogram image analysis system [39] was tested on two independent data sets to measure its ability to identify suspicious images that may merit further study by a human expert. The system operated in several steps: first, an image was pre-processed to reduce background noise and artifacts; second, the image was decomposed into a set of maps at different scale levels using a 2D discrete wavelet transform; third, whole-image statistical features were measured from each map and the best triplet of these features was input into naïve Bayes classifiers to determine if an image is normal or suspicious; fourth, several classifiers were chained together to calculate confidence levels from the normally hard classifiers.

Three network designs were tested here: a sequential series of classifiers, a vote-taking scheme of classifiers, and networks where individual classifiers were tuned to detect only calcifications or only masses. All of the networks were designed with sensitivity as the top priority over specificity, since the system is designed to be a first pass for images, so any abnormal images missed by the algorithm would not be likely re-examined by a human expert. All the networks tested provided higher sensitivity than is typically achieved in the screening clinic. Removing a large fraction of normal images from the review queue will reduce the volume of cases that must be examined and, at least statistically, should improve detection of pathology. In the best-case scenario reported here, pre-sorting the images doubled the prior probability of disease in the sorted database.

Once sensitivity is maximized, the effectiveness of a system is governed by its specificity. Here the expert reader excels, typically achieving greater than 95% specificity. The combination of a highly sensitive pre-screening tool and an expert breast screener promises to significantly enhance the overall performance of the typical screening program.

Competing interests
Financial competing interests:
EJK and MGB hold United States Patent US 2010/0310183 that deals, in part, with the material presented in this manuscript. See reference [39].
Non-financial competing interests:
The authors declare that there are no non-financial competing interests.

Authors' contributions
EJK study concept, data analysis/interpretation, prepared manuscript. MGB study concept, data analysis/interpretation, reviewed manuscript, Matlab and C++ programming. KCP study concept, data analysis/ interpretation, reviewed manuscript, feature generation and matrix size experiments. All authors are responsible for the content of the paper and approved the final draft.

Acknowledgements
Research supported by:
Canadian Breast Cancer Foundation -Atlantic Region operating grant to EK
Natural Sciences and Engineering Research Council studentships to MB, KC

Author details
[1]Discipline of Radiology, Janeway Child Health Centre, Memorial University of Newfoundland, Newfoundland A1B 3V6, Canada. [2]Prairie North Health Region, Battlefords Office, 1092 107th Street, North Battleford, Saskatchewan S9A 1Z1, Canada. [3]Radiation Oncology Department, Nova Scotia Cancer Centre, 5820 University Avenue, Halifax, Nova Scotia B3H 1V7, Canada.

References
1. Canadian-Cancer-Statistics-2012—English.pdf. Canadian Cancer Society's Advisory Committee on Cancer Statistics: *Canadian Cancer Statistics 2012.* Toronto: Canadian Cancer Society; 2013.
2. Wadden N: **Breast cancer screening in Canada: a review.** *Can Assoc Radiol J* 2005, **56**(5):271–275.
3. Wadden N, Doyle GP: **Breast cancer screening in Canada: a review (vol 56, pg 5, 2005).** *Can Assoc Radiol J* 2006, **57**(2):67.

4. Cheng HD, Shi XJ, Min R, Hu LM, Cai XR, Du HN: **Approaches for automated detection and classification of masses in mammograms.** *Pattern Recogn* 2006, **39**(4):646–668.

5. Jiang Y, Nishikawa RM, Schmidt RA, Metz CE: **Comparison of independent double readings and computer-aided diagnosis (CAD) for the diagnosis of breast calcifications.** *Acad Radiol* 2006, **13**(1):84–94.

6. Sentelle S, Sentelle C, Sutton MA: **Multiresolution-based segmentation of calcifications for the early detection of breast cancer.** *Real-Time Imaging* 2002, **8**(3):237–252.

7. Tang JS, Rangayyan RM, Xu J, El Naqa I, Yang YY: **Computer-aided detection and diagnosis of breast cancer with mammography: recent advances.** *Ieee T Inf Technol B* 2009, **13**(2):236–251.

8. Torrent A, Oliver A, Llado X, Marti R, Freixenet J: **A supervised micro-calcification detection approach in digitised mammograms.** *Ieee International Conference on Image Processing* 2010, **2010**:4345–4348.

9. Alto H, Rangayyan RM, Paranjape RB, Desautels JEL, Bryant H: **An indexed atlas of digital mammograms for computer-aided diagnosis of breast cancer.** *Ann Telecommun* 2003, **58**(5–6):820–835.

10. Andre TCSS, Rangayyan RM: **Classification of breast masses in mammograms using neural networks with shape, edge sharpness, and texture features.** *J Electron Imaging* 2006, **15**(1):013019-013019-10.

11. Freixenet J, Oliver A, Marti R, Llado X, Pont J, Perez E, Denton ERE, Zwiggelaar R: **Eigendetection of masses considering false positive reduction and breast density information.** *Med Phys* 2008, **35**(5):1840–1853.

12. Guliato D, Rangayyan RM, Adorno F, Ribeiro MMG: **Analysis and classification of breast masses by fuzzy-set-based image processing.** In *Digital Mammography.* Edited by Peitgen HO. Heidelberg: Springer; 2003:195–197.

13. Guliato D, Rangayyan RM, Carnielli WA, Zuffo JA, Desautels JEL: **Segmentation of breast tumors in mammograms by fuzzy region growing.** *P Ann Int Ieee Embs* 1998, **20**:1002–1005.

14. Guliato D, de Carvalho JD, Rangayyan RM, Santiago SA: **Feature extraction from a signature based on the turning angle function for the classification of breast tumors.** *J Digit Imaging* 2008, **21**(2):129–144.

15. Gur D, Stalder JS, Hardesty LA, Zheng B, Sumkin JH, Chough DM, Shindel BE, Rockette HE: **Computer-aided detection performance in Mammographic examination of masses: assessment1.** *Radiology* 2004, **233**(2):418–423.

16. Llado X, Oliver A, Freixenet J, Marti R, Marti J: **A textural approach for mass false positive reduction in mammography.** *Comput Med Imag Grap* 2009, **33**(6):415–422.

17. Rangayyan RM, Ayres FJ, Desautels JEL: **A review of computer-aided diagnosis of breast cancer: Toward the detection of subtle signs.** *J Franklin I* 2007, **344**(3–4):312–348.

18. Prajna S, Rangayyan RM, Ayres FJ, Desautels JEL: **Detection of architectural distortion in mammograms acquired prior to the detection of breast cancer using texture and fractal analysis - art. no. 691529.** *P Soc Photo-Opt Ins* 2008, **6915**:91529.

19. Astley SM: **Computer-aided detection for screening mammography.** *Acad Radiol* 2004, **11**(10):1139–1143.

20. Gilbert FJ, Astley SM, Gillan MG, Agbaje OF, Wallis MG, James J, Boggis CR, Duffy SW, Group CI: **Single reading with computer-aided detection for screening mammography.** *New Engl J Med* 2008, **359**(16):1675–1684.

21. Padmanabhan S, Sundararajan R: *Texture and statistical analysis of mammograms: A novel method to detect tumor in Breast Cells.* Machine Vision and Image Processing (MVIP), 2012 International Conference on: 14–15 Dec. 2012 2012; 2012:157–160.

22. Choi JY, Kim DH, Choi SH, Ro YM: **Multiresolution local binary pattern texture analysis for false positive reduction in computerized detection of breast masses on mammograms.** *Proc Spie* 2012, **8315**:83152B-7.

23. Choi JY, Ro YM: **Multiresolution local binary pattern texture analysis combined with variable selection for application to false-positive reduction in computer-aided detection of breast masses on mammograms.** *Phys Med Biol* 2012, **57**(21):7029–7052.

24. Azavedo E, Zackrisson S, Mejare I, Heibert Arnlind M: **Is single reading with computer-aided detection (CAD) as good as double reading in mammography screening? A systematic review.** *BMC Med Imaging* 2012, **12**:22.

25. Houssami N, Given-Wilson R: **Incorporating new technologies into clinical practice without evidence of effectiveness in prospective studies: computer-aided detection (CAD) in breast screening reinforces the need for better initial evaluation.** *Breast* 2007, **16**(3):219–221.

26. Heath M, Bowyer K, Kopans D: *The digital database for screening mammography.* Madison: Medical Physics Publishing; 2001.

27. Heath M, Bowyer K, Kopans D, Kegelmeyer P Jr, Moore R, Chang K, Munishkumaran S: *Current status of the digital database for screening mammography.* Digital Mammography edn: Springer; 1998:457–460.

28. Heath M, Bowyer K, Kopans D, Moore R, Kegelmeyer P: **The digital database for screening mammography.** In *Proceedings of the 5th international workshop on digital mammography.* 2000:212–218.

29. Suckling J, Parker J, Dance D, Astley S, Hutt I, Boggis C, Ricketts I, Stamatakis E, Cerneaz N, Kok S-L: *The mammographic image analysis society digital mammogram database.* 1994.

30. Sonka M: *Image processing, analysis, and machine vision.* Mason, OH: Thomson: International student edn; 2007.

31. Cui J, Loewy J, Kendall EJ: **Automated search for arthritic patterns in infrared spectra of synovial fluid using adaptive wavelets and fuzzy C-means analysis.** *IEEE Transactions on Bio-Medical Engineering* 2006, **53**(5):800–809.

32. Cheng HD, Cai XP, Chen XW, Hu LM, Lou XL: **Computer-aided detection and classification of microcalcifications in mammograms: a survey.** *Pattern Recogn* 2003, **36**(12):2967–2991.

33. Ferreira CB, Borges DL: **Analysis of mammogram classification using a wavelet transform decomposition.** *Pattern Recogn Lett* 2003, **24**:973–982.

34. Taylor P, Given-Wilson R, Champness J, Potts HWW, Johnston K: **Assessing the impact of CAD on the sensitivity and specificity of film readers.** *Clin Radiol* 2004, **59**(12):1099–1105.

35. Rangayyan RM, Nguyen TM, Ayres FJ, Nandi AK: **Effect of pixel resolution on texture features of breast masses in mammograms.** *J Digit Imaging* 2010, **23**(5):547–553.

36. Coldman AJ, Major D, Doyle GP, D'yachkova Y, Phillips N, Onysko J, Shumak R, Smith NE, Wadden N: **Organized breast screening programs in Canada: effect of radiologist reading volumes on outcomes1.** *Radiology* 2006, **238**(3):809–815.

37. Elmore JG, Armstrong K, Lehman CD, Fletcher SW: **Screening for breast cancer.** *Jama-J Am Med Assoc* 2005, **293**(10):1245–1256.

38. Fenton JJ, Abraham L, Taplin SH, Geller BM, Carney PA, D'Orsi C, Elmore JG, Barlow WE: **Effectiveness of computer-aided detection in community mammography practice.** *J Natl Cancer Inst* 2011, **103**(15):1152–1161.

39. Kendall EJ, Barnett MG: **Image analysis.** 2010. In. vol. 12808099. US.

6

Real-time ultrasound elastography in 180 axillary lymph nodes: elasticity distribution in healthy lymph nodes and prediction of breast cancer metastases

Sebastian Wojcinski[1*†], Jennifer Dupont[2†], Werner Schmidt[3], Michael Cassel[4] and Peter Hillemanns[1]

Abstract

Background: To determine the general appearance of normal axillary lymph nodes (LNs) in real-time tissue sonoelastography and to explore the method's potential value in the prediction of LN metastases.

Methods: Axillary LNs in healthy probands (n=165) and metastatic LNs in breast cancer patients (n=15) were examined with palpation, B-mode ultrasound, Doppler and sonoelastography (assessment of the elasticity of the cortex and the medulla). The elasticity distributions were compared and sensitivity (SE) and specificity (SP) were calculated. In an exploratory analysis, positive and negative predictive values (PPV, NPV) were calculated based upon the estimated prevalence of LN metastases in different risk groups.

Results: In the elastogram, the LN cortex was significantly harder than the medulla in both healthy (p=0.004) and metastatic LNs (p=0.005). Comparing healthy and metastatic LNs, there was no difference in the elasticity distribution of the medulla (p=0.281), but we found a significantly harder cortex in metastatic LNs (p=0.006). The SE of clinical examination, B-mode ultrasound, Doppler ultrasound and sonoelastography was revealed to be 13.3%, 40.0%, 14.3% and 60.0%, respectively, and SP was 88.4%, 96.8%, 95.6% and 79.6%, respectively. The highest SE was achieved by the disjunctive combination of B-mode and elastographic features (cortex >3mm in B-mode or blue cortex in the elastogram, SE=73.3%). The highest SP was achieved by the conjunctive combination of B-mode ultrasound and elastography (cortex >3mm in B-mode and blue cortex in the elastogram, SP=99.3%).

Conclusions: Sonoelastography is a feasible method to visualize the elasticity distribution of LNs. Moreover, sonoelastography is capable of detecting elasticity differences between the cortex and medulla, and between metastatic and healthy LNs. Therefore, sonoelastography yields additional information about axillary LN status and can improve the PPV, although this method is still experimental.

Keywords: Breast ultrasound, Axillary lymph nodes, Sonoelastography, Real-time tissue elastography, Cancer detection, Elasticity imaging, HI-RTE, Lymph node metastases

* Correspondence: s@wojcinski.de
†Equal contributors
[1]Hannover Medical School, Department for Obstetrics and Gynecology, OE 6410, Carl-Neuberg-Straße 1, Hannover 30625, Germany
Full list of author information is available at the end of the article

Background

The prediction of axillary lymph node (LN) status remains an important issue in the preoperative assessment of breast cancer patients. Sentinel node biopsy (SNB) is the standard option for women that are staged with a negative nodal status [1-5]. Nevertheless, if axillary metastases are suspected, the success of SNB may be impaired. These patients should still receive axillary LN dissection (ALND) [6,7]. The procedure of radical ALND implies a significant increase in morbidity, such as lymphedema or paresthesia of the arm [8]. Provided that the preoperative assessment was correct, the precision of histological staging by SNB is very high and postoperative morbidity is significantly minimized [9]. Recently, omission of radical ALND in certain cases of positive sentinel nodes has been discussed [10,11].

However, the diagnostic precision of the preoperative assessment of the axillary LN status is far from perfect. Palpation of the axilla lacks sensitivity (SE) as only vast metastases are clinically apparent. Mammography does not fully cover the axillary region and the prediction of the malignant or benign character of LNs is not possible. On the other hand, B-mode ultrasound is known to be a precise method for the examination of the axilla with a SE of 45-73% and a specificity (SP) of 44-100%, depending on the distinct B-mode criteria that are investigated [12,13]. Other imaging methods such as computer tomography (CT), magnetic resonance imaging (MRI), scintimammography and positron emission tomography (PET) have been investigated, but they have all demonstrated no relevant clinical advantage in the evaluation of the axilla. Additionally, they are overly expensive and labor-intensive [14-19].

Therefore, ultrasound remains the most suitable imaging method to assess axillary LNs, although the diagnostic accuracy is still unsatisfactory [20]. Technical advances like sonoelastography, tissue harmonic imaging and increasing frequencies may allow a better differentiation of benign and malignant masses [21-23]. Concerning the evaluation of breast lesions, sonoelastography has demonstrated an improved diagnostic performance when combining this method with B-mode ultrasound [22,24-26]. Sonoelastography has also been performed on cervical [27-29], mediastinal [30,31], celiac or mesenteric [32,33] and inguinal [34] LNs.

However, to the best of our knowledge, no data concerning sonoelastography of axillary LNs were published prior to the studies of Choi et al. (n=64) and Taylor et al. (n=50) in 2011 [35,36]. Therefore, our current results from 165 healthy and 15 metastatic LNs may expand the knowledge in this field of research to a certain degree.

Our primary study objective was to determine the typical color distributions of healthy LNs in the elastogram.

The secondary study objective was an exploratory analysis of the method/s potential value in the prediction of LN metastases when used as an adjunct to conventional B-mode ultrasound.

Materials and methods

Our study was carried out at the Breast Cancer Center in the University Hospital of Saarland, Homburg/Saar, Germany. The responsible ethics committee did not require additional approval for this non-interventional study design. The study cohort (n=180 LNs) was recruited from patients who attended the outpatient service of our institution.

Healthy patients with no suspicious findings in the breast examination were eligible for the control group (group 1, n=165 LNs). In these patients, we performed the experimental sonoelastography of a randomly chosen axillary LN. Patients with a history of breast surgery concerning a larger resection volume, inflammatory conditions of the breast or systemic infections and skin disorders were excluded.

Patients with histologically-proven breast cancer before treatment were potentially eligible for group 2. In these patients, we performed experimental sonoelastography of an ipsilateral axillary LN. These breast cancer patients (n=33) were scheduled to undergo surgery of the breast and the axilla. Concerning the previously studied LN, we used a skin marker for identification and correlated the pathological size with the ultrasonographic size in order to ensure that this was a representative specimen. Eighteen patients had benign axillary LNs on histological examination. These patients were excluded from analysis. The remaining fifteen patients showed metastases in the previously examined LN. These patients were assigned to the metastatic group (group 2, n=15 LNs).

Ultrasound examinations and image analysis

The routine examinations were performed by the author SW, a DEGUM (Deutsche Gesellschaft für Ultraschall in der Medizin, German society for ultrasound in medicine) level I certified senior physician in gynecology with four years experience in breast ultrasound [37]. The elastograms were obtained by the author JD, a doctoral fellow at our institution. All examinations were performed with the Hitachi EUB-8500 ultrasound system (Hitachi Medical Systems GmbH, Wiesbaden, Germany) using the Hitachi EUP-L54M probe (50 mm, 6–13 MHz) and the integrated elastography module [38].

First, each LN was measured in two planes (i.e. three axes). Furthermore, we determined the dimension of the cortex and the medulla and performed color Doppler ultrasound. Pathological vascularization was defined as the presence of neoangiogenesis disrupting the capsule of the LN or an increased vascularization of the cortex. Next, experimental sonoelastography was carried out. The region of interest for the elastogram was chosen to encompass a maximum of 30% LN tissue and a minimum of 70% encircling tissue.

Image analysis was conducted by JD. As the analysis was performed before surgery, JD had no information about the final histological diagnosis in group 2. The B-mode and Doppler images of each LN were described by standard methods [39]. Concerning the elastogram, the elasticity distribution of the cortex and medulla were described as the predominant color of the particular anatomical region (red, yellow, green, turquoise or blue).

Sonoelastography

Dynamic real-time examinations using ultrasound to access the compressibility of breast lesions were introduced in the 1980s [40]. Today, numerous ultrasound manufacturers offer solutions that include elastography modules in the various ultrasound platforms. The principle of sonoelastography is that the tissue is subjected to a stress (i.e. compression) and the resulting strain (i.e. displacement) is assessed. Typically, the stress is applied by compressing the tissue with the ultrasound probe (freehand/handheld elastography). In addition, the newly developed method of shear wave elastography is under clinical evaluation [41]. This method utilizes an acoustic push pulse (vertically directed) to induce an elastic shear wave (horizontally directed) that propagates through the tissue. The velocity of the shear wave is measured by detection pulses and provides a semi-quantitative measurement of tissue stiffness [42]. In our study, we applied handheld sonoelastography

(Hitachi real-time tissue elastography, HI-RTE). This technology provides color elastograms, in which increasing tissue hardness appears as red, green and blue in ascending order on a continuous scale [Figures 1, 2, 3, 4, 5 and 6]. Therefore, the examiner receives information about the mechanical properties of the tissue.

Statistical analysis

Microsoft® Office Excel® 2007 (Microsoft Corporation) was used for data collection. The analysis was performed with MedCalc® 7.6 statistical software (MedCalc Software bvba, Belgium). The Student's t-test was used for continuous data and comparison of means. Ultrasonographic features of benign and malignant LNs were compared using Fisher's exact test for univariate distributions. The predominant colors in the elastograms were compared using Yates' chi-square test for multivariate distributions of categorical data. When Yates' chi-square test was found to be significant, pairwise comparisons were performed using Fisher's exact test. For the calculation of 95% confidence levels we used Newcombe intervals with continuity correction [43]. Specimen histology was the gold standard for the definition of metastatic LNs. Statistical significance was assumed at p<0.05 for all tests.

Results

We analyzed 165 healthy LNs (group 1) and 15 metastatic LNs (group 2). The breast cancer patients (group 2) were significantly older (58.3 ± 7.4 versus 50.2 ± 12.9 years, p=0.017), and had a significantly higher body mass index (28.0 ± 5.2 versus 24.8 ± 4.5 kg/m^2, p=0.012) than the healthy probands (group 1). There was no significant difference between the groups regarding the clinical presentation of the LNs (i.e. palpable mass 13.3% versus

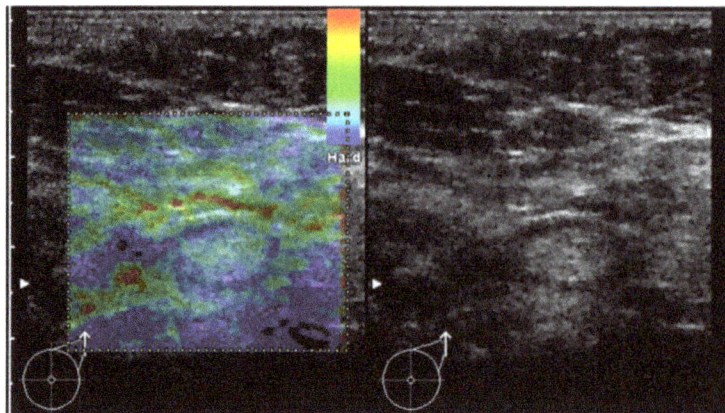

Figure 1 Example for B-mode ultrasound and elastogram of a healthy LN. In B-mode ultrasound the LN exhibits no criteria for malignancy. The predominant color of the medulla is green (with smaller areas of turquoise) and the cortex is mainly blue. Applying the criterion of a blue cortex, this case would be a false-positive.

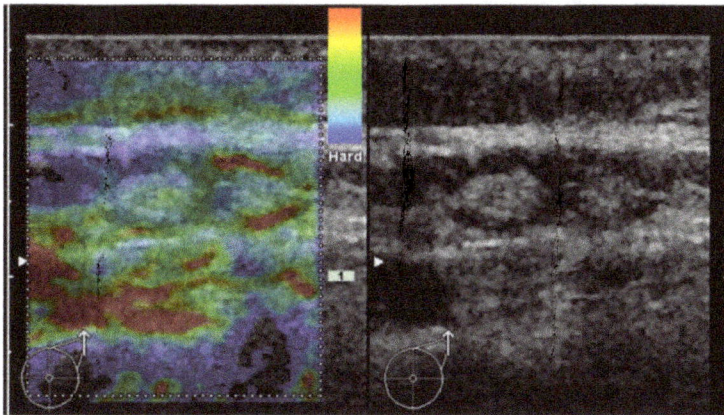

Figure 2 Example for B-mode ultrasound and elastogram of a healthy LN. In B-mode ultrasound the LN exhibits no criteria for malignancy. The predominant color of the medulla is turquoise (with smaller areas of green) and the cortex is mainly green. Applying the criterion of a blue cortex, this case would be a true-negative.

11.6%, p=0.690, and painful palpation 0% versus 2.4%, p=1.000).

B-mode features and Doppler features of healthy and metastatic lymph nodes

Regarding the horizontal size of the LNs and the diameter of the medulla, there were no significant differences between the groups. Nevertheless, the vertical dimension of metastatic LNs was significantly higher (9.2mm versus 7.2mm, p=0.013). Focusing on the cortex, we found a significantly broader cortex for the metastatic LNs (4.2mm versus 1.4mm, p<0.001). Consequently, the cortex-to-medulla-ratio as well as the vertical-to-horizontal-size were significantly higher in the metastatic group (p<0.001 and p=0.002, respectively). A cortex greater than 3mm was found in only 3.1% of the healthy LNs, compared to 40.0% of the metastatic LNs (p<0.001). The results are shown in Table 1.

Elastograms of healthy and metastatic lymph nodes

Focusing on the group of healthy LNs (n=165), the predominant color of the cortex was yellow in 1.2%, green in 13.9%, turquoise in 64.2% and blue in 20.6% of the cases respectively, and never red [Table 2]. The medulla exhibited a similar distribution of the colors (3.0%, 15.8%, 73.9% and 73.2%, respectively, never red) [Table 3]. Nevertheless, the cortex and medulla color distributions were significantly different in the multivariate analysis (p=0.004), and the pairwise comparison revealed that the cortex was significantly more often described as blue (i.e. hard) than the medulla (p<0.001).

Focusing on the group of metastatic LNs (n=15), the predominant color of the cortex was either turquoise (40.0%) or blue (60.0%) but never yellow, green or red [Table 2]. The medulla was yellow in 6.7%, green in 33.3%, turquoise in 53.3% and blue in 6.7% of cases, respectively [Table 3]. Accordingly, the difference between

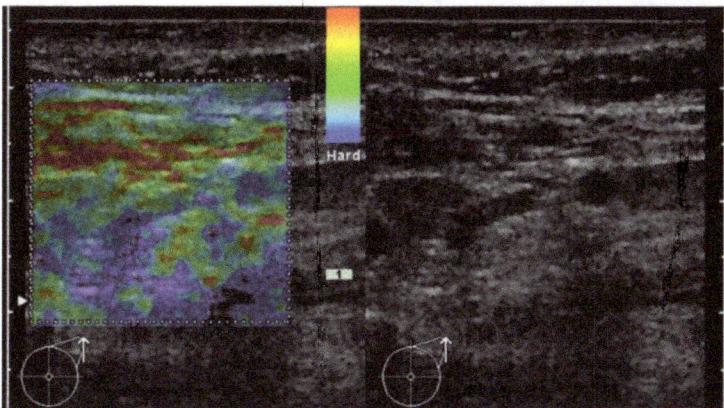

Figure 3 Example for B-mode ultrasound and elastogram of a healthy, reactive LN. In B-mode ultrasound the cortex of the LN is slightly enlarge (maximum ~2.5mm). The predominant color of the medulla is green (with smaller areas in other shades) and the cortex is mainly blue (with smaller areas of green). Applying the criterion of a blue cortex, this case would be a false-positive.

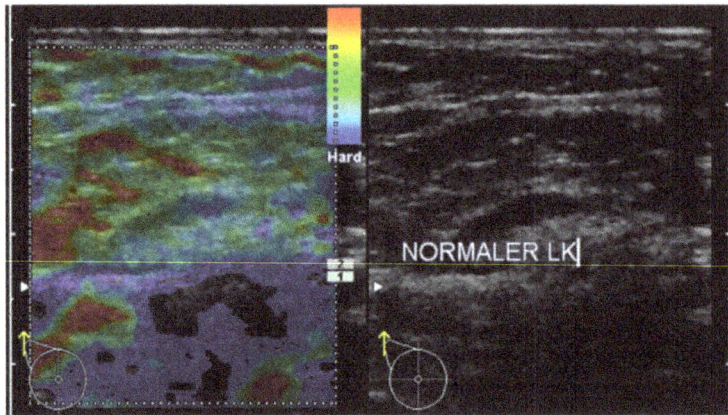

Figure 4 Example for B-mode ultrasound and elastogram of a healthy, reactive LN. In B-mode ultrasound, the cortex of the LN is slightly enlarged (maximum ~3.5mm). The predominant color of the medulla is turquoise (to green) and the cortex is mainly green. Applying the criterion of a blue cortex, this case would be a true-negative.

the cortex and the medulla was statistically significant in the multivariate analysis (p=0.005).

Comparing the two groups, there was no difference regarding the color distribution of the medulla [Table 3]. However, we found a significant difference regarding the color distribution of the cortex (p=0.005). Compared to healthy LNs, the cortex of metastatic LNs was significantly more often blue (60.0% versus 20.6%, p=0.005) [Table 2].

Sensitivity and specificity of B-mode ultrasound, Doppler ultrasound, sonoelastography and clinical examination

Analyzing the performance of single criteria, a cortex broader than 3mm in B-mode ultrasound yielded an excellent specificity (96.8%) and a low sensitivity (40.0%). Concerning sonoelastography, we applied the criterion of a blue cortex and achieved a well-balanced specificity of 79.6% and a sensitivity of 60.0%.

In order to explore the combinations of different ultrasound criteria, we combined the B-mode feature "cortex broader than 3mm" and the elastographic feature "blue cortex". In the disjunctive combination (LNs that fulfill at least one criterion were regarded as positive), the specificity was 77.5% and the sensitivity was higher than with any other criterion, namely 73.3%. In the conjunctive combination (only LNs that fulfill both criteria were regarded as positive), the specificity reached an excellent level of 99.3% (higher than with any other criterion) and the sensitivity was 26.7% [Table 4].

Model calculation concerning the diagnostic performance of B-mode ultrasound and sonoelastography

Calculation of the negative and positive predictive values (NPV, PPV) should be based on the particular prevalence in the observed collective. The prevalence of LN metastases in individual subgroups is dependent on the

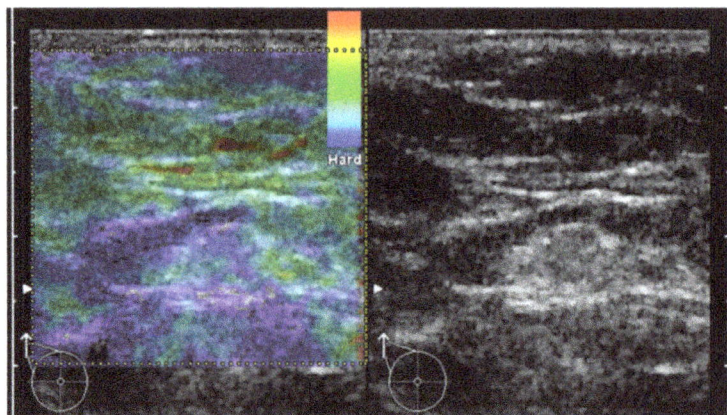

Figure 5 Example for B-mode ultrasound and elastogram of a metastatic LN. In B-mode ultrasound, the cortex of the LN is slightly enlarged (maximum ~3.5mm). The predominant color of the medulla is turquoise (to green) and the cortex is mainly blue. Applying the criterion of a blue cortex, this case would be a true-positive.

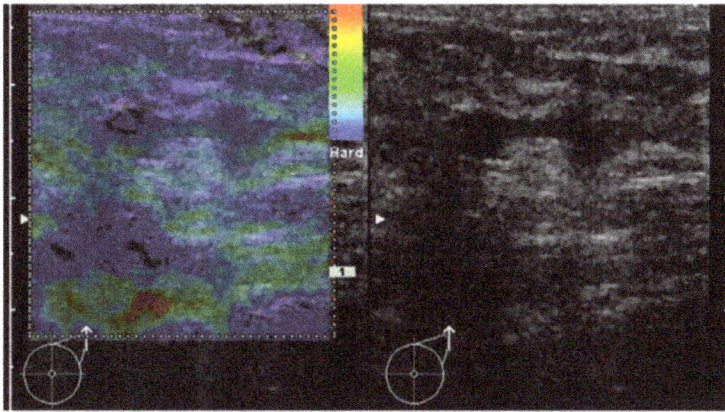

Figure 6 Example for B-mode ultrasound and elastogram of a metastatic LN. In B-mode ultrasound, the cortex of the LN is slightly enlarged (maximum ~3.0mm). The predominant color of the medulla is turquoise and cortex is mainly blue. Applying the criterion of a blue cortex, this case would be a true-positive.

tumor stage, among other factors [44-46]. In mixed collectives, the prevalence of LN metastases is estimated to be about 45% [47], which is concordant with our collective (45.5%). In particular, tumors categorized as T1 show LN metastases in about 25.9% of cases, whereas in T2 tumors, LN metastases occur in about 48.2% [48]. Based on the prevalence of LN involvement within these two risk groups, the following predictive values result:

In T1 tumors (with an estimated prevalence of LN metastases of 25.9%), the best B-mode criterion (cortex >3mm) can be expected to yield a PPV of about 81% and an NPV of ~82%. The conjunctive combination with the best elastographic criterion (blue cortex) leads to an improved PPV of ~93% with little effect on the NPV (~79%).

In T2 tumors (with an estimated prevalence of LN metastases of 48.2%), B-mode ultrasound can be expected to have a PPV of ~92% and a NPV of ~63%. The conjunctive combination with sonoelastography improves the PPV (~97%), but also impairs the NPV (~59%).

Discussion

Sonoelastography only offers a relative measurement of tissue stiffness and is dependent on the surrounding tissue [49]. We propose a relatively simple criterion (i.e. blue cortex) as the most suitable predictor of malignancy in LNs. The fact that the cortex of metastatic LNs is significantly harder than the cortex of healthy LNs is reflected in the predominance of the colors blue and turquoise in the elastograms. Applying this single criterion, the examination with sonoelastography resulted in an SE of 60.0% and an SP of 79.6%.

However, the combination of various criteria from several imaging methods is known to improve the performance. This principle is also used in breast diagnostics,

Table 1 B-mode features and Doppler sonography of healthy and metastatic LNs (mean ± standard deviation, n.s. = not significant, LN = lymph node)

LN characteristics	Group 1 healthy LNs	Group 2 metastatic LNs	p
n	165	15	
Distance from the skin (mm)	13.5 ± 5.1	15.5 ± 3.0	n.s. (0.126)
Horizontal size (mm)	15.8 ± 6.4	14.4 ± 7.0	n.s. (0.406)
Vertical size (mm)	7.2 ± 3.0	9.2 ± 3.5	0.013
Vertical-to-horizontal-size (ratio)	0.50 ± 0.24	0.70 ±0.26	0.002
Cortex (mm)	1.4 ± 0.7	4.2 ± 4.7	<0.001
Medulla (mm)	4.8 ± 2.4	4.1 ± 2.1	n.s. (0.299)
Cortex-to-medulla (ratio)	0.39 ± 0.31	1.22 ± 1.75	<0.001
Cortex >3mm	3.1%	40.0%	<0.001
Architectural distortions	0.6%	40.0%	<0.001
Pathologic vascularization	4.4%	14.3%	n.s. (0.109)

Table 2 Predominant color of the cortex in sonoelastography with respect to healthy and metastatic LNs

Cortex	Group 1 healthy LNs n=165	Group 2 metastatic LNs n=15	p (pairwise comparison)
red (soft)	0%	0%	n.a.
yellow	1.2%	0%	n.s. (1.000)
green	13.9%	0%	n.s. (0.223)
turquoise	64.2%	40.0%	n.s. (0.093)
blue (hard)	20.6%	60.0%	0.001
p-value (multivariate analysis)	0.006		

The cortex of metastatic LNs is significantly harder and therefore significantly more often described as blue than the cortex of healthy LNs. (n.s. = not significant, n.a. = not applicable, LN = lymph node).

when different ultrasound features of a lesion are combined, or mammography and MRI are added [50]. Consequently, we combined our best B-mode criterion and the most plausible elastographic criterion in order to investigate the effect on SE and SP. The conjunctive combination of B-mode and sonoelastography resulted in an improved performance. Due to the high specificity of the method, the PPV increased, while the effect on the NPV was only marginal and without clinical relevance.

However, a false negative preoperative evaluation usually results in the resection of a metastatic involved sentinel node. This scenario implies no relevant risk to the patient. On the other hand, a false positive evaluation of axillary LN status may result in an unnecessary axillary dissection instead of sentinel node biopsy with a potentially increased morbidity. Therefore, a beneficial effect of the complementary use of sonoelastography is very likely. We propose that these aspects should be investigated further.

Literature overview

Concerning breast masses, a scoring system (the so-called Tsukuba Elasticity Score, Itoh Score or Elasticity Score) is commonly used, which refers to the distribution of different colors within a lesion [51]. Obviously, this scoring system was developed for breast lesions and is not applicable to LNs.

For the elastographic assessment of cervical LNs, Lyshchik et al. determined an individual four-point rating scale including the visibility, relative brightness, margin regularity, and margin definition of the LNs in the elastogram. In the evaluation of 141 patients, they described an SP of 98%, an SE of 85% and an accuracy of 92% [27].

Saftiou et al. reported on cervical, mediastinal and abdominal LNs examined with endoscopic ultrasound elastography. The evaluation of the pictures was performed using a pattern analysis with RGB channel histograms. In their collective study of 42 LNs, they achieved an SP of 94.4% and an SE of 91.7% [52].

Taylor et al. performed sonoelastography in 50 breast cancer patients. They evaluated the LNs in the elastogram with either an individual visual scoring system or an individual strain scoring system. The authors described an SE and SP of 76% and 78% for conventional ultrasound, 90% and 86% for visual scoring, and 100% and 48% for strain scoring, respectively [36].

Alam et al. published data on cervical LNs in 85 patients. The authors analyzed the distribution and percentage of the LN area with high elasticity (i.e. hard, blue), with pattern 1 being an absent or very small hard area and pattern 5 indicating a hard area occupying the entire LN. The cutoff line for reactive versus metastatic was set between patterns 2 and 3. The authors reported an SE of 83% and an SP of 100% [28].

Choi et al. modified this system and classified 64 axillary LNs using a 4-point color scale based on the percentage and distribution of the LN areas with high elasticity (i.e. hard, blue). They achieved an SE of 80.7% and an SP of 66.7% [35]. These results do not fully comply with the previously described studies and our own

Table 3 Predominant color of the medulla in sonoelastography with respect to healthy and metastatic LNs

Medulla	Group 1 Healthy LNs n=165	Group 2 Metastatic LNs n=15	p (pairwise comparison)
red (soft)	0%	0%	n.a.
yellow	3.0%	6.7%	n.a.
green	15.8%	33.3%	n.a.
turquoise	73.9%	53.3%	n.a.
blue (hard)	7.3%	6.7%	n.a.
p-value (multivariate analysis)	n.s. (0.281)		

There is no difference between the two groups. (n.s. = not significant, n.a. = not applicable as the multivariate analysis was negative, LN = lymph node).

Table 4 Sensitivity and specificity of conventional ultrasound, Doppler and sonoelastography for the assessment of axillary LNs including conjunctive and disjunctive combinations (95% confidence intervals in brackets)

Prediction of LN status	Sensitivity	Specificity
B-Mode-US: Cortex >3mm	40.0	96.8
	(17.5-67.1)	(92.5-98.8)
Doppler-US: Pathologic vessels	14.3	95.6
	(2.5-43.9)	(90.8-98.1)
Clinical examination: Palpable LNs	13.3	88.4
	(2.3-41.6)	(82.3-92.7)
Elastogram: Cortex "blue"	60.0	79.6
	(32.9-82.5)	(72.2-85.5)
Disjunctive combination: Cortex >3mm or "blue" in the elastogram	73.3	77.5
	(44.8-91.1)	(69.8-83.7)
Conjunctive combination: Cortex >3mm and "blue" in the elastogram	26.7	99.3
	(8.9-55.2)	(95.8-100.0)

results, as a high SP and a moderate SE is usually observed in elastography.

Generally, the performance of sonoelastography is remarkably good in studies from the literature. Nevertheless, we have to consider that these data are from dissimilar, small patient collectives, the LNs are examined in different regions of the body, and the methods show relevant variations. Therefore, more advanced comparisons of the data are not possible.

Despite these reports, we have chosen a different approach for the evaluation of the elastograms, as we propagate the idea that the cortex and the medulla of an LN should be evaluated separately. Furthermore, we tried to avoid cumbersome scoring systems. For the evaluation of the elastograms we used a simple 5-point color scale describing the predominant color of the distinct structure (red, yellow, green, turquoise, or blue) as it appears in the elastogram.

Our approach is concordant with the preliminary results of Giovannini et al., who investigated LNs with endoscopic sonoelastography in 49 patients. The authors described a high SE (100%) and a moderate SP (50%) for sonoelastography using the criterion of a homogeneously blue cortex [33].

Metastases develop preferentially in the LN cortex and cause tissue alterations. As demonstrated by our results, sonoelastography seems to be capable of detecting these minute changes in elasticity distribution, although the LN cortex only constitutes a tissue structure of a few millimeters in size.

Another option for the interpretation of elastograms is the calculation of the strain-ratio [24,25]. This mode has

not been systematically analyzed in LNs and could be a matter for future research.

Limitations of our study

The main limitation of our study is that we have no validated criteria for the description of LNs in the elastogram. Accordingly, the analysis of the predominant color is, to a certain degree, observer-dependent, as it is based on image interpretation. Nevertheless, the evaluation of B-mode images is also observer-dependent and a matter of subjective interpretation. To minimize this limitation, we chose a simplified evaluation algorithm based on five categories (predominant color described as red, yellow, green, turquoise, or blue). The analysis of inter-observer concordance could be a matter for future research.

Furthermore, the still image of the elastogram is randomly depicted by the examiner during the real-time examination. This implies the risk of an observation bias. Nevertheless, this is unavoidable and has proven stable results in previous elastographic studies of LNs [52].

Finally, the analysis of SP, PPV and NPV is limited by the fact, that a group of healthy women is probably not the optimal choice for the control group, as lymph node morphology may differ even between healthy women and node negative breast cancer patients. Furthermore, there are vast confidence intervals around parameter estimated due to the small sample size. Further studies with larger collectives consisting exclusively of breast cancer patients may yield more accurate results.

Conclusion

- The cortex of healthy LNs is typically harder (i.e. has a higher elasticity) than the medulla.
- The cortex of malignant LNs is typically harder (i.e. has a higher elasticity) than the medulla.
- Comparing healthy LNs and metastatic LNs, the cortex of metastatic LNs is significantly harder (i.e. has a higher elasticity) than the cortex of healthy LNs.
- The definition of a blue cortex in the elastogram as a criterion for malignancy is feasible.
- Concerning the prediction of LN status, the combination of B-mode ultrasound with sonoelastography may be superior to B-mode ultrasound alone.
- The best specificity (99.3%) may be achieved by conjunctively combining B-mode ultrasound with the elastogram (cortex >3mm and cortex blue), although the sensitivity is low in this setting (26.7%).
- The conjunctive combinations of B-mode ultrasound and sonoelastography may improve the PPV (i.e. reduced false positive rate), but there may

be an impairment of the NPV (i.e. increased false negative rate).

– Sonoelastography of axillary LNs must still be regarded as an experimental method. Nevertheless, in the hands of an experienced sonographer, the method of real-time sonoelastography may provide useful information about axillary LNs even today.

Abbreviations
ALND: Axillary lymph node dissection; CT: Computer tomography; LN: Lymph node; MRI: Magnetic resonance imaging; n.a.: not applicable; n.s.: not significant; NPV: Negative predictive value; PET: Positron emission tomography; PPV: Positive predictive value; SE: Sensitivity; SNB: Sentinel node biopsy; SP: Specificity.

Competing interests
The author's declare that they have no competing interests.

Authors' contributions
SW contributed to the conception and design of the study and WS provided methodological advice. JD performed the ultrasound examinations and data collection. SW and JD contributed to the analysis and interpretation of the data and the writing of the manuscript. MC contributed to the writing and the reviewing of the manuscript. FD, PH and SW conducted the final review of the data and the manuscript. SW, JD, WS and MC were employees at the University Hospital of Saarland at the time of the study. All authors read and approved the final manuscript.

Acknowledgements
Publication costs were covered by a grant of the DFG (German Research Foundation) within the project "Open Access Publications" at MHH (Hannover Medical School, Germany).

Author details
[1]Hannover Medical School, Department for Obstetrics and Gynecology, OE 6410, Carl-Neuberg-Straße 1, Hannover 30625, Germany. [2]Main-Taunus-Kreis Hospital, Department for Obstetrics and Gynecology, Bad Soden, Germany. [3]University Hospital of Saarland, Department for Obstetrics and Gynecology, Homburg/Saar, Germany. [4]University of Potsdam, Center for Sports Medicine, Recreational and High Performance Sports, Potsdam, Germany.

References
1. Krag D, Weaver D, Ashikaga T, Moffat F, Klimberg VS, Shriver C, Feldman S, Kusminsky R, Gadd M, Kuhn J, Harlow S, Beitsch P: The sentinel node in breast cancer–a multicenter validation study. N Engl J Med 1998, 339(14):941–6.
2. Kuehn T, Bembenek A, Decker T, Munz DL, Sautter-Bihl ML, Untch M, Wallwiener D: Consensus committee of the german society of, senology: a concept for the clinical implementation of sentinel lymph node biopsy in patients with breast carcinoma with special regard to quality assurance. Cancer 2005, 103(3):451–61.
3. Veronesi U, Galimberti V, Zurrida S, Pigatto F, Veronesi P, Robertson C, Paganelli G, Sciascia V, Viale G: Sentinel lymph node biopsy as an indicator for axillary dissection in early breast cancer. Eur J Cancer 2001, 37(4):454–8.
4. Veronesi U, Paganelli G, Galimberti V, Viale G, Zurrida S, Bedoni M, Costa A, de Cicco C, Geraghty JG, Luini A, Sacchini V, Veronesi P: Sentinel-node biopsy to avoid axillary dissection in breast cancer with clinically negative lymph-nodes. Lancet 1997, 349(9069):1864–7.
5. Giuliano AE, Haigh PI, Brennan MB, Hansen NM, Kelley MC, Ye W, Glass EC, Turner RR: Prospective observational study of sentinel lymphadenectomy without further axillary dissection in patients with sentinel node-negative breast cancer. J Clin Oncol 2000, 18(13):2553–9.
6. Esen G, Gurses B, Yilmaz MH, Ilvan S, Ulus S, Celik V, Farahmand M, Calay OO: Gray scale and power doppler US in the preoperative evaluation of axillary metastases in breast cancer patients with no palpable lymph nodes. Eur Radiol 2005, 15(6):1215–23.
7. The NCCN Clinical Practice Guidelines in Oncology^{TM}BREAST CANCER (V.2.2012).: © 2010 National Comprehensive Cancer Network, Inc; [http://www.nccn.org]
8. Lucci A, McCall LM, Beitsch PD, Whitworth PW, Reintgen DS, Blumencranz PW, Leitch AM, Saha S, Hunt KK, Giuliano AE: American college of surgeons oncology, group: surgical complications associated with sentinel lymph node dissection (SLND) plus axillary lymph node dissection compared with SLND alone in the american college of surgeons oncology group trial Z0011. J Clin Oncol 2007, 25(24):3657–63.
9. Kocak Z, Overgaard J: Risk factors of arm lymphedema in breast cancer patients. Acta Oncol 2000, 39(3):389–92.
10. Giuliano AE, Hunt KK, Ballman KV, Beitsch PD, Whitworth PW, Blumencranz PW, Leitch AM, Saha S, McCall LM, Morrow M: Axillary dissection vs no axillary dissection in women with invasive breast cancer and sentinel node metastasis: a randomized clinical trial. JAMA 2011, 305(6):569–75.
11. Giuliano AE, Han SH: Local and regional control in breast cancer: role of sentinel node biopsy. Adv Surg 2011, 45:101–16.
12. Nori J, Vanzi E, Bazzocchi M, Bufalini FN, Distante V, Branconi F, Susini T: Role of axillary ultrasound examination in the selection of breast cancer patients for sentinel node biopsy. Am J Surg 2007, 193(1):16–20.
13. Alvarez S, Anorbe E, Alcorta P, Lopez F, Alonso I, Cortes J: Role of sonography in the diagnosis of axillary lymph node metastases in breast cancer: a systematic review. AJR Am J Roentgenol 2006, 186(5):1342–8.
14. March DE, Wechsler RJ, Kurtz AB, Rosenberg AL, Needleman L: CT-pathologic correlation of axillary lymph nodes in breast carcinoma. J Comput Assist Tomogr 1991, 15(3):440–4.
15. Bonnema J, van Geel AN, van Ooijen B, Mali SP, Tjiam SL, Henzen-Logmans SC, Schmitz PI, Wiggers T: Ultrasound-guided aspiration biopsy for detection of nonpalpable axillary node metastases in breast cancer patients: new diagnostic method. World J Surg 1997, 21(3):270–4.
16. Lam WW, Yang WT, Chan YL, Stewart IE, Metreweli C, King W: Detection of axillary lymph node metastases in breast carcinoma by technetium-99m sestamibi breast scintigraphy, ultrasound and conventional mammography. Eur J Nucl Med 1996, 23(5):498–503.
17. Mumtaz H, Hall-Craggs MA, Davidson T, Walmsley K, Thurell W, Kissin MW, Taylor I: Staging of symptomatic primary breast cancer with MR imaging. AJR Am J Roentgenol 1997, 169(2):417–24.
18. Mussurakis S, Buckley DL, Horsman A: Prediction of axillary lymph node status in invasive breast cancer with dynamic contrast-enhanced MR imaging. Radiology 1997, 203(2):317–21.
19. Uematsu T, Sano M, Homma K: In vitro high-resolution helical CT of small axillary lymph nodes in patients with breast cancer: correlation of CT and histology. AJR Am J Roentgenol 2001, 176(4):1069–74.
20. Tateishi T, Machi J, Feleppa EJ, Oishi R, Furumoto N, McCarthy LJ, Yanagihara E, Uchida S, Noritomi T, Shirouzu K: In vitro B-mode ultrasonographic criteria for diagnosing axillary lymph node metastasis of breast cancer. J Ultrasound Med 1999, 18(5):349–56.
21. Hahn M, Roessner L, Krainick-Strobel U, Gruber IV, Kramer B, Gall C, Siegmann KC, Wallwiener D, Kagan KO: [Sonographic criteria for the differentiation of benign and malignant breast lesions using real-time spatial compound imaging in combination with XRES adaptive image processing]. Ultraschall in der Medizin 2012, 33(3):270–4.
22. Wojcinski S, Farrokh A, Weber S, Thomas A, Fischer T, Slowinski T, Schmidt W, Degenhardt F: Multicenter study of ultrasound real-time tissue elastography in 779 cases for the assessment of breast lesions: improved diagnostic performance by combining the BI-RADS(R)-US classification system with sonoelastography. Ultraschall in der Medizin 2010, 31(5):484–91.
23. Schulz-Wendtland R, Bock K, Aichinger U, de Waal J, Bader W, Albert US, Duda VF: [Ultrasound examination of the breast with 7.5 MHz and 13 MHz-transducers: scope for improving diagnostic accuracy in complementary breast diagnostics?]. Ultraschall in der Medizin 2005, 26(3):209–15.
24. Farrokh A, Wojcinski S, Degenhardt F: [Diagnostic value of strain ratio measurement in the differentiation of malignant and benign breast lesions]. Ultraschall in der Medizin 2011, 32(4):400–5.
25. Thomas A, Degenhardt F, Farrokh A, Wojcinski S, Slowinski T, Fischer T: Significant differentiation of focal breast lesions: calculation of strain ratio in breast sonoelastography. Acad Radiol 2010, 17(5):558–63.

26. Sadigh G, Carlos RC, Neal CH, Dwamena BA: Ultrasonographic differentiation of malignant from benign breast lesions: a meta-analytic comparison of elasticity and BIRADS scoring. *Breast Cancer Res Treat* 2012, **133**(1):23–35.

27. Lyshchik A, Higashi T, Asato R, Tanaka S, Ito J, Hiraoka M, Insana MF, Brill AB, Saga T, Togashi K: Cervical lymph node metastases: diagnosis at sonoelastography–initial experience. *Radiology* 2007, **243**(1):258–67.

28. Alam F, Naito K, Horiguchi J, Fukuda H, Tachikake T, Ito K: Accuracy of sonographic elastography in the differential diagnosis of enlarged cervical lymph nodes: comparison with conventional B-mode sonography. *AJR Am J Roentgenol* 2008, **191**(2):604–10.

29. Bhatia KS, Cho CC, Yuen YH, Rasalkar DD, King AD, Ahuja AT: Real-time qualitative ultrasound elastography of cervical lymph nodes in routine clinical practice: interobserver agreement and correlation with malignancy. *Ultrasound Med Biol* 2010, **36**(12):1990–7.

30. Tan R, Xiao Y, He Q: Ultrasound elastography: its potential role in assessment of cervical lymphadenopathy. *Acad Radiol* 2010, **17**(7):849–55.

31. Janssen J, Dietrich CF, Will U, Greiner L: Endosonographic elastography in the diagnosis of mediastinal lymph nodes. *Endoscopy* 2007, **39**(11):952–7.

32. Giovannini M, Hookey LC, Bories E, Pesenti C, Monges G, Delpero JR: Endoscopic ultrasound elastography: the first step towards virtual biopsy? preliminary results in 49 patients. *Endoscopy* 2006, **38**(4):344–8.

33. Giovannini M, Thomas B, Erwan B, Christian P, Fabrice C, Benjamin E, Genevieve M, Paolo A, Pierre D, Robert Y, Walter S, Hanz S, Carl S, Christoph D, Pierre E, Jean-Luc VL, Jacques D, Peter V, Andrian S: Endoscopic ultrasound elastography for evaluation of lymph nodes and pancreatic masses: a multicenter study. *World J Gastroenterol* 2009, **15**(13):1587–93.

34. Aoyagi S, Izumi K, Hata H, Kawasaki H, Shimizu H: Usefulness of real-time tissue elastography for detecting lymph-node metastases in squamous cell carcinoma. *Clin Exp Dermatol* 2009, **34**(8):e744–7.

35. Choi JJ, Kang BJ, Kim SH, Lee JH, Jeong SH, Yim HW, Song BJ, Jung SS: Role of sonographic elastography in the differential diagnosis of axillary lymph nodes in breast cancer. *J Ultrasound Med* 2011, **30**(4):429–36.

36. Taylor K, O'Keeffe S, Britton PD, Wallis MG, Treece GM, Housden J, Parashar D, Bond S, Sinnatamby R: Ultrasound elastography as an adjuvant to conventional ultrasound in the preoperative assessment of axillary lymph nodes in suspected breast cancer: a pilot study. *Clin Radiol* 2011, **66**(11):1064–71.

37. *DEGUM (Deutsche Gesellschaft für Ultraschall in der Medizin).* Mehrstufenkonzept Mammasonographie; [http://www.degum.de/Mehrstufenkonzept_Mammasonogra.634.0.html].

38. Frey H, Ignee A, Dietrich CF: Elastographie, ein neues bildgebendes verfahren. *Endosk heute* 2006, **19**:117–120. 117.

39. Stavros AT: *Breast ultrasound.* 1st edition. Philadelphia, PA: Lippincott Williams & Wilkins; 2004.

40. Ueno E, Tohno E, Soeda S, Asaoka Y, Itoh K, Bamber JC, Blaszczyk M, Davey J, McKinna JA: Dynamic tests in real-time breast echography. *Ultrasound Med Biol* 1988, **14**(Suppl 1):53–7.

41. Evans A, Whelehan P, Thomson K, Brauer K, Jordan L, Purdie C, McLean D, Baker L, Vinnicombe S, Thompson A: Differentiating benign from malignant solid breast masses: value of shear wave elastography according to lesion stiffness combined with greyscale ultrasound according to BI-RADS classification. *Br J Cancer* 2012, **107**(2):224–9.

42. Friedrich-Rust M, Nierhoff J, Lupsor M, Sporea I, Fierbinteanu-Braticevici C, Strobel D, Takahashi H, Yoneda M, Suda T, Zeuzem S, Herrmann E: Performance of acoustic radiation force impulse imaging for the staging of liver fibrosis: a pooled meta-analysis. *J Viral Hepat* 2012, **19**(2):e212–9.

43. Newcombe RG: Interval estimation for the difference between independent proportions: comparison of eleven methods. *Stat Med* 1998, **17**(8):873–90.

44. Tan LG, Tan YY, Heng D, Chan MY: Predictors of axillary lymph node metastases in women with early breast cancer in singapore. *Singapore Med J* 2005, **46**(12):693–7.

45. Chan GS, Ho GH, Yeo AW, Wong CY: Correlation between breast tumour size and level of axillary lymph node involvement. *Asian J Surg* 2005, **28**(2):97–9.

46. UICC: *TNM Classification of Malignant Tumours.* Hoboken, NJ: John Wiley & Sons; 2002.

47. Chua B, Ung O, Taylor R, Boyages J: Is there a role for axillary dissection for patients with operable breast cancer in this era of conservatism? *ANZ J Surg* 2002, **72**(11):786–792.

48. Yip CH, Taib NA, Tan GH, Ng KL, Yoong BK, Choo WY: Predictors of axillary lymph node metastases in breast cancer: is there a role for minimal axillary surgery? *World J Surg* 2009, **33**(1):54–57.

49. Wojcinski S, Cassel M, Farrokh A, Soliman AA, Hille U, Schmidt W, Degenhardt F, Hillemanns P: Variations in the elasticity of breast tissue during the menstrual cycle determined by real-time sonoelastography. *J Ultrasound Med* 2012, **31**(1):63–72.

50. Mendelson EB, Baum JK, Berg WA, Merritt CR, Rubin E: BI-RADS: Ultrasound. In *In In Breast Imaging Reporting and Data System: ACR BI-RADS - Breast Imaging Atlas*. Edited by D'Orsi CJ, Mendelson EB, Ikeda DM. Reston, VA: American College of Radiology; 2002.

51. Itoh A, Ueno E, Tohno E, Kamma H, Takahashi H, Shiina T, Yamakawa M, Matsumura T: Breast disease: clinical application of US elastography for diagnosis. *Radiology* 2006, **239**(2):341–50.

52. Saftoiu A, Vilmann P, Hassan H, Gorunescu F: Analysis of endoscopic ultrasound elastography used for characterisation and differentiation of benign and malignant lymph nodes. *Ultraschall in der Medizin* 2006, **27**(6):535–42.

7

Sentinel nodes identified by computed tomography-lymphography accurately stage the axilla in patients with breast cancer

Kazuyoshi Motomura[1*], Hiroshi Sumino[2], Atsushi Noguchi[2], Takashi Horinouchi[2] and Katsuyuki Nakanishi[2]

Abstract

Background: Sentinel node biopsy often results in the identification and removal of multiple nodes as sentinel nodes, although most of these nodes could be non-sentinel nodes. This study investigated whether computed tomography-lymphography (CT-LG) can distinguish sentinel nodes from non-sentinel nodes and whether sentinel nodes identified by CT-LG can accurately stage the axilla in patients with breast cancer.

Methods: This study included 184 patients with breast cancer and clinically negative nodes. Contrast agent was injected interstitially. The location of sentinel nodes was marked on the skin surface using a CT laser light navigator system. Lymph nodes located just under the marks were first removed as sentinel nodes. Then, all dyed nodes or all hot nodes were removed.

Results: The mean number of sentinel nodes identified by CT-LG was significantly lower than that of dyed and/or hot nodes removed (1.1 vs 1.8, p <0.0001). Twenty-three (12.5%) patients had ≥2 sentinel nodes identified by CT-LG removed, whereas 94 (51.1%) of patients had ≥2 dyed and/or hot nodes removed (p <0.0001). Pathological evaluation demonstrated that 47 (25.5%) of 184 patients had metastasis to at least one node. All 47 patients demonstrated metastases to at least one of the sentinel nodes identified by CT-LG.

Conclusions: CT-LG can distinguish sentinel nodes from non-sentinel nodes, and sentinel nodes identified by CT-LG can accurately stage the axilla in patients with breast cancer. Successful identification of sentinel nodes using CT-LG may facilitate image-based diagnosis of metastasis, possibly leading to the omission of sentinel node biopsy.

Keywords: Sentinel node, Breast cancer, Computed tomography, Lymphography, Staging

Background

Sentinel node biopsy has been established as a standard of care in the treatment of breast cancer. This technique represents a minimally invasive, highly accurate method of axillary staging and is an alternative to conventional axillary lymph node dissection [1-5]. Controversy exists regarding the several technical and clinical aspects of sentinel node biopsy. One of the most important issues is how many and which axillary lymph nodes need to be removed as sentinel nodes for accurate axillary staging. Sentinel node biopsy using dye and/or radioisotopes often results in the identification and removal of multiple nodes as sentinel nodes, although most of these nodes could be non-sentinel nodes because the dye or radioisotope may migrate from sentinel nodes into additional non-sentinel nodes. The excision and examination of multiple sentinel nodes reduces the false negative rate, but removal of a large number of sentinel nodes increases morbidity and is time-consuming [6]. While some researchers have suggested that all dyed and/or radioactive nodes should be removed [7,8], others have proposed that the sentinel node biopsy procedure should be stopped after some lymph nodes or all nodes with radioactive counts greater than 10% of the hottest node have been removed [9-14].

Recently, sentinel nodes have been reported to be well-identified using computed tomography-lymphography (CT-LG) in patients with breast cancer [15-19]. Lymph

* Correspondence: motomurak@hotmail.com
[1]Departments of Surgery, Osaka Medical Center for Cancer and Cardiovascular Diseases, 1-3-3 Nakamichi, Higashinari-ku 537-8511 Osaka, Japan
Full list of author information is available at the end of the article

flow and sentinel nodes were successfully visualized by interstitial injection of CT contrast agent.

This study investigated whether CT-LG can distinguish sentinel nodes from non-sentinel nodes by visualization of the lymphatic channel and whether sentinel nodes identified by CT-LG can accurately stage the axilla in patients with breast cancer.

Methods
Patient selection
One hundred and eighty-four consecutive patients with clinical T1-2 breast cancers and clinically negative nodes who underwent sentinel node biopsy at Osaka Medical Center for Cancer and Cardiovascular Diseases between February 2008 and December 2010 were enrolled in this study. Patients with nonpalpable breast cancer, prior axillary surgery or pregnancy were excluded. Patients with a contraindication to CT or a known allergy to the contrast agent were also excluded. The institutional review board of Osaka Medical Center for Cancer and Cardiovascular Diseases approved the study, and written consent was obtained from all patients.

Sentinel node localization using CT-LG
Interstitial CT-LG was performed using a multidetector row helical CT scanner (Light Speed VCT; GE Healthcare, Milwaukee, WI, USA). Contiguous 1.25-mm-thick CT images from the upper thorax to axillary regions were obtained once before administration of the contrast agent. CT scanning with a detector of 0.625 mm, 64 rows was operated at 120 kV, 300 to 400 Auto-mA, 35 cm field of view, 512 x 512 matrix, section spacing of 1 mm, and table speed of 1.55 mm/0.5 sec.

Transaxial CT images were reconstructed with a 1.25-mm pitch and slice thickness of 0.3 mm. 3D CT images were reconstructed from the post-contrast CT images at each time point with volume-rendering techniques and, if necessary, a workstation (GE Advantage Workstation, version 4.3; GE Healthcare) was used to further examine lymph flow and sentinel nodes (Figure 1). Each patient was placed in the supine position and their arms were elevated. After local anesthesia with subcutaneous injection of 2 ml of 2% procaine hydrochloride, a 6-ml dose of iopamidol (Iopamiron 370; Bayer Schering Pharma, Osaka, Japan) was injected intradermally into the skin overlying the breast tumors and into the subareolar skin. A CT scan was performed after massaging the injection site of iopamidol for one minute. A localizing marker, which is usually used for CT-guided lung nodule biopsy, was attached to the skin at the axilla to identify the sentinel node location over the skin (Figure 2) [20]. Sentinel nodes were identified as the first stained nodes on the lymphatic flow from the injection sites of the contrast agent.

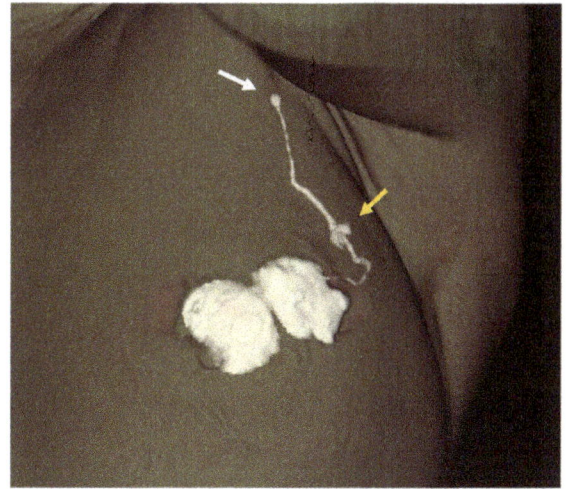

Figure 1 Three-dimensional computed tomography-lymphography (CT-LG) reconstructed from the first post-contrast images. Contrast agent was injected intradermally into the skin overlying the breast tumor and the subareolar skin. Lymphatic vessels drained into a single axillary sentinel node (yellow arrow). CT-LG can visualize lymph flow and can distinguish sentinel nodes from non-sentinel nodes (white arrow).

The sentinel node location was identified on the CT image and was indicated precisely by the crossing point of the localizing marker and the CT plane lights. The site was marked on the skin surface using an oil pen (Figure 3).

Surgery
Sentinel node biopsy was performed as described previously [21-23]. In brief, intradermal or intradermal and

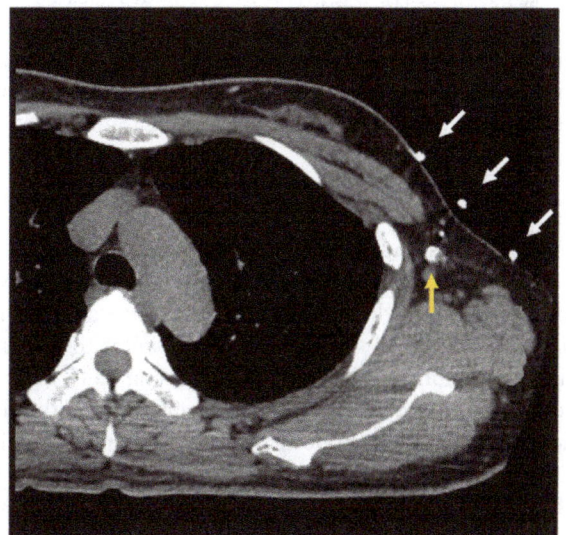

Figure 2 Sentinel node (yellow arrow) identified by axial computed tomography with localizing marker (white arrows).

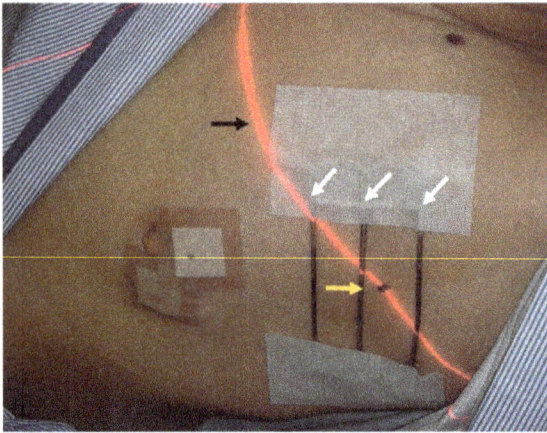

Figure 3 The sentinel node was indicated precisely by the crossing point of the localizing marker (white arrows) and the computed tomography plane lights (black arrow). The site was marked on the skin surface using an oil pen (yellow arrow).

subareolar injection of 0.3 mL of 37 MBq (1 mCi) Tc-99 m tin colloid the day before surgery and peritumoral or intradermal and subareolar injection of 5 mL indocyanine green (ICG, Diagnogreen 0.5%; Daiichi Pharmaceutical Co. Ltd., Nihonbashi, Tokyo, Japan) 10 minutes before surgery were performed, and then the injection site was massaged manually for one minute. Lymphoscintigraphy was performed 2–3 hours after the radioisotope injection.

Breast surgery was performed before axillary surgery in all patients to minimize the influence of radioactivity from the injection site [21-23]. For surgery, the elevated arm was placed as close as possible in the same position as during CT marking. Hot nodes were identified using a gamma probe (neo2000; Neoprobe Corporation, Dublin, OH, USA). Dyed and/or hot nodes located just under the markers using CT images were defined as sentinel nodes and were removed first. All dyed nodes or all nodes with an ex vivo radioisotope count of twofold or greater than the axillary background were then removed.

Histopathology

Sentinel nodes and dyed and/or hot nodes were serially sectioned at 2 mm intervals. Hematoxylin and eosin sections of these nodes were prepared from each 2-mm slice. An additional 4-μm section was cut and stained with immunohistochemistry (IHC) using the avidin-biotinylated peroxidase complex technique with the mouse monoclonal antibody against cytokeratin (NCL-CK19; Novocastra Laboratories Ltd., Newcastle, UK or AE1/AE3; Thermoelectron Corp., Waltham, MA, USA). Nodes with isolated tumor cells identified by IHC were considered to be metastasis negative in this study, according to the tumor node metastasis categories defined

in the 6th edition of the Union Internacional Contra la Cancrum TNM categories [24].

Statistical analysis

Fisher's exact test and paired t-test was used for statistical analysis. Differences were considered to be significant when $P < 0.05$.

Results

The mean age of the 184 patients was 55.7 (range, 31–79) years old and the mean tumor size was 20.8 (range, 0.2-90) mm. Patient and tumor characteristics are summarized in Table 1. The mean number of sentinel nodes identified by CT-LG was significantly lower than that of dyed and/or hot nodes removed (1.1 vs 1.8, p <0.0001). One hundred sixty-one patients (87.5%) had 1 sentinel node identified by CT-LG removed, 21 (11.4%) had 2 sentinel nodes removed, and 2 patients (1.1%) had 3

Table 1 Patient characteristics

	No. of patients	%
Age, years		
<50	56	30.4
≥50	128	69.6
Tumor size, cm		
≤2	114	62.0
>2, ≤5	65	35.3
>5	5	
Tumor location		
Upper outer	101	54.9
Upper inner	35	19.0
Lower outer	26	14.1
Lower inner	9	4.9
Central	10	5.4
Multicentric	3	1.6
Tumor histology		
Invasive ductal	161	87.5
Invasive lobular	8	4.3
Ductal carcinoma in situ	10	5.4
Others	5	2.7
Type of surgery		
Lumpectomy	178	96.7
Mastectomy	6	3.3
Estrogen receptor		
Positive	150	81.5
Negative	34	18.5
HER-2/neu		
Positive	28	15.2
Negative	156	84.8

sentinel nodes removed. Twenty-three (12.5%) patients had ≥2 sentinel nodes identified by CT-LG removed, whereas 94 (51.1%) of patients had ≥2 dyed and/or hot nodes removed (p <0.0001). Pathologic evaluation demonstrated that 47 (25.5%) of 184 patients had metastasis to at least one node. Three hundred twenty-eight dyed and/or hot nodes were removed, of which 57 (17.4%) had metastatic deposits. Two hundred eleven sentinel nodes were removed, of which 52 (24.6%) had metastatic deposits. Sixteen (30.8%) had micrometastases and 36 (69.2%) had macrometastases. All 47 patients demonstrated metastases to at least one of the sentinel nodes identified by CT-LG. No patient with negative sentinel nodes had metastases in other dyed and/or hot nodes.

CT-LG could visualize lymph flow and accurately identify sentinel nodes in 179 (97.3%) of 184 patients (Figure 1). In 4 of the other 5 patients, only one sentinel node was identified and it was not necessary to distinguish sentinel nodes from non-sentinel nodes by visualizing lymph flow. In one patient, two nodes were identified and they could not be distinguished. No extra-axillary sentinel nodes, such as internal mammary or supraclavicular sentinel nodes, were identified. Hot spots could be identified over the skin using a gamma probe on all markers of the sentinel node location by CT-LG. There were no adverse events associated with CT-LG.

Discussion

Sentinel node biopsy using dye and radioisotopes often results in the removal of multiple sentinel nodes. It remains unclear how many and which lymph nodes must be removed as sentinel nodes for accurate axillary staging. Removing only the first node identified or removing only the hottest node may not complete the sentinel node biopsy. Wong et al. reported a false-negative rate of 14.4% if only the first node had been taken [25]. Martin et al. demonstrated that the positive sentinel node was not the most radioactive node in 20% of cases with multiple sentinel nodes, and the false-negative rate was likely to be much higher (12%) if only the most radioactive sentinel node was removed [26]. Some researchers recommend that all lymph nodes above a pre-defined threshold of the ex vivo count of the hottest sentinel node should be removed. The 10% rule is one of the most common guidelines to define a radioactive sentinel node and dictates removal of all sentinel node with counts >10% of the most radioactive node. Martin et al. demonstrated that the false-negative rate would be 13% if only the hottest node was removed and 5.8% if the 10% rule was applied [13]. Sixty percent of patients had >1 sentinel node removed and the mean number of sentinel nodes per patient was 1.96. Chung et al. reported that only 1.7% of all sentinel node-positive patients had positive sentinel nodes with counts <10% radioactive

counts of the hottest node [14]. Sixty-five percent of patients had >1 sentinel node removed. More than one sentinel node needs to be removed in many patients according to the 10% rule. Others recommended that the procedure can be stopped after a certain number of lymph nodes have been removed. Zervos et al. found 98% of positive sentinel nodes were found in the first three nodes removed [9]. McCarter et al. reported that 98% of positive sentinel nodes were found when the first three nodes were removed [7]. Shrenk et al. found 99% of positive sentinel nodes within the first two nodes and 100% of positive nodes within the first three nodes [8]; however, they both concluded that all dyed and/or hot nodes should be removed to decrease the false-negative rate. Chagper et al. found that only 89.7% of positive sentinel nodes was identified within the first three nodes and did not recommend removing only three sentinel nodes because of a high false-negative rate of 10.3% [27]. Zakaria et al. demonstrated that 98% of patients with positive nodes were found by the third sentinel node, and 100% were found by the fourth sentinel node [10]. Yi et al. demonstrated that >99% of positive sentinel nodes were identified in one of the first five lymph nodes removed [11]. Woznick et al. reported that all positive sentinel nodes were identified within the first six nodes removed [12]. Removal of many more nodes was associated with a lower false-negative rate, but could worsen the morbidity of the sentinel node biopsy. Wilke et al. demonstrated an increased incidence of axillary seroma and wound infection when more than four sentinel nodes were removed [6].

In the present study, we demonstrated that sentinel nodes could be successfully identified in 183 of 184 patients and metastases could be detected in all 47 patients with positive nodes. CT-LG could visualize lymph flow and accurately distinguished sentinel nodes from dyed and/or hot non-sentinel nodes (Figure 1). Overall, 87.5% of patients had only one sentinel node removed; 12.5% of patients required removal of ≥2 sentinel nodes, whereas 51.1% of patients required removal of ≥2 dyed and/or nodes, which was statistically significant (p <0.0001). Increased operative time, procedure and pathology cost, and complication rate are associated with the removal of larger numbers of sentinel nodes [6]. It is advantageous to remove only one lymph node as a sentinel node if these nodes do not reduce mapping accuracy. Although four CT studies were performed per patient in this study to clarify which CT studies were really required, a single post-contrast CT scan may be sufficient because the first contrast CT image was able to identify lymphatic channels and sentinel nodes accurately. A further study is required to confirm the hypothesis. Another advantage of CT-LG is that we can identify how many and which node should be removed as sentinel nodes preoperatively. Moreover, we can also identify the location of sentinel nodes, including the depth from the skin, and in surrounding organs such as the chest wall, muscle and vessels according to the appearance of the axial CT and 3D-CT images (Figures 1 and 2). Some multiple sentinel nodes, which may be missed when sentinel node biopsy is performed using dye and/or radioisotopes without CT-LG because they are located far from other nodes and influenced by radioactivity from the injection site, could be accurately identified using CT-LG (Figure 4). Furthermore, axial CT and 3D-CT images enabled the demonstration of the shapes and sizes of sentinel nodes (Figures 1 and 4). The use of 3D images is useful for identification and removal during sentinel node biopsy.

On the other hand, our study had a few limitations, including that the false negative rate of this procedure for axillary staging could not be shown because axillary lymph node dissection was not performed. Sentinel node biopsy has now become the standard of care and it is impracticable to perform axillary lymph node dissection after sentinel node biopsy for sentinel node-negative patients, even in the trial setting. However, all 47 patients with positively dyed and/or hot nodes demonstrated metastases to at least one of the sentinel nodes identified by CT-LG and no patient with negative sentinel nodes had metastases in other dyed and/or hot nodes; therefore, the diagnostic accuracy of sentinel nodes for axillary staging is similar to that of sentinel nodes identified by dye and radioisotopes, demonstrated in our previous

study with 100% sensitivity, 100% specificity, and 100% accuracy [21]. Intradermal injection of enhanced agents cannot identify extra-axillary sentinel nodes, but removal of sentinel nodes in such a region has not been performed recently. Chagper et al. demonstrated that axillary sentinel nodes are usually identified even when lymphoscintigraphy shows drainage to the internal mammary nodes alone [28].

Lymphoscintigraphy can sometimes show several hot nodes and lymphatic flow before sentinel node biopsy [29]; however, it is not easy to clearly distinguish sentinel nodes from non-sentinel nodes in many cases because of unclear lymph flow images and only identification of the hottest node in spite of the existence of more than one hot node. CT-LG can identify sentinel nodes clearly. Moreover, if sentinel nodes accurately be diagnosed using imaging, even sentinel node biopsy can be omitted. CT itself is reported to be insufficient to evaluate the presence of metastases in sentinel nodes [30]. We recently tried to perform MR imaging with superparamagnetic iron oxide enhancement for the accurate detection of metastases in sentinel nodes localized by CT-LG in patients with breast cancer [31]. The sensitivity, specificity, and accuracy of MR imaging for the diagnosis of sentinel node metastases were 84.0%, 90.9%, and 89.2%, respectively. In 4 of 10 patients with micrometastases, metastases were not detected, but all 15 patients with macrometastases were successfully identified. This promising procedure may avoid even sentinel node biopsy when the sentinel node is diagnosed as disease-free on MR imaging.

Conclusions

CT-LG could distinguish sentinel nodes from non-sentinel nodes, and sentinel nodes accurately staged the axilla in patients with breast cancer. Applying this procedure may end the dispute regarding how many and which axillary lymph nodes need to be removed as sentinel nodes for accurate axillary staging. Successful identification of sentinel nodes using CT-LG may facilitate image-based diagnosis of metastasis, possibly leading to the omission of sentinel node biopsy.

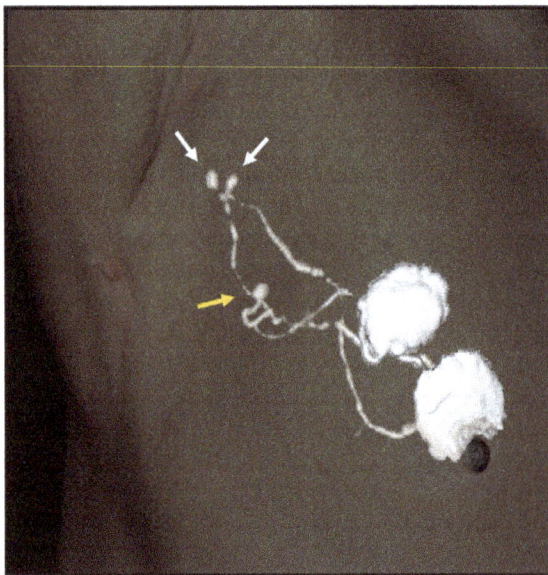

Figure 4 Three sentinel nodes were identified by computed tomography -lymphography (CT-LG). One (yellow arrow) might have been missed when sentinel node biopsy was performed without CT-LG because it was located far from the other two nodes (white arrows) and was influenced by radioactivity from the injection site.

Abbreviations
CT: Computed tomography; MR: Magnetic resonance; CT-LG: Computed tomography-lymphography; ICG: Indocyanine green; IHC: Immunohistochemistry.

Competing interests
The authors declare that they have no competing interests.

Authors' contributions
KM contributed to the conception and design of the study, data analysis and drafted the manuscript. HS contributed the analysis and interpretation of the data of CT. AN provided methodological advice. TH and KN contributed to the conception and design of the study, analysis and interpretation of the data. All authors read and approved the final manuscript.

Acknowledgment
This work was supported in part by the National Cancer Center Research and Development Fund (22–38).

Author details
[1]Departments of Surgery, Osaka Medical Center for Cancer and Cardiovascular Diseases, 1-3-3 Nakamichi, Higashinari-ku 537-8511Osaka, Japan. [2]Departments of Radiology, Osaka Medical Center for Cancer and Cardiovascular Diseases, 1-3-3 Nakamichi, Higashinari-ku 537-8511Osaka, Japan.

References

1. Giuliano AE, Kirgan DM, Guenther JM, Morton DL: **Lymphatic mapping and sentinel lymphadenectomy for breast cancer.** *Ann Surg* 1994, 220:391–401.
2. Giuliano AE, Jones RC, Brennan M, Statman R: **Sentinel lymphadenectomy in breast cancer.** *J Clin Oncol* 1997, 15:2345–2350.
3. Motomura K, Inaji H, Komoike Y, Kasugai T, Nagumo S, Noguchi S, Koyama H: **Sentinel node biopsy in breast cancer patients with clinically negative lymph-nodes.** *Breast Cancer* 1999, 6:259–262.
4. Krag D, Weaver D, Ashikaga T, Moffat F, Klimberg VS, Shriver C, Feldman S, Kusminsky R, Gadd M, Kuhn J, Harlow S, Beitsch P: **The sentinel node in breast cancer: a multicenter validation study.** *N Engl J Med* 1998, 339:941–946.
5. Veronesi U, Paganelli G, Galimberti V, Viale G, Zurrida S, Bedoni M, Costa A, de Cicco C, Geraghty JG, Luini A, Sacchini V, Veronesi P: **Sentinel-node biopsy to avoid axillary dissection in breast cancer with clinically negative lymph-nodes.** *Lancet* 1997, 349:1864–1867.
6. Wilke LG, McCall LM, Posther KE, Whitworth PW, Reintgen DS, Leitch AM, Gabram SG, Lucci A, Cox CE, Hunt KK, Herndon JE 2nd, Giuliano AE: **Surgical complications associated with sentinel lymph node biopsy: results from a prospective international cooperative group trial.** *Ann Surg Oncol* 2006, 13:491–500.
7. McCarter MD, Yeung H, Fey J, Borgen PI, Cody HS 3rd: **The breast cancer patient with multiple sentinel nodes: when to stop?** *J Am Coll Surg* 2001, 192:692–697.
8. Schrenk P, Rehberger W, Shamiyeh A, Wayand W: **Sentinel node biopsy for breast cancer: does the number of sentinel nodes removed have an impact on the accuracy of finding a positive node?** *J Surg Oncol* 2002, 80:130–136.
9. Zervos EE, Badgwell BD, Abdessalam SF, Farrar WB, Walker MJ, Yee LD, Burak WE Jr: **Selective analysis of the sentinel node in breast cancer.** *Am J Surg* 2001, 182:372–376.
10. Zakaria S, Degnim AC, Kleer CG, Diehl KA, Cimmino VM, Chang AE, Newman LA, Sabel MS: **Sentinel lymph node biopsy for breast cancer: how many nodes are enough?** *J Surg Oncol* 2007, 96:554–559.
11. Yi M, Meric-Bernstam F, Ross MI, Akins JS, Hwang RF, Lucci A, Kuerer HM, Babiera GV, Gilcrease MZ, Hunt KK: **How many sentinel lymph nodes are enough during sentinel lymph node dissection for breast cancer?** *Cancer* 2008, 113:30–37.
12. Woznick A, Franco M, Bendick P, Benitez PR: **Sentinel lymph node dissection for breast cancer: how many nodes are enough and which technique is optimal?** *Am J Surg* 2006, 191:330–333.
13. Martin RC 2nd, Edwards MJ, Wong SL, Tuttle TM, Carlson DJ, Brown CM, Noyes RD, Glaser RL, Vennekotter DJ, Turk PS, Tate PS, Sardi A, Cerrito PB, McMasters KM: **Practical guidelines for optimal gamma probe detection of sentinel lymph nodes in breast cancer: results of a multi-institutional study. For the University of Louisville breast cancer study group.** *Surgery* 2000, 128:139–144.
14. Chung A, Yu J, Stempel M, Patil S, Cody H, Montgomery L: **Is the "10% rule" equally valid for all subsets of sentinel-node-positive breast cancer patients?** *Ann Surg Oncol* 2008, 15:2728–2733.
15. Suga K, Ogasawara N, Okada M, Matsunaga N: **Interstitial CT lymphography-guided localization of breast sentinel lymph node: preliminary results.** *Surgery* 2003, 133:170–179.
16. Tangoku A, Yamamoto S, Suga K, Ueda K, Nagashima Y, Hida M, Sato T, Sakamoto K, Oka M: **Sentinel lymph node biopsy using computed tomography-lymphography in patients with breast cancer.** *Surgery* 2004, 135:258–265.
17. Suga K, Yuan Y, Okada M, Matsunaga N, Tangoku A, Yamamoto S, Oka M: **Breast sentinel lymph node mapping at CT lymphography with iopamidol: preliminary experience.** *Radiology* 2004, 230:543–552.
18. Yamamoto S, Maeda N, Tamesa M, Nagashima Y, Suga K, Oka M: **Sentinel lymph node detection in breast cancer patients by real-time virtual sonography constructed with three-dimensional computed tomography-lymphography.** *Breast J* 2010, 16:4–8.
19. Minohata J, Takao S, Hirokaga K: **Sentinel lymph node biopsy using CT lymphography in breast cancer.** *Breast Cancer* 2011, 18:129–136.
20. Ohno Y, Hatabu H, Takenaka D, Higashino T, Watanabe H, Ohbayashi C, Sugimura K: **CT-guided transthoracic needle aspiration biopsy of small (< or = 20 mm) solitary pulmonary nodules.** *AJR Am J Roentgenol* 2003, 180:1665–1669.
21. Motomura K, Inaji H, Komoike Y, Hasegawa Y, Kasugai T, Noguchi S, Koyama H: **Combination technique is superior to dye alone in identification of the sentinel node in breast cancer patients.** *J Surg Oncol* 2001, 76:95–99.
22. Motomura K, Komoike Y, Hasegawa Y, Kasugai T, Inaji H, Noguchi S, Koyama H: **Intradermal radioisotope injection is superior to subdermal injection for the identification of the sentinel node in breast cancer patients.** *J Surg Oncol* 2003, 82:91–96.
23. Motomura K, Nagumo S, Komoike Y, Koyama H, Inaji H: **Accuracy of imprint cytology for intraoperative diagnosis of sentinel node metastases in breast cancer.** *Ann Surg* 2008, 247:839–842.
24. American Joint Committee on Cancer: **Breast.** In *AJCC Cancer Staging Handbook.* 6th edition. Edited by Greene FL, Page DL, Fleming ID, Fritz AG, Balch CM, Haller DG, *et al.* New York: Springer; 2002:155–181.
25. Wong SL, Edwards MJ, Chao C, Tuttle TM, Noyes RD, Carlson DJ, Cerrito PB, McMasters KM: **Sentinel lymph node biopsy for breast cancer: impact of the number of sentinel nodes removed on the false-negative rate.** *J Am Coll Surg* 2001, 192:684–689.
26. Martin RC, Fey J, Yeung H, Borgen PI, Cody HS 3rd: **Highest isotope count does not predict sentinel node positivity in all breast cancer patients.** *Ann Surg Oncol* 2001, 8:592–597.
27. Chagpar AB, Scoggins CR, Martin RC 2nd, Carlson DJ, Laidley AL, El-Eid SE, McGlothin TQ, McMasters KM: **Are 3 sentinel nodes sufficient?** *Arch Surg* 2007, 142:456–459.
28. Chagpar AB, Kehdy F, Scoggins CR, Martin RC 2nd, Carlson DJ, Laidley AL, El-Eid SE, McGlothin TQ, Noyes RD, Ley PB, Tuttle TM, McMasters KM: **Effect of lymphoscintigraphy drainage patterns on sentinel lymph node biopsy in patients with breast cancer.** *Am J Surg* 2005, 190:557–562.
29. Uren RF, Howman-Giles RB, Chung D, Thompson JF: **Role of lymphoscintigraphy for selective sentinel lymphadenectomy.** *Cancer Treat Res* 2005, 127:15–38.
30. Yuen S, Yamada K, Goto M, Sawai K, Nishimura T: **CT-based evaluation of axillary sentinel lymph node status in breast cancer: value of added contrast-enhanced study.** *Acta Radiol* 2004, 45:730–737.
31. Motomura K, Ishitobi M, Komoike Y, Koyama H, Noguchi A, Sumino H, Kumatani Y, Inaji H, Horinouchi T, Nakanishi K: **SPIO-enhanced magnetic resonance imaging for the detection of metastases in sentinel nodes localized by computed tomography lymphography in patients with breast cancer.** *Ann Surg Oncol* 2011, 18:3422–3429.

Correlation between the area of high-signal intensity on SPIO-enhanced MR imaging and the pathologic size of sentinel node metastases in breast cancer patients with positive sentinel nodes

Kazuyoshi Motomura[1][*], Tetsuta Izumi[2], Souichirou Tateishi[2], Hiroshi Sumino[2], Atsushi Noguchi[2], Takashi Horinouchi[2] and Katsuyuki Nakanishi[2]

Abstract

Background: We previously demonstrated that superparamagnetic iron oxide (SPIO)-enhanced MR imaging is promising for the detection of metastases in sentinel nodes localized by CT-lymphography in patients with breast cancer. The purpose of this study was to determine the predictive criteria of the size of nodal metastases with SPIO-enhanced MR imaging in breast cancer, with histopathologic findings as reference standard.

Methods: This study included 150 patients with breast cancer. The patterns of SPIO uptake for positive sentinel nodes were classified into three; uniform high-signal intensity, partial high-signal intensity involving ≥50% of the node, and partial high-signal intensity involving <50% of the node. Imaging results were correlated with histopathologic findings.

Results: Thirty-three pathologically positive sentinel nodes from 30 patients were evaluated. High-signal intensity patterns that were uniform or involved ≥50% of the node were observed in 23 nodes that contained macro-metastases and no node that contained micro-metastases, while high-signal intensity patterns involving <50% of the node were observed in 2 nodes that contained macro-metastases and 8 nodes that contained micro-metastases. When the area of high-signal intensity was compared with the pathological size of the metastases, a pathologic >2 mm sentinel node metastases correlated with the area of high-signal intensity, however, a pathologic ≤2 mm sentinel node metastases did not.

Conclusions: High-signal intensity patterns that are uniform or involve ≥50% of the node are features of nodes with macro-metastases. The area of high-signal intensity correlated with the pathological size of metastases for nodes with metastases >2 mm in this series.

Keywords: Sentinel node, Breast cancer, Magnetic resonance imaging, Computed tomography, Superparamagnetic iron oxide, Nodal enhancement pattern, Lymph node metastasis

Background

Sentinel node biopsy is emerging as an alternative to axillary lymph node dissection for patients with breast cancer with clinically negative nodes [1-5]. It is associated with less morbidity, such as lymph edema and neuropathies, than axillary lymph node dissection, but with high

* Correspondence: motomurak@hotmail.com
[1]Department of Surgery, Osaka Medical Center for Cancer and Cardiovascular Diseases, 1-3-3 Nakamichi, Higashinari-ku, Osaka 537-8511, Japan
Full list of author information is available at the end of the article

accuracy in the prediction of axillary nodal status; however, it still involves a surgical procedure with associated morbidity. Overall, 2-7% of patients are reported to have lymphedema even after sentinel node biopsy [6-8].

Recently, intravenously administered ultrasmall superparamagnetic iron oxide (USPIO)-enhanced MR imaging has been reported to be promising for the diagnosis of lymph node metastases as a noninvasive method. Some researchers have already evaluated nodal staging in various tumors [9-11]. Harisinghani et al. demonstrated a sensitivity of 100% with a specificity of 95.7% for nodal staging using USPIO-enhanced MR imaging in 80 patients with prostate cancer [9]. Rockall et al. reported that the sensitivity for nodal staging using USPIO-enhanced MR imaging in 768 lymph nodes from 44 patients with endometrial or cervical cancer was 100%, significantly higher than the conventional method using size criteria, which has a sensitivity of 27% [10]. Stets et al. reported an accuracy of 87%, sensitivity of 81%, and specificity of 92% using USPIO-enhanced MR imaging for axillary lymph node metastases in 52 lymph nodes from 9 patients with breast cancer [11]. A recent meta-analysis demonstrated that USPIO-enhanced MR imaging is sensitive and specific, and superior to other modalities in the detection of nodal metastases for various malignancies [12].

We previously assessed MR imaging using interstitial injection of superparamagnetic iron oxide (SPIO) enhancement for the detection of metastases in sentinel nodes which were localized by CT-lymphography (CT-LG) in patients with breast cancer [13]. We demonstrated that SPIO-enhanced MR imaging accurately stages the axilla and may avoid even sentinel node biopsy in patients with breast cancer.

In the present study, we investigated the correlation between the area of high-signal intensity on SPIO-enhanced MR imaging and the pathologic size of sentinel node metastases in breast cancer patients with pathologically positive sentinel nodes for determining the predictive criteria of the size of nodal metastases.

Patients and methods

Patient selection

One hundred and fifty consecutive patients with clinical T1-2 breast cancers and clinically negative nodes who underwent sentinel node biopsy at Osaka Medical Center for Cancer and Cardiovascular Diseases between January 2008 and November 2009 were enrolled in this study. Patients with nonpalpable breast cancer, prior axillary surgery or who were pregnant were excluded. Patients with a contraindication to CT or MR imaging, or a known allergy to the contrast agents were also excluded. The institutional review board of Osaka Medical Center for Cancer and Cardiovascular Diseases approved the study, and written consent was obtained from all patients.

Sentinel node localization using CT-LG

Interstitial CT-LG was performed using a multidetector row helical CT scanner (Light Speed VCT; GE Healthcare, Milwaukee, WI, USA). Contiguous 1.25-mm-thick CT images from the upper thorax to axillary regions were obtained once before administration of the contrast agent. CT scanning with a detector of 0.625 mm, 64 rows was operated at 120 kV, 300 to 400 Auto-mA, 35 cm field of

view, 512 × 512 matrix, section spacing of 1 mm, and a table speed of 1.55 mm/0.5 sec.

Transaxial CT images were reconstructed with a 1.25-mm pitch and slice thickness of 0.3 mm. Each patient was placed in the supine position. Three small plastic bullets were placed as landmarks on the upper chest wall on the skin for a merged image of the CT-LG and axial MR image. First, their arms were placed in an elevated position. After local anesthesia with a subcutaneous injection of 2 ml of 2% procaine hydrochloride, 6 ml iopamidol (Iopamiron 370; Bayer Schering Pharma, Osaka, Japan) was injected intradermally into the skin overlying the breast tumor and into the subareolar skin. A CT scan was performed after massaging the iopamidol injection site for one minute. Second, a CT scan was performed in the adducted arm position. Finally, their arms were placed in an elevated position again, and a localizing marker, which is usually used for CT-guided lung nodule biopsy, was attached to the skin at the axilla to identify the sentinel node location over the skin [14]. The sentinel node location was identified on the CT image and was indicated precisely by the crossing point of the localizing marker and the CT plane lights. The site was marked on the skin surface using an oil pen.

3D-CT images were reconstructed from the post-contrast CT images at each time point with volume-rendering techniques and, if necessary, a workstation (GE Advantage Workstation, version 4.3; GE Healthcare, Milwaukee, WI, USA) was used to further examine lymph flow and the sentinel node (Figure 1a).

MR imaging

MR images were obtained using a 1.5 T imaging system (Sonata/Symphony; Siemens, Erlangen, Germany) with a 12-channel matrix body coil. T1-weighted axial images were obtained from the upper thorax to axillary lesions (repetition time in msec (TR), 140; echo time in msec (TE), 1.88; slice width, 4 mm; interslice gap, 0 mm; number of acquisitions, one; field of view, 28 × 28 cm; matrix, 141 × 256); T2-weighted axial images were obtained through the axilla (TR, 4,000; TE, 85 effective time; echo train length, 11; slice width, 4 mm; interslice gap, 0 mm; number of acquisitions, one; field of view, 25 × 25 cm; matrix, 250 × 384). Additional nodal imaging sequences included T2*-weighted gradient echo images in the axial plane (TR, 613; TE, 30; flip angle, 30; slice width, 4 mm; interslice gap, 0 mm; number of acquisitions, one; field of view, 25 × 25 cm; matrix, 230 × 384).

Each patient was placed in the supine position in the adducted arm position. A 40 μl aliquot of SPIO (Resovist; FUJIFILM RI Farma Co., Ltd., Kyobashi, Tokyo), containing 1.115 mg iron, was diluted in 20 ml normal saline. After local anesthesia with subcutaneous injection of 2 ml of 2% procaine hydrochloride, 6 ml SPIO, containing 0.3345 mg iron, was injected intradermally into

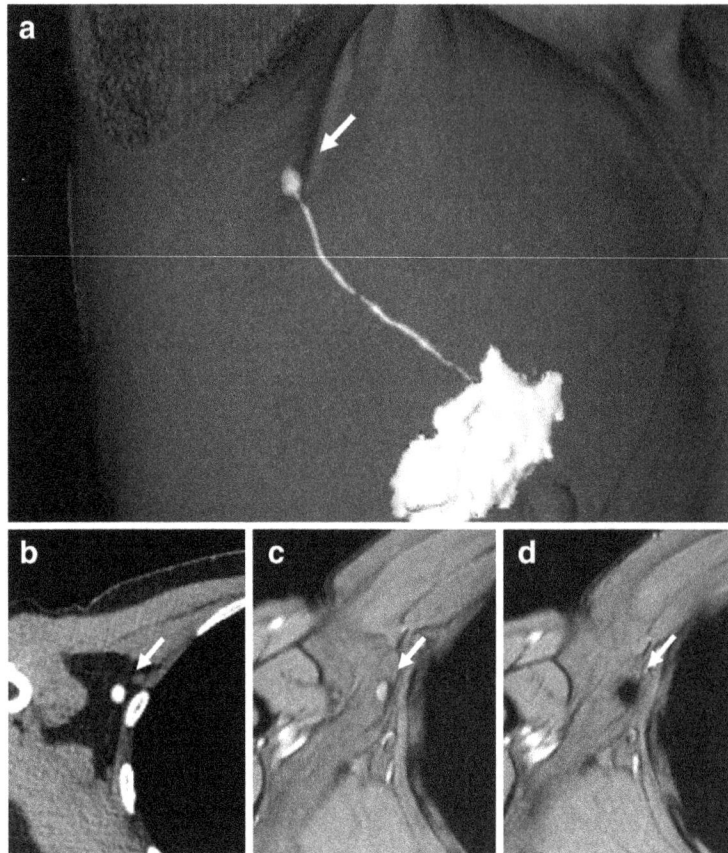

Figure 1 Sentinel node localization using CT-lymphography and SPIO-enhanced MR imaging for diagnosis. Three-dimensional CT-lymphography reconstructed from the first post-contrast images **(a)**. Lymphatic vessels drained into a single axillary sentinel node (arrow). Images of CT-lymphography **(b)** and T2*-weighted axial MR images **(c)** at the same level were compared to specify the node (arrow) on T2*-weighted axial MR imaging corresponding to the sentinel node (arrow) identified by CT-lymphography. The node (arrow) showed high-signal intensity before administration of superparamagnetic iron oxide (SPIO). **(d)** After administration of SPIO, the node showed homogenous low signal intensity and was diagnosed as benign (arrow).

the skin overlying the breast tumor and into the subareolar skin. The injection sites of SPIO were gently massaged for one minute. At 18 to 24 hours after the administration of SPIO, the T1-, T2- and T2*-weighted sequences used for interpretation of the lymph node status were repeated. The MR imaging interval was determined by referring to the report of the study using USPIO [15]. T1-weighted and T2-weighted images were used for anatomic localization; the T1-weighted image in particular allows the shape and size of nodes clearly.

Images of the CT-LG (Figure 1b) and T2*-weighted axial MR images (Figure 1c) in the adducted arm position at the same level were compared to specify the node on T2*-weighted axial MR imaging corresponding to the sentinel node identified by CT-LG. If necessary, a merged image of the CT-LG and T2*-weighted axial MR images was obtained on a workstation (PEGASYS; ADAC, Milpitas, CA, USA), with the help of small plastic bullets.

Nodes were evaluated on pre- and post-SPIO images by 1 reader (K.M.). Visual analysis was based on the diagnostic guidelines previously reported by Anzai et al. [16]. In brief, a node was considered non-metastatic if it showed homogeneous low-signal intensity (Figure 1d) and metastatic if the entire node or more than 50% of the node has high-signal intensity on post-SPIO MR imaging compared with the signal intensity on pre-SPIO images. A node was considered possibly metastatic if less than 50% of the node has high-signal intensity [16]. In this study, patterns of SPIO uptake for positive sentinel nodes were classified into three referring to the guideline [16]; uniform high-signal intensity, partial high-signal intensity involving more than 50% of the node, and partial high-signal intensity involving less than 50% of the node (Figures 2, 3 and 4).

Surgery

Sentinel node biopsy was performed as described previously [17-19]. In brief, intradermal or intradermal and

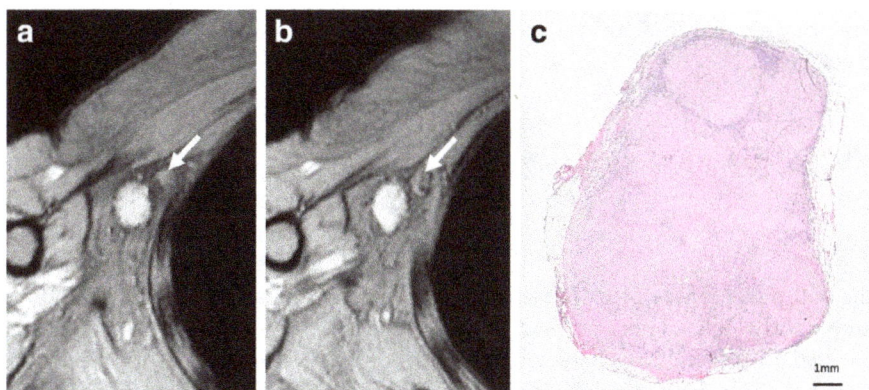

Figure 2 Pattern of uniform high-signal intensity on SPIO-enhanced MR imaging. (a) The node (arrow) showed high-signal intensity before administration of superparamagnetic iron oxide (SPIO). **(b)** After administration of SPIO, the node showed uniform high-signal intensity and was diagnosed as malignant (arrow). **(c)** Histological findings confirmed it as malignant. This node was almost entirely replaced by metastatic tissue.

subareolar injection of 0.3 ml of 37 MBq (1 mCi) Tc-99 m tin colloid the day before surgery and peritumoral or intradermal and subareolar injection of 5 ml indocyanine green (ICG, Diagnogreen 0.5%; Daiichi Pharmaceutical Co. Ltd., Nihonbashi, Tokyo, Japan) 10 minutes before surgery were performed, and then the injection site was massaged manually for one minute. Lymphoscintigraphy was performed 2–3 hours after the radioisotope injection.

Breast surgery was performed before axillary surgery in all patients to minimize the influence of radioactivity from the injection site [17-19]. Hot nodes were identified using a gamma probe (neo2000; Neoprobe Corporation, Dublin, OH, USA). Dyed and/or hot nodes located just under the markers using CT images were defined as sentinel nodes and were removed.

Histopathology

Sentinel nodes were serially sectioned at 2 mm intervals. Hematoxylin and eosin sections of these nodes were prepared from each 2-mm slice. When these nodes were tumor-negative in paraffin sections, an additional 4-μm section was cut and stained with immunohistochemistry (IHC) using the avidin-biotinylated peroxidase complex technique with the mouse monoclonal antibody against cytokeratin (NCL-CK19; Novocastra Laboratories Ltd., Newcastle, UK or AE1/AE3; Thermoelectron Corp., Waltham, MA, USA). On the basis of the 6th edition of the Union Internacional Contra la Cancrum TNM categories, metastatic nodes were categorized according to the degree of metastatic burden as follows: macrometastases (>2 mm) and micrometastases (0.2 to 2.0 mm). Nodes with isolated tumor cells identified by IHC were considered to be

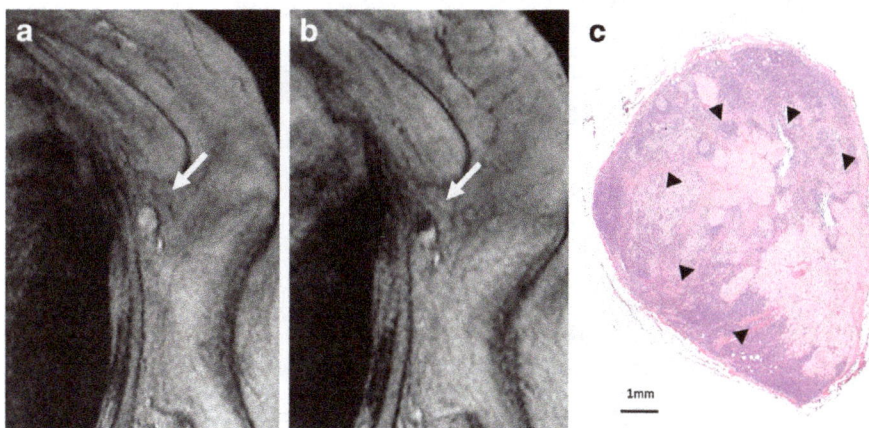

Figure 3 Pattern of partial high-signal intensity involving more than 50% of the node on SPIO-enhanced MR imaging. (a) The node showed high-signal intensity before administration of superparamagnetic iron oxide (SPIO). **(b)** After administration of SPIO, the node showed partial high-signal intensity involving more than 50% and was diagnosed as malignant (arrow). **(c)** Histological findings showed the presence of macro-metastases within the node (arrowheads).

metastasis-negative [20]. The long axis of the area of high-signal intensity was compared with the pathological size of the metastases.

Statistical analysis

Spearman's rank-order correlation was used for statistical analysis.

Results

The mean age of the 150 patients was 56.0 (range, 31–79) years and the mean pathologic tumor size was 19.4 (range, 0.2–60) mm. Patient and tumor characteristics are summarized in Table 1. The mean number of sentinel nodes identified by CT-LG was 1.15 (range 1–3). The mean size of sentinel nodes was 9.6 (range, 4–25) mm. Thirty-three pathologically positive sentinel nodes from 30 patients were evaluated. Four false-negative patients were excluded. Three patterns of SPIO uptake were demonstrated for positive sentinel nodes. Six nodes (18.2%) showed uniform high-signal intensity, 17 nodes (51.5%) showed partial high-signal intensity involving more than 50% of the node, and 10 nodes (30.3%) showed partial high-signal intensity involving less than 50% of the node. High-signal intensity patterns that were uniform or involved more than 50% of the node were observed in 23 nodes that contained macro-metastases and no node that contained micro-metastases, while high-signal intensity patterns involving less than 50% of the node were observed in 2 nodes that contained macro-metastases and 8 nodes that contained micro-metastases. When the area of high-signal intensity was compared with the pathological size of the metastases, a pathologic >2 mm sentinel node metastases correlated with the area of high-signal intensity, however, a

pathologic ≤2 mm sentinel node metastases did not. ($r_s = 0.482$, p = 0.015; $r_s = 0.309$, p = 0.457, respectively).

Discussion

The patterns of contrast enhancement have been demonstrated to distinguish between malignant and benign lymph nodes using USPIO-enhanced MR images [16]. A lymph node with an area of high-signal intensity encompassing the entire node or a portion of it was considered metastatic according to the diagnostic guidelines for USPIO-enhanced MR imaging, which are based on qualitative analysis of the results [16]. If there is no blackening of the node or if the node is hyperintense to surrounding tissue, or the node has central high-signal with darkening along the peripheral rim, or partial darkening whereby more than 50% of the node has an area of high-singal intensity, a node is diagnosed as metastatic. If less than 50% of the node has high-signal intensity, it is possibly metastatic. If the node has overall dark signal intensity, it is diagnosed as non-metastatic. A larger area of high-signal intensity within the node was reported to be more likely to be metastatic on USPIO-enhanced MR imaging. Lahaye et al. reported that an estimated area of high-signal intensity within the node that was more than 30% was highly predictive of a metastatic node, with a sensitivity of 93% and a specificity of 96% in patients with primary rectal cancer [21]. They demonstrated that the most accurate and practical predictive criterion is the estimation of the percentage of high-signal intensity within the node on USPIO-enhanced MR imaging. In the present study, we classified the patterns of SPIO uptake for positive sentinel nodes into three; uniform high-signal intensity, partial

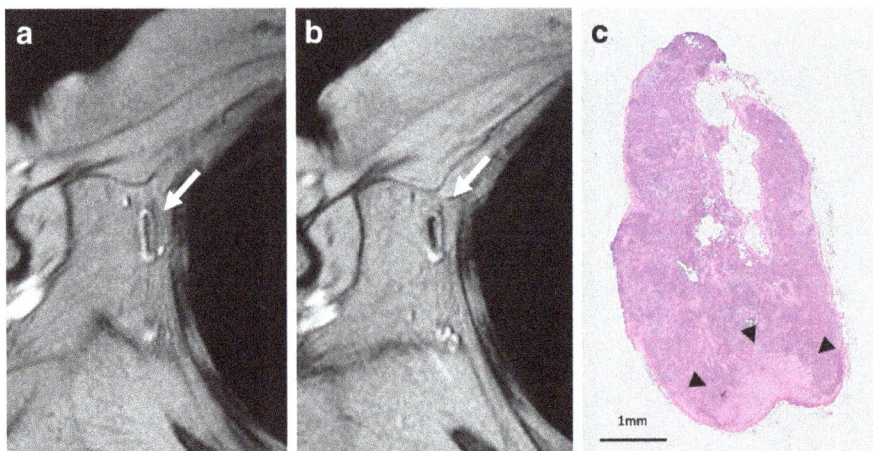

Figure 4 Pattern of partial high-signal intensity involving less than 50% of the node on SPIO-enhanced MR imaging. (a) The node showed high-signal intensity before administration of superparamagnetic iron oxide (SPIO). **(b)** After administration of SPIO, the node showed partial high-signal intensity involving less than 50% and was diagnosed as malignant (arrow). **(c)** Histological findings showed the presence of micro-metastases within the node (arrowheads).

Table 1 Patient characteristics

	No. of patients	%
Age, years		
<50	45	30.0
≥50	105	70.0
Tumor size, cm		
≤2	95	63.3
>2, ≤5	53	35.3
>5	2	1.3
Tumor location		
Upper outer	82	54.7
Upper inner	30	20.0
Lower outer	24	16.0
Lower inner	4	2.7
Central	8	5.3
Multicentric	2	1.3
Tumor histology		
Invasive ductal	132	88.0
Invasive lobular	7	4.7
Ductal carcinoma in situ	7	4.7
Others	4	2.7
Type of surgery		
Lumpectomy	146	96.7
Mastectomy	4	3.3
Estrogen receptor		
Positive	123	82.0
Negative	27	18.0
HER-2/neu		
Positive	19	12.7
Negative	131	87.3

high-signal intensity involving more than 50% of the node, and partial high-signal intensity involving less than 50% of the node. We demonstrated that high-signal intensity patterns that were uniform or involved more than 50% of the node were observed in nodes with macro-metastases (Figures 2 and 3). High signal intensity patterns involving less than 50% of the node were often observed in nodes with micro-metastases (Figure 4). When the area of high-signal intensity was compared with the pathological size of the metastases, a pathologic > 2 mm sentinel node metastases correlated with the area of high-signal intensity, however, a pathologic ≤ 2 mm sentinel node metastases did not. The size of small metastatic foci could not be assessed because MR imaging had limited resolution in the present setting. It may be difficult to detect micro-metastases with a section thickness of 4 mm at this resolution on 1.5 T MR images. Interstitial administration of SPIO

leads to excessive dosage or a high concentration of SPIO, which may conceal some micro-metastatic foci, resulting in underestimation of the size of metastatic foci, while the fatty hilum of a node, which coexists with metastases, may mimic a metastatic deposit, resulting in overestimation of the size of the metastatic foci. In our previous study, MR imaging with interstitial injection of SPIO was evaluated for the detection of metastases in sentinel nodes, which were localized by CT-LG in 102 patients with breast cancer [13]. The sensitivity, specificity, and accuracy of MR imaging for the diagnosis of sentinel node metastases were 84%, 91%, and 89%, respectively. In 40% of patients with micro-metastases, metastases were not detected, but all patients with macro-metastases were successfully identified. False negatives may be due to micro-metastases. Of the 7 false-positive results, 6 were due to a prominent fatty hilum. False positives may be due to prominent fatty tissue and insufficient transition of SPIO to sentinel nodes. Fat-saturated images, a 3 T MR system and special coil for MR imaging may be needed to clearly identify small metastatic foci.

However, the clinical implication of micro-metastases is debatable. De Boer et al. reported that the presence of both isolated tumor cells and micro-metastases was associated with reduced disease-free survival among patients who did not receive systemic adjuvant therapy [22]. In patients with isolated tumor cells and micro-metastases who received adjuvant therapy, disease-free survival was improved. In the systematic review, the presence of micro-metastases in axillary lymph nodes detected on single-section examination was associated with poorer disease-free and overall survival [23], while Hansen et al. reported that patients with micro-metastases do not have a worse disease-free or overall survival than sentinel node-negative patients [24]. Whether intensive identification of the existence of small disease foci is needed in clinical practice is an urgent problem.

There were some limitations to our study. There was a relatively small number of metastatic nodes in our series. This was due to the selection of patients with T1-2 breast cancers and clinically negative nodes, who do not have many metastatic axillary nodes. In addition, it is unclear whether the 50% cut-off value was appropriate. The 50% cut-off value was applied according to the diagnostic guidelines for USPIO-enhanced MR imaging, and for high-signal intensity in which more than 50% of the node was observed in sentinel nodes with macro-metastases [16]. A larger study is needed to find the most appropriate cut-off value to confirm the results of our study.

Conclusions

High-signal intensity patterns that are uniform or involve more than 50% of the node are features of nodes with macro-metastases. The area of high-signal intensity correlated with the pathological size of metastases for nodes with metastases >2 mm in this series.

Abbreviations

SPIO: Superparamagnetic iron oxide; USPIO: Ultrasmall superparamagnetic iron oxide; CT: Computed tomography; MR: Magnetic resonance; CT-LG: Computed tomography-lymphography; TR: Repetition time; TE: Echo time; ICG: Indocyanine green; IHC: Immunohistochemistry.

Competing interests

The authors declare that they have no competing interests.

Authors' contributions

KM contributed to the conception and design of the study, data analysis and drafted the manuscript. TI and SH contributed the analysis and interpretation of the data of MR imaging. HS contributed the analysis and interpretation of the data of CT. AN provided methodological advice. TH and KN contributed to the conception and design of the study, analysis and interpretation of the data. All authors read and approved the final manuscript.

Acknowledgments

This work was supported in part by the National Cancer Center Research and Development Fund (22–38).

Author details

[1]Department of Surgery, Osaka Medical Center for Cancer and Cardiovascular Diseases, 1-3-3 Nakamichi, Higashinari-ku, Osaka 537-8511, Japan. [2]Department of Radiology, Osaka Medical Center for Cancer and Cardiovascular Diseases, Osaka, Japan.

References

1. Giuliano AE, Kirgan DM, Guenther JM, Morton DL: Lymphatic mapping and sentinel lymphadenectomy for breast cancer. Ann Surg 1994, 220:391–401.
2. Giuliano AE, Jones RC, Brennan M, Statman R: Sentinel lymphadenectomy in breast cancer. J Clin Oncol 1997, 15:2345–2350.
3. Motomura K, Inaji H, Komoike Y, Kasugai T, Nagumo S, Noguchi S, Koyama H: Sentinel node biopsy in breast cancer patients with clinically negative lymph-nodes. Breast Cancer 1999, 6:259–262.
4. Krag D, Weaver D, Ashikaga T, Moffat F, Klimberg VS, Shriver C, Feldman S, Kusminsky R, Gadd M, Kuhn J, Harlow S, Beitsch P: The sentinel node in breast cancer: a multicenter validation study. N Engl J Med 1998, 339:941–946.
5. Veronesi U, Paganelli G, Galimberti V, Viale G, Zurrida S, Bedoni M, Costa A, de Cicco C, Geraghty JG, Luini A, Sacchini V, Veronesi P: Sentinel-node biopsy to avoid axillary dissection in breast cancer with clinically negative lymph-nodes. Lancet 1997, 349:1864–1867.
6. Wilke LG, McCall LM, Posther KE, Whitworth PW, Reintgen DS, Leitch AM, Gabram SG, Lucci A, Cox CE, Hunt KK, Herndon JE 2nd, Giuliano AE: Surgical complications associated with sentinel lymph node biopsy: results from a prospective international cooperative group trial. Ann Surg Oncol 2006, 13:491–500.
7. Lucci A, McCall LM, Beitsch PD, Whitworth PW, Reintgen DS, Blumencranz PW, Leitch AM, Saha S, Hunt KK, Giuliano AE: American College of Surgeons Oncology Group: Surgical complications associated with sentinel lymph node dissection (SLND) plus axillary lymph node dissection compared with SLND alone in the American College of Surgeons Oncology Group Trial Z0011. J Clin Oncol 2007, 25:3657–3663.
8. McLaughlin SA, Wright MJ, Morris KT, Sampson MR, Brockway JP, Hurley KE, Riedel ER, Van Zee KJ: Prevalence of lymphedema in women with breast cancer 5 years after sentinel lymph node biopsy or axillary dissection: objective measurements. J Clin Oncol 2008, 26:5213–5219.
9. Harisinghani MG, Barentsz J, Hahn PF, Deserno WM, Tabatabaei S, van de Kaa CH, de la Rosette J, Weissleder R: Noninvasive detection of clinically occult lymph-node metastases in prostate cancer. N Engl J Med 2003, 348:2491–2499.
10. Rockall AG, Sohaib SA, Harisinghani MG, Babar SA, Singh N, Jeyarajah AR, Oram DH, Jacobs IJ, Shepherd JH, Reznek RH: Diagnostic performance of nanoparticle-enhanced magnetic resonance imaging in the diagnosis of lymph node metastases in patients with endometrial and cervical cancer. J Clin Oncol 2005, 23:2813–2821.
11. Stets C, Brandt S, Wallis F, Buchmann J, Gilbert FJ, Heywang-Köbrunner SH: Axillary lymph node metastases: a statistical analysis of various parameters in MRI with USPIO. J Magn Reson Imaging 2002, 16:60–68.
12. Will O, Purkayastha S, Chan C, Athanasiou T, Darzi AW, Gedroyc W, Tekkis PP: Diagnostic precision of nanoparticle-enhanced MRI for lymph-node metastases: a meta-analysis. Lancet Oncol 2006, 7:52–60.
13. Motomura K, Ishitobi M, Komoike Y, Koyama H, Noguchi A, Sumino H, Kumatani Y, Inaji H, Horinouchi T, Nakanishi K: SPIO-enhanced magnetic resonance imaging for the detection of metastases in sentinel nodes localized by computed tomography lymphography in patients with breast cancer. Ann Surg Oncol 2011, 18:3422–3429.
14. Ohno Y, Hatabu H, Takenaka D, Higashino T, Watanabe H, Ohbayashi C, Sugimura K: CT-guided transthoracic needle aspiration biopsy of small (< or = 20 mm) solitary pulmonary nodules. AJR Am J Roentgenol 2003, 180:1665–1669.
15. Hudgins PA, Anzai Y, Morris MR, Lucas MA: Ferumoxtran-10, a superparamagnetic iron oxide as a magnetic resonance enhancement agent for imaging lymph nodes: a phase 2 dose study. AJNR Am J Neuroradiol 2002, 23:649–656.
16. Anzai Y, Piccoli CW, Outwater EK, Stanford W, Bluemke DA, Nurenberg P, Saini S, Maravilla KR, Feldman DE, Schmiedl UP, Brunberg JA, Francis IR, Harms SE, Som PM, Tempany CM, Group: Evaluation of neck and body metastases to nodes with ferumoxtran 10-enhanced MR imaging: phase III safety and efficacy study. Radiology 2003, 228:777–788.
17. Motomura K, Inaji H, Komoike Y, Hasegawa Y, Kasugai T, Noguchi S, Koyama H: Combination technique is superior to dye alone in identification of the sentinel node in breast cancer patients. J Surg Oncol 2001, 76:95–99.
18. Motomura K, Komoike Y, Hasegawa Y, Kasugai T, Inaji H, Noguchi S, Koyama H: Intradermal radioisotope injection is superior to subdermal injection for the identification of the sentinel node in breast cancer patients. J Surg Oncol 2003, 82:91–96.
19. Motomura K, Nagumo S, Komoike Y, Koyama H, Inaji H: Accuracy of imprint cytology for intraoperative diagnosis of sentinel node metastases in breast cancer. Ann Surg 2008, 247:839–842.
20. American Joint Committee on Cancer, et al: Breast. In AJCC Cancer Staging Handbook. 6th edition. Edited by Greene FL, Page DL, Fleming ID, Fritz AG, Balch CM, Haller DG. New York: Springer; 2002:155–181.
21. Lahaye MJ, Engelen SM, Kessels AG, de Bruïne AP, von Meyenfeldt MF, van Engelshoven JM, van de Velde CJ, Beets GL, Beets-Tan RG: USPIO-enhanced MR imaging for nodal staging in patients with primary rectal cancer: predictive criteria. Radiology 2008, 246:804–811.
22. de Boer M, van Deurzen CH, van Dijck JA, Borm GF, van Diest PJ, Adang EM, Nortier JW, Rutgers EJ, Seynaeve C, Menke-Pluymers MB, Bult P, Tjan-Heijnen VC: Micrometastases or isolated tumor cells and the outcome of breast cancer. N Engl J Med 2009, 361:653–663.
23. de Boer M, van Dijck JA, Bult P, Borm GF, Tjan-Heijnen VC: Breast cancer prognosis lymph node metastases, isolated tumor cells, and micrometastases. J Natl Cancer Inst 2010, 102:410–425.
24. Hansen NM, Grube B, Ye X, Turner RR, Brenner RJ, Sim MS, Giuliano AE: Impact of in the sentinel node of patients with invasive breast cancer. J Clin Oncol 2009, 27:4679–4684.

Magnetic resonance imaging-radioguided occult lesion localization (ROLL) in breast cancer using Tc-99m macro-aggregated albumin and distilled water control

Fernanda Philadelpho Arantes Pereira[1,2,3*], Gabriela Martins[2,3], Maria Julia Gregorio Calas[1,2], Maria Veronica Fonseca Torres de Oliveira[4,5], Emerson Leandro Gasparetto[1,3] and Lea Mirian Barbosa da Fonseca[4,5]

Abstract

Background: Magnetic resonance imaging (MRI) guided wire localization presents several challenges apart from the technical difficulties. An alternative to this conventional localization method using a wire is the radio-guided occult lesion localization (ROLL), more related to safe surgical margins and reductions in excision volume. The purpose of this study was to establish a safe and reliable magnetic resonance imaging-radioguided occult lesion localization (MRI-ROLL) technique and to report our initial experience with the localization of nonpalpable breast lesions only observed on MRI.

Methods: Sixteen women (mean age 53.2 years) with 17 occult breast lesions underwent radio-guided localization in a 1.5-T MR system using a grid-localizing system. All patients had a diagnostic MRI performed prior to the procedure. An intralesional injection of Technetium-99m macro-aggregated albumin followed by distilled water was performed. After the procedure, scintigraphy was obtained. Surgical resection was performed with the help of a gamma detector probe. The lesion histopathology and imaging concordance; the procedure's positive predictive value (PPV), duration time, complications, and accuracy; and the rate of exactly excised lesions evaluated with MRI six months after the surgery were assessed.

Results: One lesion in one patient had to be excluded because the radioactive substance came back after the injection, requiring a wire placement. Of the remaining cases, there were four malignant lesions, nine benign lesions, and three high-risk lesions. Surgical histopathology and imaging findings were considered concordant in all benign and high-risk cases. The PPV of MRI-ROLL was greater if the indication for the initial MR examination was active breast cancer. The median procedure duration time was 26 minutes, and all included procedures were defined as accurate. The exact and complete lesion removal was confirmed in all (100%) patients who underwent six-month postoperative MRI (50%).

Conclusions: MRI-ROLL offers a precise, technically feasible, safe, and rapid means for performing preoperative MRI localizations in the breast.

Keywords: Magnetic resonance imaging (MRI), MR-guided interventional procedures, Nuclear medicine, Radioisotopes, Breast cancer

* Correspondence: fephila@gmail.com
[1]Department of Radiology, Federal University of Rio de Janeiro, Rua Prof. Rodolpho Paulo Rocco 255, Cidade Universitária, Rio de Janeiro, RJ 21941-617, Brazil
[2]Department of Breast Imaging, Clínica de Diagnóstico por Imagem (CDPI), Av. Ataulfo de Paiva 669, 2nd floor, Leblon, Rio de Janeiro, RJ 22440-032, Brazil
Full list of author information is available at the end of the article

Background

Magnetic resonance imaging (MRI) of the breast has proven to be a valuable complement to the conventional techniques, including mammography, ultrasonography, and physical examination, for breast cancer detection, diagnosis, staging, and treatment follow-up [1]. In addition, MRI is able to detect lesions that are not visible on these conventional techniques in 10-39% of cases [2]. In patients with proven breast cancer, MRI can detect additional ipsilateral cancer sites in 6-34% of cases and unsuspected contralateral cancer in 4-24% of cases [3-5]. However, as the reported specificity of breast MRI (37–97%) is lower than its high sensitivity (94-100%), suspicious lesions detected by MRI must be confirmed histologically [3].

When suspicious, enhancing breast lesions are detected solely with MRI, MRI-guided biopsy techniques are used for accurate sampling of the lesions and for histopathological analysis. MRI-guided tissue sampling of these "MRI-only observed lesions" can be accomplished by needle localization followed by surgical excision, by MRI-guided large-core needle biopsy, or through vacuum biopsy [1,6]. For an interventional procedure to be clinically useful, factors such as safety, accuracy, availability, cost, patient preference, and surgeon's request should be considered [7]. MRI-guided needle localization is a well-known and widely utilized technique for tissue sampling, especially for breast lesions that are difficult to access [1,6-8].

Until now, MRI-guided needle localization has been performed through the deployment of a wire. While the accuracy of needle and wire placement is important with any means of guidance, it is particularly important for MRI-guided procedures because lesion retrieval cannot be verified with radiography of the lumpectomy specimen, as the lesion is commonly only visible *in vivo* after the intravenous administration of a gadolinium-based contrast material [9]. Although excisional biopsy after MRI-guided wire localization has proven to be a successful method for obtaining adequate material for pathological evaluation, this technique is associated with several challenges apart from the technical difficulties [10-12], including the accordion effect, which leads to a final wire position that is not the ideal after breast decompression; wire displacement and migration; wire breakage; difficulties related to establishing surgical access to the lesion; infection; and bleeding. Nevertheless, its main disadvantage is the high incidence of residual disease (up to 51% at the biopsy site) [12-15].

An alternative to this conventional localization method using a wire is the radio-guided occult lesion localization (ROLL), which consists of an intratumoral injection of Technetium-99m (Tc-99m) macro-aggregated albumin (MAA). On the day of surgery, a portable gamma probe guides the biopsy, providing a practical and precise method for locating the intratumor injection site. In the last years, this technique has been proposed by many different studies as being the best option for the localization of non-palpable breast lesions guided by mammography or ultrasonography [12,16-19], resulting in correct localization in more than 90% of cases. It has also been associated with a higher prevalence of safe surgical margins, improved cosmetic outcome, and less postoperative pain, in addition to reductions in excision volume and more accurate lesion centricity within the surgical specimen [7,12-20].

Although ROLL has been used for more than 10 years for mammography- and ultrasonography-guided localizations, to the best of our knowledge, there is only one study in the literature describing the use of radioactive substances in MRI-guided localizations using a different technique than the one described here [7]. Hence, this study was designed to establish a safe and reliable technique and to report our initial experience with MRI-ROLL of nonpalpable breast lesions only observed on MRI.

Methods

Study population and lesion characteristics

From May 2011 to July 2012, this study prospectively enrolled 16 women with 17 breast lesions. One lesion in one patient was excluded from the study because the procedure was unsuccessful, and a wire was required. As a result, the study included 15 patients (age range, 38–78 years; mean age, 53.3 years) with 16 breast lesions.

All patients had a diagnostic MRI performed prior to the procedure, showing lesions not identified by mammography or ultrasonography, even by "second look" ultrasonography. The size range of these 16 lesions was 0.6-4.0 cm (median, 1 cm). Eleven lesions (68.75%) were located in the left breast, and five lesions (31.25%) were located in the right breast.

The ACR BI-RADS-MRI Lexicon was used to classify the morphological and dynamic characteristics of the lesions [21]. Eight of the 16 lesions (50%) were non-mass enhancement-type lesions, and the remaining eight (50%) were mass-type lesions. From the eight non-mass enhancement lesions, three showed focal distribution, three ductal distribution, one segmental distribution, and one linear distribution. From the eight mass lesions, six had oval shape and smooth margins, one had a lobulated shape and smooth margins, and one had irregular shape and margins. Most lesions had either moderate or early marked enhancement. The delayed enhancement pattern analyzed in the mass lesions showed plateau curves in three out of the eight lesions and washout curves in the remaining five lesions. The BI-RADS classifications were BI-RADS 4 for 14 of the 16 lesions and BI-RADS 3, which signifies a likely benign lesion, for 2 of the 16 lesions.

Indications for the previous MRI examinations were problem-solving in nine cases, a present history of ipsilateral or contralateral breast cancer in three cases, a previous personal history of breast cancer in one case, search for an occult primary tumor in one patient with an altered axillary lymph node, and integrity of breast implants in two cases.

Our institutional review (CEP HUCFF/FM) board approved the study, and all patients gave their informed consent.

MRI-ROLL technique

All MRI-ROLL were performed by one of three radiologists (FPAP, GM, MJGC) who were experts in breast imaging, including MRI-guided breast procedures, using a 1.5-T MR System (Signa Excite HD, GE Healthcare, Milwaukee, WI) with the patient positioned prone in a dedicated 8-channel breast coil. The breast undergoing localization was placed in the coil using a grid-localizing system. First, the medial aspect of the breast was positioned flush against a compression plate or a grid, depending on whether the access to the lesion was lateral or medial, respectively. A lateral grid or compression plate, also depending on whether the access was lateral or medial, respectively, was then firmly adjusted to fully compress and immobilize the breast. A vitamin E capsule was used as a fiducial marker and was taped to the grid over the expected lesion site, which was determined based on review of the diagnostic MR images.

First, a localizing sequence was acquired, and the volume of interest was selected to include the compression device and the vitamin E marker. Then, a sagittal T1-weighted 3D fat-suppressed gradient-echo sequence (flip angle, 15°; bandwidth, 41.67 MHz; matrix size, 220 × 220; field of view, 220 mm; number of excitations, 1; slice thickness, 2 mm; intersection gap, 0 mm) was repeated before and after the rapid bolus injection of 0.1 mmol/L of gadoterate meglumine (Dotarem, Guerbet, Roissy, France) per kilogram of body weight, followed by 20 mL of saline, until the enhancing lesion was visualized. The acquisition time, which was approximately 1 min per sequence, varied depending on the size of the breast and the area covered.

The images were reviewed. A cursor was placed over the lesion on the monitor, and its relationship to the skin surface and the vitamin E marker was determined by manually scrolling through sequential sagittal slices. The grid of the compression device was evident as low-signal-intensity lines on the skin surface due to pressure indentation. The plastic of the compression device was not visible on MRI. The vitamin E capsule was identified as an area of high signal intensity on the skin surface. The skin entry site was determined based on visual assessment of the location of the lesion with respect to the grid lines using the vitamin E capsule as a guide. The depth of the lesion from the skin surface was calculated as the difference between the depth of the skin surface and the depth of the sagittal slice containing the lesion.

After calculating the entrance site and lesion depth, the patient was withdrawn from the magnet. The skin overlying the lesion was marked, and the skin was cleansed with alcohol and anesthetized with 1–2 mL of 1% lidocaine hydrochloride (Xylocaine, Astra USA, Westborough, MA). A needle guide block (Needle block, In Vivo, Gainesville, FL) was inserted into the grid hole overlying the anesthetized area. A needle guide with 20-gauge holes was used to anchor and stabilize the needle and to allow insertion of the needle in a straight perpendicular fashion, thereby reducing needle angulation during insertion. The MR-compatible needle (20 ga, MRI-compatible needle, EZEM, Westbury, NY) was then placed in the hole of the needle guide closest to the skin marking. We inserted the needle to the desired depth, taking into account the 1.5-cm thickness of the needle guide.

Sagittal and axial T1-weighted 3D fat-suppressed gradient-echo sequences were then obtained to document the location of the needle, with the desired depth of the tip optimally positioned within the lesion. The needle was evident as a low-signal-intensity structure with an adjacent susceptibility artifact. If the needle was too deep or too superficial, adjustments were made.

When the needle tip was within the lesion or at least within 5 mm of the lesion, a sagittal fat-suppressed T2-weighted fast spin-echo sequence (repetition time/echo time, 2300/102 ms; bandwidth, 35.7 MHz; matrix size, 256 × 224; field of view, 230 mm; number of excitations, 4; slice thickness, 2 mm; intersection gap, 0 mm; and acquisition time, 1.46 minutes) was repeated before and after the injection of the radioactive substance (Tc-99m MAA). The injected dose was 1 mCi or 37 MBq if the surgery had been performed the same day as the localization or 4 mCi or 148 MBq if the surgery had been performed the day after, followed by the administration of 1 mL of distilled water. In this sequence, the needle is also evident as a low-signal-intensity structure with an adjacent susceptibility artifact. In contrast, the water injected after the radioactive substance is evident as a high-signal-intensity area and confirms the injection of the radioactive material in the proper location within the lesion. The subtraction technique was also used as a control for the radioactive substance injection. The T2-weighted sequence obtained before the radioactive material plus water administration was subtracted from the T2-weighted sequence obtained after the radioactive substance plus water administration, and the high-signal-intensity area from the injected water was better visualized. The needle was then removed.

Immediately after localization, scintigraphy (Ventri, GE Healthcare, Milwaukee, WI) was performed to serve as a control for the presence of the radioactive substance; a two-view mammography (Lorad M-IV, Hologic, Bedford, MA) was also performed to serve as a road map for the surgeon. We were aware that the radioactive substance would not appear on the mammographic images. The report and the images obtained from the MRI localization and from the scintigraphic and mammographic control were sent to the surgeon along with the patient. A six-month follow-up MRI was suggested in the report to confirm lesion removal, mainly for benign cases.

During the surgery, a gamma probe (Johnson & Johnson, New Jersey, NY) was used to locate the maximum radioactive focus and, thus, the lesion. The complete removal of the lesion was confirmed by the absence of radioactivity in the breast tissue and by the presence of safe surgical margins. The excised tissue was sent for histopathological examination.

MRI analysis and data collection

Histopathological characteristics of the lesion were determined from the surgical pathology reports and were categorized as benign, malignant, or high-risk. MR imaging and histopathological findings were reviewed and considered concordant if the histopathological findings provided an explanation for the imaging features, particularly in the benign and high-risk lesions. The positive predictive value (PPV) of MRI-ROLL was defined as the number of cancers identified during MRI localization divided by the total number of lesions that had undergone MRI localization. The PPV was also analyzed according to the indication of the previous MRI examination, i.e., the MRI that first showed the lesion.

Breast MRI-ROLL cases were reviewed to assess the procedure time (total magnet time), complication rate, and accuracy. The procedure accuracy was measured by the distance between the needle tip and the target lesion prior to the injection of the radioactive material, by the presence of high-signal-intensity area on T2-weighted sequence and on the subtracted images in the exact location of the lesion after the water administration, and by the presence of the radioactive material in the scintigraphic control. The rate of exactly excised lesions was evaluated on the MRI obtained six months postoperatively.

Data were collected and analyzed on a computerized spreadsheet (Excel, Microsoft, Redmond, WA).

Results

Histopathological findings

A total of four malignant lesions (25%), all invasive ductal carcinomas (IDC), were verified upon histopathologic examination. The median size of the malignant lesions was 0.85 cm (range, 0.6-1.2 cm). The first carcinoma was an oval-shaped mass with smooth margins, which

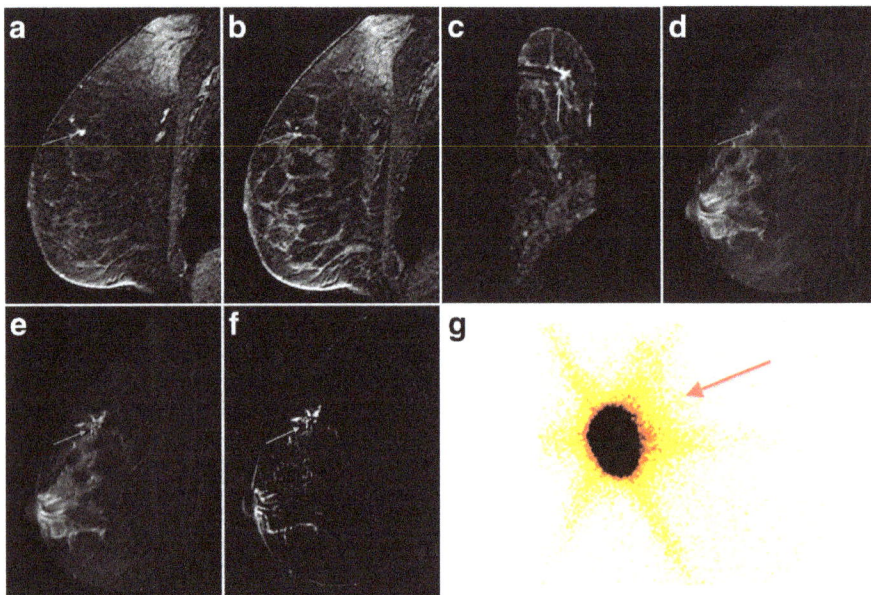

Figure 1 A 78-year-old woman with invasive ductal carcinoma (IDC) of the right breast. (a) Sagittal T1-weighted contrast-enhanced sequence shows a regular mass in the upper inner quadrant of the right breast (arrow). **(b)** Sagittal T1-weighted contrast-enhanced sequence reveals the lesion with the needle, low-signal-intensity dot, inside (arrow). **(c)** Axial T1-weighted contrast-enhanced sequence shows the needle tip close to the lesion (arrow). **(d)** Sagittal fat-suppressed T2-weighted sequence shows the exact location of the lesion after correlation with the contrast-enhanced sequences (arrow). **(e)** Sagittal T2-weighted sequence after injection of Tc-99m MAA followed by injection of 1 mL of distilled water reveals a high-signal-intensity area and confirms that the radioactive material is in the exact location of the lesion. **(f)** Sagittal T2-weighted sequence subjected to subtraction technique: the high-signal-intensity area from the water injected is visualized better (arrow). **(g)** Scintigraphic control reveals the presence of the radioactive substance (arrow).

presented a plateau curve in the delayed enhancement phase and was classified as BI-RADS 3 (Figure 1). The second, third, and forth carcinomas were non-mass-enhancement masses with linear, focal, and focal distributions, respectively (Figure 2); all three were classified as BI-RADS 4 (Tables 1 and 2).

There were nine benign lesions (56.25%) with the following classifications: fibroadenoma (n = 2), columnar cell alteration without atypia, apocrine metaplasia, adenosis (n = 2), focal florid ductal hyperplasia (n = 2), nodular florid adenosis (n = 1), intramammary lymph node (n = 1), and fat necrosis (n = 1). The median size of the benign lesions was 1.0 cm (range, 0.8-4.0 cm) (Tables 3 and 2).

Additionally, there were three high-risk lesions (23.1%) with the following classifications: intraductal papilloma (n = 1), fibroadenoma with atypia (n = 1), and atypical ductal hyperplasia (n = 1). The median size of the high-risk lesions was 0.6 cm (range, 0.6-2.8 cm) (Tables 4 and 2).

After revision, surgical histology and MR imaging findings were considered concordant in all benign and high-risk cases.

The PPV of MRI-ROLL was 25% (4/16). Importantly, the PPV was greatest if the indication for the initial MR examination was a current history of breast cancer (3/4 = 75%). Among the three carcinomas diagnosed on MRI-ROLL in women with synchronous cancer, the cancers that had MRI localization were in the ipsilateral breast in one case and in the contralateral breast in two cases (Table 1).

Procedure time, complications, accuracy, and follow-up
The median duration time to perform MRI-ROLL was 26 minutes (range, 20–37 minutes). No complications occurred during any of the interventions. However, one case had to be excluded because a hematoma formed during the needle placement and the radioactive substance came back after the injection, requiring a wire placement. Therefore, this study achieved technical success in 16/17 (94.1%) of the cases.

The tip of the needle was placed within the lesions in 12 of the 16 cases (75%) and within 0.3 cm of the edge of the lesions in the remaining four cases (25%) prior to the radioactive material injection. Because the high-signal-intensity area observed on the T2-weighted sequence and on the subtracted images was present in the exact location of the lesion after the water administration and the scintigraphic control, the radioactive material was confirmed to be present in all cases.

Exact and complete lesion removals were confirmed in all cases (100%) that underwent MRI six months postoperatively, i.e., eight of the 16 cases (50%). Four patients (25%) did not have MRIs because their surgeries had

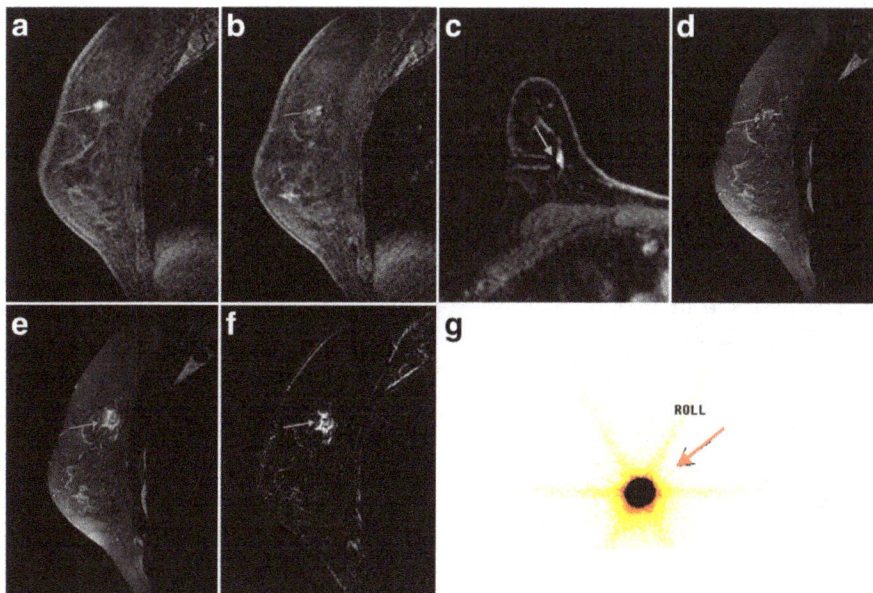

Figure 2 A 38-year-old woman with invasive ductal carcinoma (IDC) of the right breast. (a) Sagittal T1-weighted contrast-enhanced sequence shows a focal nonmass enhancement in the upper inner quadrant of the right breast (arrow). **(b)** Sagittal T1-weighted contrast-enhanced sequence reveals the lesion with the needle, low-signal-intensity dot, inside (arrow). **(c)** Axial T1-weighted contrast-enhanced sequence shows the needle tip close to the lesion (arrow). **(d)** Sagittal T2-weighted sequence shows the exact location of the lesion after correlation with the contrast-enhanced sequences (arrow). **(e)** Sagittal fat-suppressed T2-weighted sequence after injection of Tc-99m MAA followed by 1 mL of distilled water reveals a high-signal-intensity area and confirms that the radioactive material is in the exact location of the lesion. **(f)** Sagittal T2-weighted sequence subjected to subtraction technique: the high-signal-intensity area from the water injected can be visualized better (arrow). **(g)** Scintigraphic control reveals the presence of the radioactive substance (arrow).

Table 1 Malignant histopathological findings based on patient age, MRI indication, breast density, and MRI lesion characteristics

Histopathological findings	Age	MRI indication	Breast density	Morphological and dynamic characteristics of the lesions	Lesion size (cm)	BI-RADS
Invasive ductal carcinoma, grade I	51	Known contralateral breast cancer	Heterogeneously dense	Linear nonmass enhancement	1.2	4
Invasive ductal carcinoma, grade I	78	Known contralateral breast cancer	Heterogeneously dense	Oval shape and smooth margins mass, type 2 curve	0.7	3
Invasive ductal carcinoma, grade II	38	Known ipsilateral breast cancer	Extremely dense	Focal nonmass enhancement	0.6	4
Invasive ductal carcinoma, grade I	54	Problem-solving	Heterogeneously dense	Focal nonmass enhancement	1.0	4

been performed less than six months before the end of the study. The remaining four patients (25%) did not undergo MRI because the surgeon did not request it.

Discussion

Here, we present the technique and results of MRI-ROLL of suspicious breast lesions only observed on MRI. In total, we successfully performed MRI localizations of 16 breast lesions in 15 patients. Although ours was a small series, the findings suggest that this localization technique is rapid, technically successful, and accurate, without the challenges of MRI-guided wire localization.

In our study, the PPV of MRI-ROLL was 25%, which is similar to the PPV of MRI-guided wire localization [7]. The overall ratio of benign to malignant biopsies among MRI-detected lesions ranges between 1:1 and 3:1, depending on diagnostic criteria and indications, e.g., in case of a personal or a family history of breast cancer, invasive procedures are likely to be more frequently indicated [2,11]. In our study, carcinoma was revealed in women with known cancer who had been referred for MRI-guided localization for preoperative staging. Of the four carcinomas identified, one was classified as BI-RADS 3 and three as BI-RADS 4. In addition, the three BI-RADS 4 lesions exhibited morphology and enhancement characteristics that were not specific for malignancy. Even without suspicious characteristics, lesions in a patient with a present history of ipsilateral or contralateral breast cancer should be investigated and biopsied.

Our actual MRI-ROLL time was similar to the 15–59 minute time range that has been previously reported for

Table 2 BI-RADS classification and histopathological findings

	Malignant	Benign	High-risk	Total
BI-RADS 3	1	0	1	2
BI-RADS 4	3	9	2	14
Total	4	9	3	16

MRI-guided wire localization [9-11]. With more experience, we expect to perform procedures faster and utilize fewer sequences, while maintaining a high success rate.

Although we did not experience complications during the procedures, we did not succeed in one case and had to exclude it from our study. In that particular case, a hematoma formed during placement of the needle; due to the pressure caused by the hematoma, the radioactive substance could not be injected properly, therefore requiring wire placement. Injection of the radioactive substance may also be challenging when the lesion is harder or more compact.

Currently, the added benefit of MRI in the detection of clinically, mammographically, and ultrasonographically occult cancers is well known. Cancers that are only truly visible on MRI are detected in 14-35% of patients who undergo breast MRI for a variety of reasons [9]. One of the most frequently used methods for sampling MRI-detected lesions remains needle localization with a wire, either because it provides a better approach to breast lesions that are difficult to access or because it is less expensive and more available than other MRI biopsy methods. Although excisional biopsy after MRI-guided wire localization has proven to be a successful method for obtaining adequate material for pathological evaluation, the technique is associated with several disadvantages, including technical difficulties for the interventional radiologist and the surgeon, thereby limiting the success rate of the procedure and increasing the surgery duration time [2].

A potential problem with MRI-guided wire localizations is that the breast is compressed during the deployment of the wire but not during the surgical excision [11]. This deployment creates an accordion effect. The accordion effect has been a recognized explanation for partly excised or missed lesions after MRI-guided needle localizations [2,9,11,22,23]. The accordion effect in MRI-ROLL is not a considerable problem because the radioactive substance is injected on or very close to the lesion and does not change position when the compression is released. Wire displacement or migration between localization and surgery has been recognized in the MRI

Table 3 Benign histopathological findings based on patient age, MRI indication, breast density, and MRI lesion characteristics

Histopathological findings	Age	MRI indication	Breast density	Morphological and dynamic characteristics of the lesions	Lesion size (cm)	BI-RADS
Columnar cell alteration without atypia, apocrine metaplasia, adenosis	57	Integrity of breast implants	Heterogeneously dense	Segmental nonmass enhancement	3.3	4
Columnar cell alteration without atypia, apocrine metaplasia, adenosis	60	Problem-solving	Heterogeneously dense	Ductal nonmass enhancement	1.6	4
Fat necrosis	55	Previous personal history of breast cancer	Scattered fibroglandular densities	Ductal nonmass enhancement	4	4
Intramammary lymph node	53	Occult primary tumor and altered axillary lymph node	Scattered fibroglandular densities	Irregular shape and margins mass, type 3 curve	1	4
Nodular florid adenosis	42	Problem-solving	Heterogeneously dense	Oval shape and smooth margins mass, type 3 curve	1	4
Focal florid ductal hyperplasia	56	Problem-solving	Scattered fibroglandular densities	Focal nonmass enhancement	1.8	4
Focal florid ductal hyperplasia	51	Problem-solving	Scattered fibroglandular densities	Lobulated shape and smooth margins mass, type 3 curve	0.9	4
Fibroadenoma	46	Integrity of breast implants	Scattered fibroglandular densities	Oval shape and smooth margins mass, type 3 curve	1	4
Fibroadenoma	57	Problem-solving	Scattered fibroglandular densities	Oval shape and smooth margins mass, type 2 curve	0.8	4

and mammographic literature [2,9]. MRI-ROLL also solves this problem.

There was no important difference between the cost of the radioactive substance and the titanium wire. However, considering the surgical time, the preoperative wire localization can result in a higher cost to the patient.

Confirmation of lesion retrieval remains an issue in MRI-guided localization with a radioactive marker or a wire. Because the lesion does not enhance *ex vivo*, there is no possibility of direct verification that the correct area has been excised [1]. Correlation of imaging and histology plays an important role in this procedure, as in breast biopsy with any method [10,11,24]. If the pathological assessment yields a benign histology, review of the original MRI and biopsy imaging is advised to reassess the level of suspicion and adequacy of sampling. For cases that are felt to be discordant or possibly missed, repeat biopsy or surgical excision is recommended as soon as can be reasonably tolerated by the patient.

Postoperative MR imaging should be incorporated into the routine follow-up of patients who have MR imaging-guided localization to ensure lesion retrieval if the procedure yields benign findings and to assess for residual tumor if the procedure reveals breast cancer. A study analyzed postoperative MRI scans performed on 33 lesion sites, suggesting that the lesion was completely excised in 29 (87.9%), partly excised in three (9.1%), and missed in one case (3.0%) [11]. Another study reported 13.5% inadequate removal of the lesion despite correct needle positioning [2]. In our study, the exact and complete lesion removal was confirmed in all cases (100%) that underwent six-month follow up MRI. However, postoperative MR imaging was not routinely performed, although it was suggested to the surgeons in the procedure report. To this point, only half of the cases have undergone postoperative MRI.

Our study has some limitations. First, our series is relatively small. The two main reasons for the study's

Table 4 High-risk histopathological findings according to patient age, MRI indication, breast density, and MRI lesion characteristics

Histopathological findings	Age	MRI indication	Breast density	Morphological and dynamic characteristics of the lesions	Lesion size (cm)	BI-RADS
Intraductal papilloma	51	Problem-solving	Heterogeneously dense	Oval shape and smooth margins mass, type 3 curve	0.6	4
Fibroadenoma with atypia	52	Problem-solving	Heterogeneously dense	Oval shape and smooth margins mass, type 2 curve	0.6	3
Atypical ductal hyperplasia	52	Problem-solving	Heterogeneously dense	Ductal nonmass enhancement	2.8	4

small size are the following: MRI procedures continue to be expensive, and MRI-ROLL is a new technique that is not well known by mastologists. Further studies should consider increasing the sample number to improve the statistical power. Second, the water injected after the radioactive substance in the target lesion is only observed on MRI. Therefore, it is impossible to determine the exact injection site using any other imaging modality. The same occurs in the single study published in the literature regarding MRI-ROLL, in which the MRI contrast material injected after the radioactive material was only observed on MRI [7]. The scintigraphy identifies the radioactive material but does not reveal the exact injection site. Further work in this area might also include the injection of a radiographically visible marker within the lesion in addition to the injected radioactive substance, e.g., an iodinated contrast or air [25], so that the surgeon can see the location of the lesion with respect to the nipple, the chest wall, and the remainder of the breast tissue using mammography.

Conclusions

MRI-ROLL offers a relatively rapid and accurate means for performing preoperative MRI-guided localizations in the breast. The results of this preliminary study show that MRI-ROLL is technically feasible and safe. This is particularly important, as radio-guided surgery is easier to perform, allows an effective lesion resection, and leads to better cosmetic results. Larger studies and a comparison between the results of MRI-ROLL and MRI-guided wire localization are needed before this technique can become routine clinical practice.

Competing interests
No competing interests to disclose.

Authors' contributions
FPAP performed the procedures, participated in the design of the study, collected and analyzed the data, and drafted and submitted the manuscript. GM and MJGC performed the procedures and reviewed the manuscript. MVFTO participated in the procedures and reviewed the manuscript. ELG participated in the design and coordination of the study and reviewed the manuscript. LMBF conceived the study, participated in its design and coordination, and approved the final version. All authors have read and approved the final version of this manuscript.

Authors' information
LMBF, MD, PhD, Full Professor of Medical School of Federal University of Rio de Janeiro, Head of Department of Radiology of Hospital Clementino Fraga Filho (Federal University of Rio de Janeiro Hospital), Nuclear Medicine Physician of Clínica de Diagnóstico por Imagem and Hospital Samaritano, Rio de Janeiro.

Author details
[1]Department of Radiology, Federal University of Rio de Janeiro, Rua Prof. Rodolpho Paulo Rocco 255, Cidade Universitária, Rio de Janeiro, RJ 21941-617, Brazil. [2]Department of Breast Imaging, Clínica de Diagnóstico por Imagem (CDPI), Av. Ataulfo de Paiva 669, 2nd floor, Leblon, Rio de Janeiro, RJ 22440-032, Brazil. [3]Department of Magnetic Resonance Imaging, Clínica de Diagnóstico por Imagem (CDPI), Av. Ataulfo de Paiva 669, 2nd floor, Leblon, Rio de Janeiro, RJ 22440-032, Brazil. [4]Department of Nuclear Medicine, Federal University of Rio de Janeiro, Rua Prof. Rodolpho Paulo Rocco 255, Cidade Universitária, Rio de Janeiro, RJ 21941-617, Brazil. [5]Department of Nuclear Medicine, Clínica de Diagnóstico por Imagem (CDPI), Av. Ataulfo de Paiva 669, 2nd floor, Leblon, Rio de Janeiro, RJ 22440-032, Brazil.

References
1. Meeuwis C, Peters NH, Mali WP, Gallardo AM, van Hillegersberg R, Schipper ME, van den Bosch MA: **Targeting difficult accessible breast lesions: MRI-guided needle localization using a freehand technique in a 3.0 T closed bore magnet.** *Eur J Radiol* 2007, **62**(2):283–288.
2. Landheer ML, Veltman J, van Eekeren R, Zeillemaker AM, Boetes C, Wobbes T: **MRI-guided preoperative wire localization of nonpalpable breast lesions.** *Clin Imaging* 2006, **30**(4):229–233.
3. David J, Trop I, Lalonde L: **Breast procedures guided by magnetic resonance imaging.** *Can Assoc Radiol J* 2005, **56**(5):309–318.
4. Liberman L, Morris EA, Dershaw DD, Thornton CM, Van Zee KJ, Tan LK: **Fast MRI-guided vacuum-assisted breast biopsy: initial experience.** *AJR Am J Roentgenol* 2003, **181**(5):1283–1293.
5. Perlet C, Heinig A, Prat X, Casselman J, Baath L, Sittek H, Stets C, Lamarque J, Anderson I, Schneider P, Taourel P, Reiser M, Heywang-Köbrunner SH: **Multicenter study for the evaluation of a dedicated biopsy device for MR-guided vacuum biopsy of the breast.** *Eur Radiol* 2002, **12**(6):1463–1470.
6. Heywang-Köbrunner SH, Sinnatamby R, Lebeau A, Lebrecht A, Britton PD, Schreer I: **Interdisciplinary consensus on the uses and technique of MR-guided vacuum-assisted breast biopsy (VAB): results of a European consensus meeting.** *Eur J Radiol* 2009, **72**(2):289–294.
7. Yilmaz MH, Kilic F, Icten GE, Aydogan F, Ozben V, Halac M, Olgun DC, Gazioglu E, Celik V, Uras C, Altug ZA: **Radio-guided occult lesion localization for breast lesions under computed-aided MRI guidance: the first experience and initial results.** *Br J Radiol* 2012, **85**(1012):395–402.
8. van den Bosch MA, Daniel BL: **MR-guided interventions of the breast.** *Magn Reson Imaging Clin N Am* 2005, **13**(3):505–517.
9. Causer PA, Piron CA, Jong RA, Curpen BN, Luginbuhl CA, Glazier JE, Warner E, Hill K, Muldoon J, Taylor G, Wong JW, Plewes DB: **MR imaging–guided breast localization system with medial or lateral access.** *Radiology* 2006, **240**(2):369–379.
10. Liberman L: **Magnetic resonance imaging guided needle localization.** In *Breast MRI Diagnosis and Intervention.* 1st edition. Edited by Morris EA, Liberman L. New York: Springer; 2005:280–296.
11. Morris EA, Liberman L, Dershaw DD, Kaplan JB, LaTrenta LR, Abramson AF, Ballon DJ: **Preoperative MR imaging-guided needle localization of breast lesions.** *AJR Am J Roentgenol* 2002, **178**(5):1211–1220.
12. Pilkington Woll JP, Cortés Romera M, García Vicente AM, González García B, Delgado Portela M, Cordero García JM, Pardo García R, Molino Trinidad C, Soriano Castrejón AM: **Impact of radioguided occult lesion localization on the correct excision of malignant breast lesions: effect of histology and tumor size.** *Ann Nucl Med* 2011, **25**(3):197–203.
13. Paganelli G, Luini A, Veronesi U: **Radioguided occult lesion localization (ROLL) in breast cancer: maximizing efficacy, minimizing mutilation.** *Ann Oncol* 2002, **13**(12):1839–1840.
14. De Cicco C, Pizzamiglio M, Trifirò G, Luini A, Ferrari M, Prisco G, Galimberti V, Cassano E, Viale G, Intra M, Veronesi P, Paganelli G: **Radioguided occult lesion localization (ROLL) and surgical biopsy in breast cancer. Technical aspects.** *Q J Nucl Med* 2002, **46**(2):145–151.
15. Luini A, Zurrida S, Paganelli G, Galimberti V, Sacchini V, Monti S, Veronesi P, Viale G, Veronesi U: **Comparison of radioguided excision with wire localization of occult breast lesions.** *Br J Surg* 1999, **86**(4):522–525.
16. Pleijhuis RG, Graafland M, de Vries J, Bart J, de Jong JS, van Dam GM: **Obtaining adequate surgical margins in breast-conserving therapy for patients with early-stage breast cancer: current modalities and future directions.** *Ann Surg Oncol* 2009, **16**(10):2717–2730.
17. Mariscal Martínez A, Solà M, de Tudela AP, Julián JF, Fraile M, Vizcaya S, Fernández J: **Radioguided localization of nonpalpable breast cancer lesions: randomized comparison with wire localization in patients undergoing conservative surgery and sentinel node biopsy.** *AJR Am J Roentgenol* 2009, **193**(4):1001–1009.
18. Medina-Franco H, Abarca-Pérez L, García-Alvarez MN, Ulloa-Gómez JL, Romero-Trejo C, Sepúlveda-Méndez J: **Radioguided occult lesion**

localization (ROLL) versus wire-guided lumpectomy for non-palpable breast lesions: a randomized prospective evaluation. *J Surg Oncol* 2008, **97**(2):108–111.

19. Sarlos D, Frey LD, Haueisen H, Landmann G, Kots LA, Schaer G: Radioguided occult lesion localization (ROLL) for treatment and diagnosis of malignant and premalignant breast lesions combined with sentinel node biopsy: a prospective clinical trial with 100 patients. *Eur J Surg Oncol* 2009, **35**(4):403–408.

20. Thind CR, Desmond S, Harris O, Nadeem R, Chagla LS, Audisio RA: **Radio-guided localization of clinically occult breast lesions (ROLL): a DGH experience.** *Clin Radiol* 2005, **60**(6):681–686.

21. American College of Radiology (ACR): **ACR BI-RADS – magnetic resonance imaging.** In *Breast Imaging Reporting and Data System, Breast Imaging Atlas.* 1st edition. Edited by ACR. Reston, VA: American College of Radiology; 2003.

22. Bedrosian I, Schlencker J, Spitz FR, Orel SG, Fraker DL, Callans LS, Schnall M, Reynolds C, Czerniecki BJ: **Magnetic resonance imaging-guided biopsy of mammographically and clinically occult breast lesions.** *Ann Surg Oncol* 2002, **9**(5):457–461.

23. Lampe D, Hefler L, Alberich T, Sittek H, Perlet C, Prat X, Taourel P, Amaya B, Koelbl H, Heywang-Kobrunner SH: **The clinical value of preoperative wire localization of breast lesions with magnetic resonance imaging – a multicenter study.** *Breast Cancer Res Treat* 2002, **75**(2):175–179.

24. Philpotts LE: **MR intervention: indications, technique, correlation and histologic.** *Magn Reson Imaging Clin N Am* 2010, **18**(2):323–332.

25. Machado RH, Oliveira AC, Rocha AC, Landesmann MC, Martins FP, Lopes SA, Gutfilen B, da Fonseca LM: **Radioguided occult lesion localization (ROLL) and excision of breast lesions using technetium-99m-macroaggregate albumin and air injection control.** *J Exp Clin Cancer Res* 2007, **26**(3):323–327.

Diagnostic performance and inter-observer concordance in lesion detection with the automated breast volume scanner (ABVS)

Sebastian Wojcinski[1*], Samuel Gyapong[2], André Farrokh[2], Philipp Soergel[1], Peter Hillemanns[1] and Friedrich Degenhardt[2]

Abstract

Background: Automated whole breast ultrasound scanners of the latest generation have reached a level of comfortable application and high quality volume acquisition. Nevertheless, there is a lack of data concerning this technology. We investigated the diagnostic performance and inter-observer concordance of the Automated Breast Volume Scanner (ABVS) ACUSON S2000™ and questioned its implications in breast cancer diagnostics.

Methods: We collected 100 volume data sets and created a database containing 52 scans with no detectable lesions in conventional ultrasound (BI-RADS®-US 1), 30 scans with benign lesions (BI-RADS®-US 2) and 18 scans with breast cancer (BI-RADS®-US 5).
Two independent examiners evaluated the ABVS data on a separate workstation without any prior knowledge of the patients' histories.

Results: The inter-rater reliability reached fair agreement ($\kappa=0.36$; 95% confidence interval (CI): 0.19-0.53). With respect to the true category, the conditional inter-rater validity coefficient was $\kappa=0.18$ (95% CI: 0.00-0.26) for the benign cases and $\kappa=0.80$ (95% CI: 0.61-1.00) for the malignant cases.
Combining the assessments of examiner 1 and examiner 2, the diagnostic accuracy (AC), sensitivity (SE) and specificity (SP) for the experimental ABVS were AC = 79.0% (95% CI: 67.3-86.1), SE = 83.3% (95% CI: 57.7-95.6) and SP = 78.1% (% CI: 67.3-86.1), respectively.
However, after the ABVS examination, there were a high number of requests for second-look ultrasounds in up to 48.8% of the healthy women due to assumed suspicious findings in the volume data.
In an exploratory analysis, we estimated that an ABVS examination in addition to mammography alone could detect a relevant number of previously occult breast cancers (about 1 cancer in 300 screened and otherwise healthy women).

Conclusions: The ABVS is a reliable imaging method for the evaluation of the breast with high sensitivity and a fair inter-observer concordance. However, we have to overcome the problem of the high number of false-positive results. Therefore, further prospective studies in larger collectives are necessary to define standard procedures in image acquisition and interpretation. Nevertheless, we consider the ABVS as being suitable for integration into breast diagnostics as a beneficial and reliable imaging method.

Keywords: Breast cancer, Automated breast ultrasound, Automated breast volume scanner, ABVS, Inter-observer concordance, Screening

* Correspondence: s@wojcinski.de
[1]Department of OB/GYN, Hannover Medical School, OE 6410,
Carl-Neuberg-Straße 1, 30625 Hannover, Germany
Full list of author information is available at the end of the article

Background

Today, we can expect that more than one million women will be newly diagnosed with breast cancer each year [1]. The most recent data were reported in 2000, when about 400,000 women died from breast cancer, which represented 1.6 percent of all female deaths [2]. Nations with the highest cancer rates include the U.S.A, Italy, Australia, Germany, the Netherlands, Canada and France [3]. Secondary prevention, i.e. the early detection of usually curable stages of breast cancer, has moved into the very focus of all healthcare systems. While the incidence of breast cancer remains considerably high, we notice a relevant decline in cancer mortality in numerous countries. This effort can partly be explained by new and innovative therapies, but there is sound evidence that advances in early detection probably play the most decisive role [4]. Hence, the early detection of breast cancer has moved into the central focus of primary healthcare. This success could only be achieved because of improvements in imaging technologies and a higher degree of health awareness.

Breast cancer screening programs are based on radiologic examinations of the breast. Additional imaging modalities are only indicated if suspicious or unclear findings are present in the mammogram. Mammography has demonstrated excellent sensitivity, specificity and inter-observer concordance [5,6]. Nevertheless, the diagnostic accuracy of breast ultrasound and magnetic resonance imaging (MRI) is as good as mammography. However, these two modalities imply a number of major disadvantages. Breast MRI is an expensive and complex technology. Moreover, MRI has insufficient specificity and, consequently, produces a relevant number of false-positive findings. Ultrasound, on the other hand, is observer-dependent, time-consuming and the examiner has to be present at the time of image acquisition. Furthermore, only subjectively chosen screenshots from the ultrasound examination are printed and/or stored. Mammography has the advantage that the examination is rapid, standardizable and cost efficient. The generation of the mammogram can be performed by medical assistant personnel and the stored images allow second-readings and follow-ups. However, merely focusing on detection rates and diagnostic accuracy, breast ultrasound, breast MRI or even the combination of several imaging technologies may be superior to mammography alone.

So far, breast ultrasound is the most commonly accepted and reliable diagnostic method for women with clinically or radiologically suspicious breast lesions [7]. Furthermore, bilateral whole breast ultrasound has even demonstrated diagnostic advantages in screening asymptomatic women [8-12]. Nevertheless, after a comparison of the advantages and disadvantages of the various imaging techniques, mammography has become the most common, reliable and efficient screening method. This attitude in breast cancer screening may change someday, when technical advances allow further improvements of ultrasound and MRI. At this point, the concept of automated whole breast ultrasound emerges with the potential capability to overcome the inherent deficits of hand-held breast ultrasound. Automated breast scanners can be easily operated by medical assistants. The stored volume data allow comfortable and time-efficient evaluation at anytime by a medical professional. The performance of second-readings by additional examiners and follow-up evaluations are unproblematic. The concept of automated breast ultrasound dates back to the 1970s [13].

In the current report, we present data concerning an up-to-date technology in automated ultrasound, the Automated Breast Volume Scanner (ACUSON S2000™ ABVS; Siemens Medical Solutions, Inc., CA, USA). The ABVS reconstructs 3D data sets of the entire breast volume from automatically acquired B-mode images. These data can be stored and analyzed on a separate workstation.

We evaluated whether or not breast lesions, previously detected by means of conventional ultrasound, could also be detected and correctly classified by independent examiners who only used ABVS data. Furthermore, we analyzed the inter-observer concordance and performed a model calculation to scrutinize the potential implications of the ABVS in a screening setting.

Materials and methods

General design and patient database

Our study was carried out at the Franziskus Hospital Breast Cancer Center in Bielefeld, Germany, between March 2010 and July 2011. For the ultrasound examinations, we used the Siemens ACUSON S2000™ ultrasound system with the integrated ABVS (Siemens Medical Solutions, Inc., CA, USA). Patients are generally referred to our outpatient department on account of specific diagnostic queries, such as palpable breast lesions, breast pain, suspicious mammograms and intensified screening in low-risk and high-risk populations. Usually, patients receive a clinical examination, mammography and conventional breast ultrasound as the standard diagnostic methods, as well as subsequent examinations whenever necessary. Additionally, we offer an optional ABVS examination to all our patients within the routine practice of our breast cancer center. As a diagnostic standard, ultrasound pictures are categorized according to the Breast Imaging Reporting and Data System criteria of the American College of Radiology (ACR BI-RADS®-US) [14]. Study participants were recruited from this population. Patients with a final categorization of BI-RADS®-US 1, 2 or 5 in the conventional ultrasound examination were regarded as suitable for our study. BI-RADS®-US categories 0, 3 and 4 involve breast lesions of questionable dignity. As the focus of our study was on the detection of evidently benign or malignant lesions, we excluded patients with BI-RADS®-US 0, 3 and 4. Patients with a bra cup size greater than D, a history of breast surgery, inflammatory conditions of the breast, skin disorders or psychiatric disorders were also excluded. Patients who met the inclusion criteria and agreed to receive an additional ABVS examination entered our study. In this way, we performed 100 breast examinations with the ABVS and, consequently, we created a database containing 100 3D-scans with BI-RADS®-US 1, 2 or 5 findings in the volume.

All data were obtained using a standard of care clinical protocol and approved equipment. Therefore, the responsible ethics committee did not demand additional approval for this non-interventional case study. Although the requirements of individual informed consent were waived, we decided that all study participants signed an additional informed consent form before the ABVS examination.

Two independent examiners evaluated the cases from the anonymized ABVS database. We compared the performance of these two examiners (ABVS, experimental method) with each other and with the results from the conventional ultrasound (gold standard).

Technical background of the ABVS ultrasound system

For our study we used the ACUSON S2000™ ABVS (Siemens Medical Solutions, Inc., CA, USA), an ultrasound system that automatically acquires full-field volumes of the breast (Figure 1). The system is equipped with an ultra-wide linear transducer (Siemens 14L5BV, 14 MHz, 15.4 cm, and 768 piezoelectric elements). While automatically sweeping over the breast, this ultrasound probe covers a distance of 16.8 cm in approximately one minute, acquiring about 300 high-resolution slices for post-processing (resolution: axial = 0.09 mm, lateral = 0.16 mm, sagittal = 0.44 mm). These images are the source for the creation of the 3D data sets. A separate workstation provides comprehensive tools for image analysis and manipulation of the volume data (Figure 2). The secondary images are calculated from the acquisition volume in real-time. Details concerning the ABVS have been described elsewhere [15,16].

Conventional B-mode ultrasound examinations (gold standard)

Conventional B-mode ultrasound examinations were performed by the author SW, a DEGUM (Deutsche Gesellschaft für Ultraschall in der Medizin, German society for ultrasound in medicine) level II certified senior consultant in gynecology with 8 years' experience in breast ultrasound [17]. This examiner also knew the results of the other imaging modalities when available (mammography, magnetic resonance imaging) and, therefore, defined the reference standard for the interpretation of the volume data sets. The conventional ultrasound

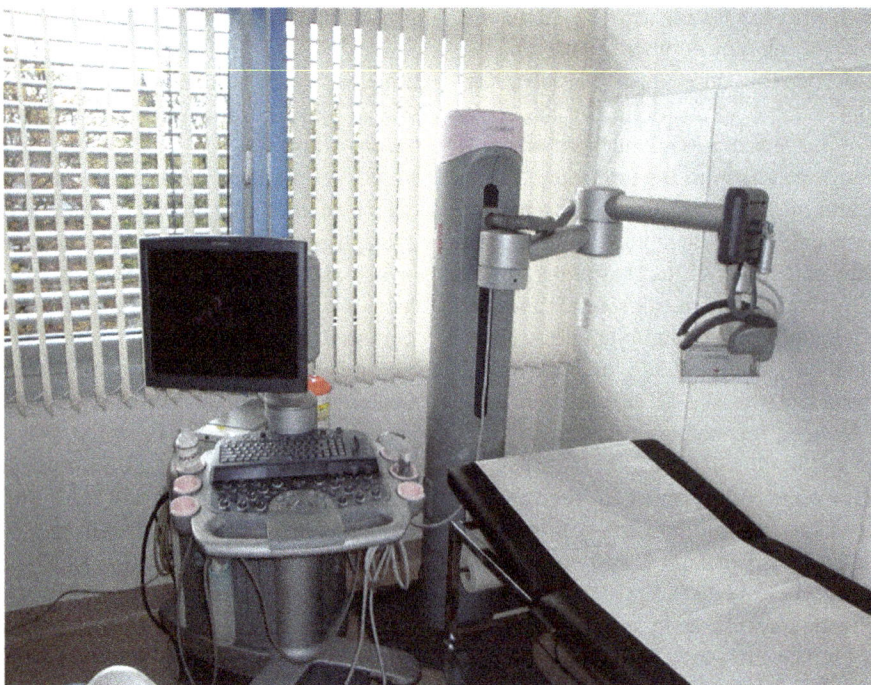

Figure 1 ACUSON S2000™ ABVS. On the left-hand side is the ACUSON S2000™ ultrasound machine, on the right-hand side is the 14L5BV volume transducer attached to a mechanical arm.

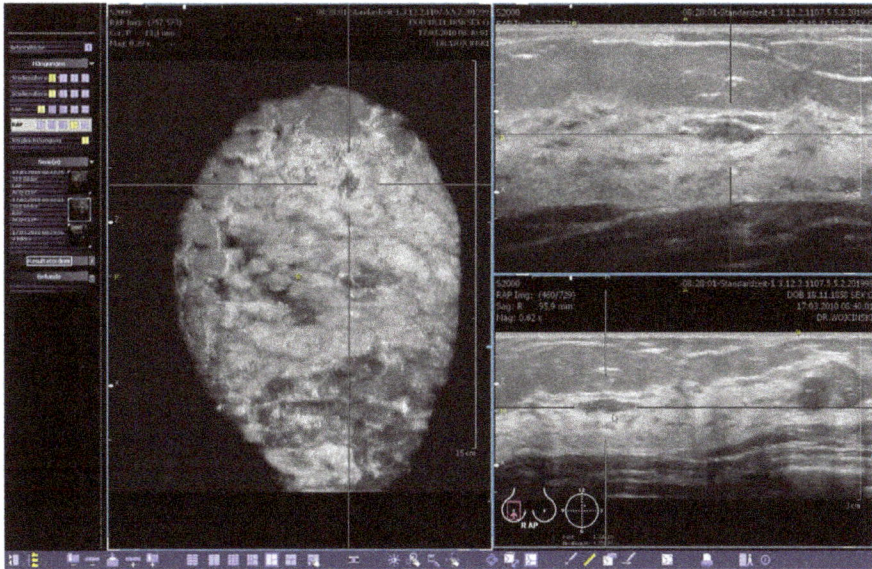

Figure 2 ABVS data on the workstation. This view provides the coronal (left), transverse (upper right) and sagittal (lower right) planes. The yellow spot marks the position of the nipple. The body marker indicates that this volume was acquired at the apex of the right breast. A plane of interest can be selected and marked by two orthogonal lines. Then, the corresponding cross-sections are calculated in real-time. Finally, the images can be optimized by adjusting magnification, brightness and contrast.

was carried out with the ACUSON S2000™ using a standard linear transducer (Siemens 18 L6 HD, 5.5-18 MHz, 5.6 cm).

After having completed these diagnostic steps, eligible patients were additionally examined using the ABVS.

According to the national regulatory authority statutes, breast US systems have to fulfill basic technical requirements and undergo regular quality control measures [18]. These standards applied to the equipment used in our study.

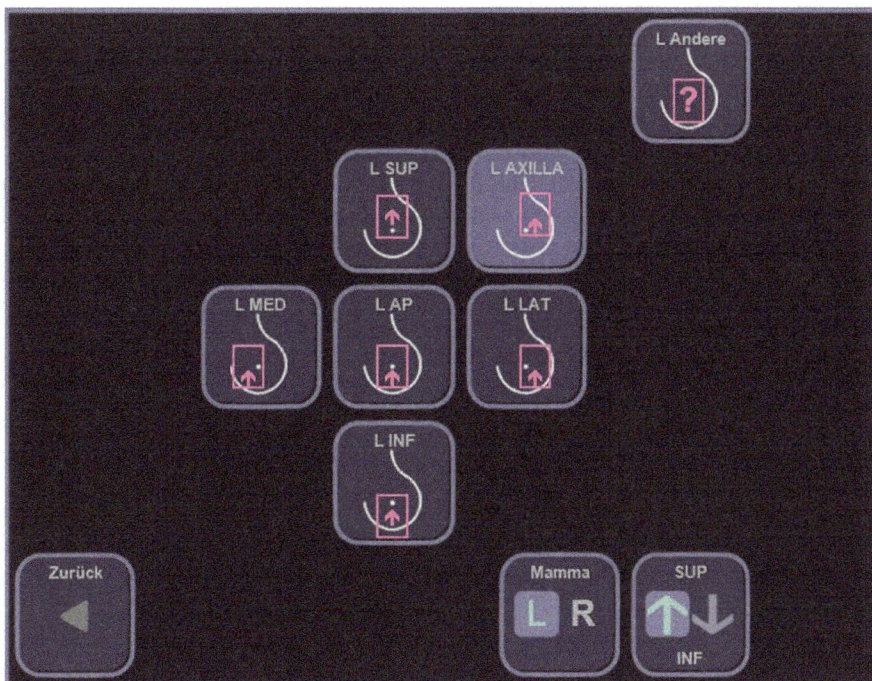

Figure 3 Predefined positions of the scanner for the left breast that are used to cover the entire volume.

ABVS examinations (experimental method)

The author SW performed the experimental ABVS examination in order to create 3D data sets. For the ABVS examination, the patients were in the supine position with the ipsilateral hand placed on the head. Depending on the size of the breast, the examiner chose the number of scans to be taken from each side. Usually, breasts with a bra cup size A or B can be fully displayed by performing two volume scans (medial and lateral, Figure 3). In larger breasts, it is frequently necessary to choose additional views (usually a separate view of the apex and the axillary process of the breast).

In order to guarantee sufficient contact with the skin, a replaceable membrane was attached to the transducer surface according to the manufacturer's instructions. Next, the transducer was positioned on the breast with slight pressure. An automated scan took between 55 and 65 seconds. Finally, the entire set of volume scans was sent to the workstation.

Interpretation of the experimental ABVS data by two independent examiners

The authors SG (examiner 1) and AF (examiner 2) performed the independent interpretation of the ABVS data sets. Both, SG and AF, are DEGUM level I certified senior residents in gynecology with 5 years' experience in breast ultrasound [17].

The independent examiners exclusively analyzed the volume data sets without any knowledge of the patients' histories, clinical findings or results of other imaging modalities. Furthermore, they had no information about the proportion of BI-RADS®-US 1, 2 and 5 cases in the database.

The following standard procedure was applied to the systematic analysis of the ABVS data: Initially, the entire volume was explored in the coronal plane moving slowly (i.e. in thin slices) from the skin to the chest wall. During this process, the examiner marked all mass lesions with the system's default tool. Next, the examiner evaluated all of the selected lesions by displaying them in the sagittal and axial planes. Finally, the examiner assigned the lesions a category according to the ACR BI-RADS®-US system. Overall interpretation times usually range from 4 to 10 min per case.

Despite the fact that the examiner knew that there were no BI-RADS®-US 0, 3 or 4 cases in the database, he was allowed to categorize lesions as BI-RADS®-US 0, 3 or 4 whenever he requested a second-look ultrasound in order to further assess uncertain lesions.

When a second-look ultrasound was requested for a lesion that eventually turned out to be benign, the result of the AVBS examination was defined as "non-concordant" (false-positive). On the other hand, when a second-look ultrasound was requested for a lesion that turned out to be malignant, the result was classified as "concordant" (true-positive) because the cancer could then be correctly detected in the subsequent conventional ultrasound (Table 1).

Statistical analysis

Microsoft® Office Excel® 2007 (Microsoft Corporation) was used for data collection.

Statistical analysis was performed by the author SW using MedCalc® 7.6 statistical software (MedCalc Software bvba, Belgium) and validated by the other authors.

In order to assess the diagnostic performance of the ABVS, we calculated sensitivity, specificity and accuracy for both examiners and used the Z-Test to compare the performance of examiner 1 with examiner 2. As our study population did not reflect the real prevalence of breast cancer, the positive and negative predictive values were estimated based on the Bayesian theorem using the reported prevalence of malignancies in screening collectives [19]. For the calculation of the 95% confidence levels, we used the Newcombe intervals with continuity correction [20].

The statistical analysis of the extent of agreement between the two raters was based on Cohen's Kappa test. For the interpretation of κ-values we used the magnitude guidelines published by Landis and Koch, who

Table 1 Methods

			Evaluation of ABVS data (experimental method)					
			BI-RADS® ABVS					
			0	1	2	3	4	5
		0	n.a.	n.a.	n.a.	n.a.	n.a.	n.a.
		1	FP	TN	TN	FP	FP	FP
Evaluation in conventional ultrasound (gold standard)	BI-RADS®-US	2	FP	TN	TN	FP	FP	FP
		3	n.a.	n.a.	n.a.	n.a.	n.a.	n.a.
		4	n.a.	n.a.	n.a.	n.a.	n.a.	n.a.
		5	TP	FN	FN	TP	TP	TP

Concerning the performance of the ABVS examination the above scheme was applied to define cases as true-positive (TP), true-negative (TN), false-positive (FP) or false-negative (FN).

characterized the values of κ<0 as indicating no agreement, κ 0–0.20 slight, κ 0.21-0.40 fair, κ 0.41-0.60 moderate, κ 0.61-0.80 substantial, and κ 0.81-1 as almost perfect agreement [21].

Furthermore, we assessed the correlation between the expected and the observed rate of second-look ultrasounds using the Chi-square test.

Statistical significance was assumed as $p < 0.05$ for all tests.

Results

In our study population, the age ranged from 19 to 86 years (median 52 years). According to the BI-RADS®-US categorization, 52% (n = 52) of our cases were assigned as BI-RADS®-US 1, 30% (n = 30) had BI-RADS®-US 2 lesions and 18% (n = 18) of the cases had BI-RADS®-US 5 lesions. All BI-RADS®-US 5 lesions were confirmed with histological specimens. The mean tumor size for malignant and benign lesions was 22.0 mm (range 13 to 55) and 16.7 mm (range 8 to 36), respectively.

Inter-rater reliability

The concordance between examiner 1 and examiner 2 concerning the correct clinical decision of whether the patient should undergo a control ultrasound due to a suspicious finding or whether the patient should be defined as healthy as there is no suspicious lesion is shown in (Table 2). The inter-rater reliability reached

Table 2 Concordance between examiner 1 and examiner 2 concerning the correct clinical decision of whether the patient should undergo a control ultrasound due to a suspicious finding in ABVS (due to BI-RADS® 0,3,4 or 5) or whether the patient should be defined as healthy as there is no suspicious lesion in ABVS (i.e. BI-RADS® 1 or 2)

		Examiner 1 (SG)		
		BI-RADS® ABVS 1 or 2 (negative)	BI-RADS® ABVS 0, 3, 4 or 5 (positive)	Total
Examiner 2 (AF)	BI-RADS® ABVS 1 or 2 (negative)	34[a]	8	42
	BI-RADS® ABVS 0, 3, 4 or 5 (positive)	25	33[a]	58
	Total	59	41	100

Distribution of cases by rater and by category. The inter-rater reliability coefficient calculates to κ = 0.36 (0.19-0.53).
[a]concordance between examiner 1 and examiner 2.

fair agreement and the Cohen's Kappa value was κ=0.36 (95% CI: 0.19-0.53).

A more detailed breakdown of the concordance between examiner 1 and examiner 2 concerning the distinct BI-RADS® category in the ABVS examination is given in (Table 3). In this analysis, the inter-rater reliability also reached fair agreement and the Cohen's Kappa value was κ = 0.27 (0.14-0.40).

Inter-rater validity

With respect to the true category (benign cases and malignant cases), the inter-rater validity coefficient calculated to κ=0.31 (95% CI: 0.21-0.41). Focusing on the benign cases (n = 82), the conditional inter-rater validity coefficient was κ=0.18 (95% CI: 0.00-0.26), indicating slight agreement. Concerning the malignant cases, we found a Cohen's Kappa value of κ=0.80 (95% CI: 0.61-1.00), indicating substantial to almost perfect agreement (Table 4).

Diagnostic performance of the ABVS

The sensitivity for examiner 1 and examiner 2 in detecting malignant lesions with the ABVS was 83.3% (95% CI: 57.7-95.6) and 100% (95% CI: 78.1-100.0), respectively. The diagnostic accuracy of the method was 71.0% (95% CI: 60.9-79.4) and 60.0% (95% CI: 49.7-69.5), respectively. The differences between examiner 1 and examiner 2 were statistically not significant. Nevertheless, specificity revealed to be quite low at 68.3% (95% CI: 57.0-77.9) and 51.2% (40.0-62.3), respectively, as there was a relevant number of requests for second-look ultrasounds or further examinations in the group of healthy patients after the evaluation of the ABVS data. As previously described in the methods, these cases had to be classified as false-positives if there was no cancer (Table 1). Moreover, specificity was significantly different between examiner 1 and examiner 2 (p = 0.001). The detailed results are shown in (Table 5).

In order to investigate the effect of a second reading of ABVS data, we performed a tentative analysis and combined the evaluations of examiner 1 and examiner 2. With respect to the low specificity, the following rules for the combination of assessments were applied: If both examiners agreed that a scan was suspicious, the evaluation was considered "positive". If both examiners agreed that a scan was unsuspicious or disagreed (and only one examiner regarded the scan as unsuspicious), the evaluation was considered "negative". In this scenario, the accuracy increased to 79.0% (95% CI: 69.5-86.3), the specificity increased to 78.1% (95% CI: 67.3-86.1) and the sensitivity remained acceptably high at 83.3% (95% CI: 57.7-95.6) (Table 6).

Rate of second-look ultrasounds

We expected 18 requests for second-look ultrasounds after the ABVS examination as there were 18 BI-RADS®-

Table 3 Concordance between examiner 1 and examiner 2 concerning the distinct BI-RADS® category in the ABVS examination

		BI-RADS® ABVS 1 (No finding)	BI-RADS® ABVS 2 (Benign finding)	BI-RADS® ABVS 0, 3 or 4 (Unclear finding)	BI-RADS® ABVS 5 (Malignant finding)	Total
	BI-RADS® ABVS 1 (No Finding)	20[a]	2	4	2	28
	BI-RADS® ABVS 2 (Benign finding)	4	8[a]	2	0	14
Examiner 2 (AF)	BI-RADS® ABVS 0, 3 or 4 (Unclear finding)	14	7	13[a]	9	43
	BI-RADS® ABVS 5 (Malignant finding)	4	0	5	6[a]	15
	Total	42	17	24	17	100

Distribution of cases by rater and by detailed BI-RADS® ABVS category. Concerning this detailed evaluation, the inter-rater reliability coefficient calculates to κ = 0.27 (0.14-0.40).
[a]concordance between examiner 1 and examiner 2.

US 5 lesions in our database of 100 cases. We did not expect requests for the other 82 cases (BI-RADS®-US 1 or 2 lesions). However, the observed rate of second-look ultrasounds was significantly high, totaling 41 for examiner 1 and 58 for examiner 2, respectively (p < 0.001).

Therefore, the rate of second-look ultrasounds in healthy women (i.e. BI-RADS®-US 1 and 2) was 31.7% for examiner 1 and 48.8% for examiner 2.

Regarding the BI-RADS®-US 1 and 2 cases separately, there was a request for a second-look ultrasound in 33.3% and 53.3% (examiner 1 and examiner 2) of the women with BI-RADS®-US 2 lesions and in 30.8% and 46.2% of the women with no breast lesions at all (i.e. BI-RADS®-US 1).

Model calculation and exploratory analysis

Based on our findings, we performed a model calculation to estimate how additional ABVS examinations could affect the detection rate of cancer in screening collectives.

As described in the literature, the prevalence of occult cancer that can be detected by additional ultrasound in women who already underwent mammography and clinical examination can be estimated to be between 0.3% and 0.4% [8-12]. Therefore, conventional ultrasound can detect one cancer in about 250 otherwise healthy women.

Using these numbers, the positive predictive value in a screening collective would calculate to 1.49% and the negative predictive value to 99.91%, respectively. Therefore, the new false-negative rate in a diagnostic setting using the ABVS would be about 0.09% instead of 0.4% (Table 7).

If 10,000 women were additionally screened with the ABVS, we could expect 2,219 positive scans resulting in the same number of second-look-ultrasounds, finally leading to 33 detected cancers. Therefore, one cancer would

Table 4 Distribution of cases by rater, reported and true categories

	Examiner 1 ABVS negative		Examiner 1 ABVS positive		Total
	Examiner 2 ABVS negative	Examiner 2 ABVS positive	Examiner 2 ABVS negative	Examiner 2 ABVS positive	
Benign cases (conventional ultrasound negative)	34[a]	22	8	18[a]	82
Malignant cases (conventional ultrasound positive)	0[a]	3	0	15[a]	18
Total	34	25	8	33	100

The inter-rater validity coefficient calculates to κ = 0.31 (95% CI: 0.21-0.41). The conditional inter-rater validity coefficient is κ=0.18 (95% CI: 0.00-0.26) for the benign cases and κ=0.80 (95% CI: 0.61-1.00) for the malignant cases.
[a]concordance between examiner 1 and examiner 2.

Table 5 Performance of examiner 1 and examiner 2 using the ABVS data to classify the breast either healthy (BI-RADS® 1or 2) or suspicious of malignancy (BI-RADS® 0, 3, 4, or 5)

	Examiner 1 (SG)	Examiner 2 (AF)	p
Sensitivity	83.3%	100%	n.s. (0.059)
	(57.7-95.6)	(78.1-100)	
Specificity	68.3%	51.2%	0.001
	(57.0-77.9)	(40.0-62.3)	
Accuracy	71.0%	60.0%	n.s. (0.102)
	(60.9-79.4)	(49.7-69.5)	

be detected in 67 second-look ultrasounds. 7,781 scans would be negative, and only seven cancers would be missed in this group (Figure 4).

Discussion
Primum non nocere
Innovative features for existing medical imaging modalities and even entirely new imaging technologies are constantly being developed [22,23]. Boosted by the industry, these technical novelties are rapidly made available for inpatient and outpatient care. Nevertheless, the new technologies often lack standardized imaging methodology evaluation and validation studies [24]. Therefore, the distinct indications for these methods, their definite diagnostic spectrum and, even more, their potential risk for the patient remain unclear to a certain degree. A universal principle for medical practice is "primum non nocere!" translated as "first, do no harm!" [25]. We bear this in mind when we address medical malpractice related to therapeutic interventions. However, malpractice can also occur in diagnostic procedures. The wrong interpretation of diagnostic findings, deficits in image acquisition, and, in particular, the wrong indication for a potentially beneficial examination may harm the patient in terms of unnecessary biopsies or overlooked breast cancer. Finally, the attending physician is charged with applying any new method with discernment. A prerequisite for this responsible utilization of new technologies is a profound knowledge of the powers and limitations of the same. Therefore, we encourage the reader to regard any

new imaging technology critically until evident data has demonstrated a benefit for the patient beyond all doubt. Concerning the ABVS, such definite data is missing in the literature, but we regard our own results as a first approach to approve the ABVS for routine diagnostics.

Performance of the ABVS in our study and in the literature
The focus of our current study was on the inter-rater agreement concerning the evaluation of ABVS data. We were able to demonstrate fair agreement for both the classification into the categories "positive/negative" ($\kappa=0.36$) and the detailed classification according to the BI-RADS® system ($\kappa=0.27$). Nevertheless, this performance could be improved. The conditional inter-rater validity coefficients for benign and malignant cases revealed that the concordance is almost perfect for the malignant cases ($\kappa=0.80$), but only slight for the benign cases ($\kappa=0.18$). These results correlate with the experience, that both examiners reached high sensitivity (83.3% and nominally 100%, respectively), but lower specificity (68.3% and 51.2%). In other words, the detection of malignant lesions can be precisely performed with the ABVS. Cancers are rarely missed with this technology. The examiners agree in those cases in which a suspicious lesion is present in the volume data. On the other hand, the examiners tend to suspect doubtful lesions even in the normal breast tissue of healthy women. Consequently, the ABVS has a low specificity and a high false-positive detection rate. This condition impairs the conditional inter-rater validity for the benign cases and leads to a high number of unnecessary second-look ultrasounds. In fact, when the ABVS system is used, we lose the ability to immediately further explore a questionable lesion by modifying factors such as compression, the orientation of the probe and the machine's setting whilst acquiring the image in real-time. Ultrasound techniques such Doppler imaging or sonoelastography cannot be used either. Because the examiners cannot rely on standardized interpretation criteria or rules how to handle technical artifacts in the volume data, they seem to prefer false positive evaluation rather than missing a malignant lesion. Nevertheless, with accumulating data, growing experience and better diagnostic criteria this problem may be solved.

Table 6 Estimation of the performance of the ABVS in a scenario, where second-reading of the data is performed

	At least one examiners judges ABVS as normal (negative)	Both examiners concordantly suspicious ABVS (positive)	Total
Benign cases (conventional ultrasound negative)	64[a]	18[b]	82
Malignant cases (conventional ultrasound positive)	3[b]	15[a]	18
Total	67	33	100

Sensitivity, specificity and accuracy calculate to 83.3%, 78.0% and 79.0%, respectively. For the evaluation of the second-reading the following rules were applied: If both examiners agreed that a scan was suspicious, the evaluation was considered "positive". If both examiners agreed that a scan was unsuspicious or disagreed and only one examiner regarded the scan as unsuspicious, the evaluation was considered "negative".
[a]"true" evaluation.
[b]"false" evaluation.

Table 7 Model calculation

	Interpretation of the ABVS data by 2 raters
Performance of the ABVS in our study collective (n = 100)	
Prevalence of disease	18.00%
SE	83.33%
SP	78.05%
Rate of second look ultrasounds in healthy women (=100%-SP)	21.95%
Estimated performance of the ABVS in a screening collective of asymptomatic women[1]	
Prevalence of disease[2]	0.40%
PPV[3]	1.49%
NPV[3]	99.91%
FNR[3,4]	0.09%

Based on our data concerning the performance with two examiners (second-reading of the ABVS data sets), the effect in a screening setting was estimated.
(SE = sensitivity; SP = specificity; PPV = positive predictive value; NPV = negative predictive value; FNR = false negative rate).
[1]Asymptomatic women are defined as women, who have a normal mammogram and exhibit no symptoms
[2]As described in the literature, the prevalence of occult carcinomas that can be detected by conventional breast ultrasound can be estimated to be about 0.4%. This value resembles the theoretical false negative rate (FNR) of clinical examination and mammography alone.
[3]The new performance values of the ABVS are based upon the estimated prevalence of 0.4% in a screening collective.
[4]The new false negative rate is based upon a combination of clinical examination, mammography and ABVS in a screening collective.

The consequence of a false positive result is the performance of an unnecessary second-look ultrasound, which is expensive, time-consuming and frustrating for both the patient and the medical professional. However, this second-look ultrasound implies no direct harm for the patient. A false-negative result may have a more serious implication as the diagnosis of malignancy is delayed, with a potentially worse clinical outcome for the patient.

In conclusion, as the false-negative rate is low we assume high patient safety and encourage the clinical use of the ABVS for breast diagnostics.

There is only limited data in the literature describing the inter-observer concordance in lesion detection with the ABVS:

In 2011, Shin et al. reported on 55 women with 145 breast masses who were examined with handheld ultrasound and the ABVS [26]. Five radiologists reviewed the volume data and detected between 74% and 88% of the lesions. Substantial agreement was found for BI-RADS® final assessment category (κ = 0.63).

Recently, Golatta et al. published data on 84 single breast examinations in 42 women [27]. Six breast diagnostic specialists interpreted the 3D-images. Based on

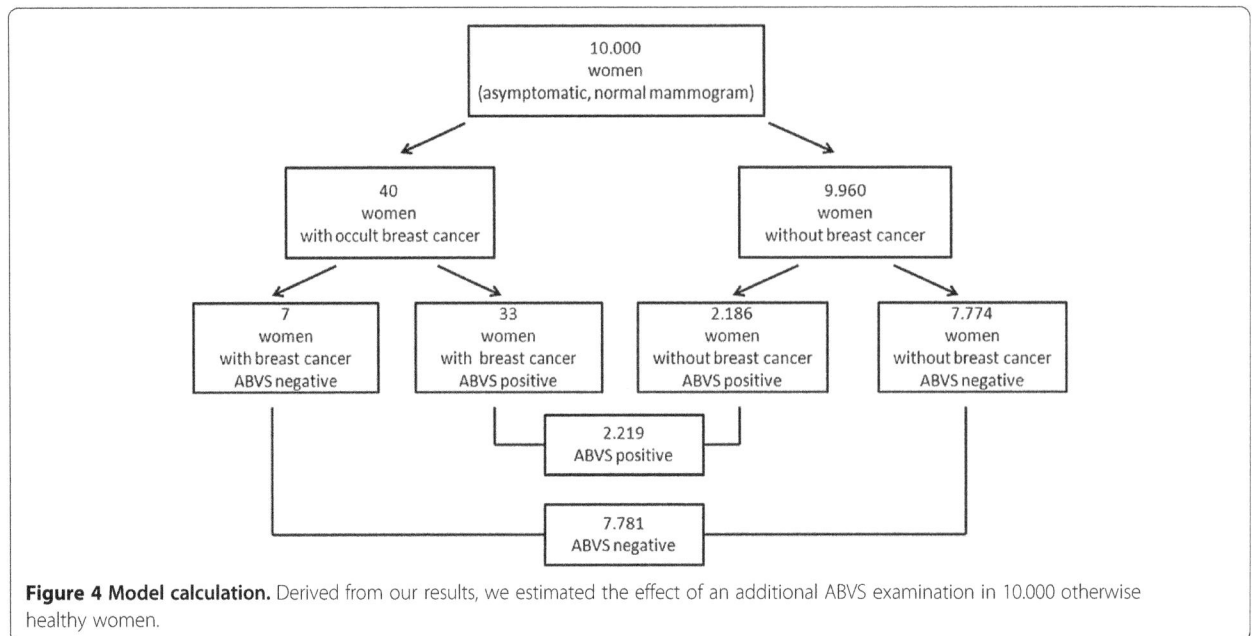

Figure 4 Model calculation. Derived from our results, we estimated the effect of an additional ABVS examination in 10.000 otherwise healthy women.

the BI-RADS® classification the multiple kappa coefficient was κ = 0.35.

In our analysis, we found fair agreement between the two examiners, which correlates with the latter results (κ = 0.27). However, more data is needed to evaluate the performance of the ABVS in breast imaging convincingly.

Moreover, there are several reports comparing the ABVS with hand-held ultrasound [15,28-31]:

The first detailed description of the technical background and performance of the ABVS was published by our study group in 2011 [15]. In 2011, 50 ABVS datasets were evaluated by an independent examiner and accuracy, sensitivity and specificity were calculated as 66.0% (95% CI: 52.9-79.1), 100% (95% CI: 73.2-100) and 52.8% (95% CI: 35.7-69.2), respectively. Concerning these variables, our current study yielded comparable results (Table 5). Nevertheless, as both studies were conducted in the same institution, a comparison with the results from other study groups will be of greater interest.

In 2012, Lin et al. published data on 81 patients and compared ABVS to handheld ultrasound. The authors described a perfect sensitivity for both methods (ABVS: 100%, hand-held ultrasound: 100%), high specificity (95.0% and 85.0%, respectively) and, consequently, a high diagnostic accuracy (97.1% and 91.4%, respectively) [28]. This performance appears extraordinarily high. We suggest that further standardized studies in larger collectives should investigate if these expectations can be fulfilled.

In the same year, Wang HY et al. studied 239 lesions in 213 women who were scheduled to undergo biopsy. In this study, ABVS was similar to hand-held ultrasound in terms of sensitivity (ABVS: 95.3%, hand-held ultrasound: 90.6%), specificity (80.5% and 82.5%, respectively), and accuracy (85.8% and 85.3%, respectively) [29].

Recently, Wang ZL et al. published data on 153 patients with 165 breast lesions. The patients underwent mammography, ABVS and hand-held ultrasound. The authors reported no significant differences between ABVS and conventional ultrasound concerning sensitivity (ABVS: 96.1%, hand-held ultrasound: 93.2%), specificity (91.9% and 88.7%, respectively), and accuracy (94.5% and 91.5%, respectively) [30,31].

Compared to our data, there is a discrepancy mainly concerning the specificity, which was lower in our investigation (Table 8). Actually, we had a relevant number of healthy women without breast lesions (i.e. BI-RADS®-US 1) in our collective. This condition automatically increases the false-positive rate and actually reduces specificity.

Hence, the main difference of our study design in comparison to the above-mentioned studies is that we did not focus on the evaluation of known lesions alone, but also on the detection. Therefore, our examiners did not know whether there was a lesion in the particular volume or not. In the studies from the literature, the

Table 8 Data in the literature concerning sensitivity (SE) and specificity (SP) of the ABVS

Author	N	SE	SP
Wojcinski et al. 2011 [15]	50[a]	100%	52.8%
Lin et al. 2012 [28]	81[b]	100%	95.0%
Wang HY et al. 2012 [29]	239[c]	95.3%	80.5%
Wang ZL et al. 2012 [30]	165[c]	96.1%	91.9%
Current study, Examiner 1	100[a]	83.3%	68.3%
Current study, Examiner 2	100[a]	100%	51.2%

[a]volume data sets (including scans without lesions, BI-RADS®-US 1).
[b]patients.
[c]lesions.

examiners were well aware, that there is definitely a lesion in the volume that requires biopsy (i.e. BI-RADS® 3 and above). This knowledge certainly has an influence on the evaluation of the lesion and the overall performance of the ABVS.

Our interpretation: the almost perfect performance of the ABVS as described in the literature is only valid for collectives of women with already pre-diagnosed breast lesions. In realistic collectives that also involve women without breast lesions (i.e. BI-RADS®-US 1) or with clearly benign breast lesions (i.e. BI-RADS®-US 2), our data may be more convincing.

Concerning the inter-observer agreement, Zhang et al. published data on 234 breast lesions from 208 patients who were examined with the ABVS [32]. Zhang et al. investigated the inter-observer agreement concerning the description of known breast masses according to the BI-RADS®-US lexicon. They found substantial agreement for lesion shape, orientation, margin, echo pattern, posterior acoustic features, calcification and final assessment, and fair agreement for retraction phenomenon and lesion boundary, respectively. Our study design did not focus the detailed description of lesions, but we showed fair agreement for the detection of breast masses. This aspect was not analyzed by Zhang et al.

Furthermore, there are reports in the literature about the ABVS that concentrate on the optimal scanning technique [16], the accuracy of measuring the cancer extent [33] and the detection of lesions located behind the nipple [34].

Limitations of our study and limitations of the ABVS

All previously mentioned studies have the essential limitation of unicentric design and small patient collectives. This limitation also applies to our current study. Future study concepts should include multicenter design and larger, well-defined patient populations as described elsewhere [15]. Furthermore, we compared only two examiners. Although the results demonstrated fair agreement, the concordance should be confirmed with more observers. Another limitation of our study is the selection of the study population and the resulting concentration on BI-RADS®-US 1, 2 and 5 lesions which causes a certain bias. Therefore, the proportion of cases to controls is not representative of the whole population and BI-RADS®-US 0, 3 and 4 lesions are missing in the study population. We attempted to overcome this limitation by conducting a model calculation. Although this approach is statistically correct, it must be considered that, due to the small sample size and the vague estimation of the prevalence, the results must be carefully interpreted.

Moreover, the technology of the ABVS has some limitations per se. As previously described in the literature, automated breast ultrasound is limited in women with macromastia and pronounced ptosis [15,16]. In addition, the ABVS is not capable of scanning the axillary region. Today, sentinel node biopsy is the standard therapy for women that were preoperatively staged with a negative nodal status, which requires ultrasound of the axilla [35]. Furthermore, lymph node alterations may be the first sign in mammographically and/or sonographically occult breast cancer or other malignant diseases [36,37]. Therefore, additional conventional ultrasound of the axilla would be necessary after a suspicious ABVS scan.

Furthermore, we presume that even with optimal scanning technique the peripheral areas of the breast parenchyma are not fully covered by the ABVS. Additionally, shadowing artifacts occur in the retroareolar region and to a certain extent in the remaining breast volume. Therefore, a certain proportion of breast parenchyma may be lost in the volume data. This may reduce the diagnostic potential in comparison to hand-held ultrasound.

Future implications of the ABVS

Finally, we have to discuss the question of which role the ABVS could play in future breast cancer diagnosis and breast cancer screening. Conventional hand-held breast ultrasound has a commonly accepted role as a complementary method to mammography, by adding to the diagnostic accuracy. Despite the well-known advantages, conventional breast ultrasound is a time-consuming, examiner-dependent and therefore costly procedure. Furthermore, breast cancer screening with additional breast ultrasound in low-risk women has not been established, as data concerning an effect on the overall survival is missing. Nevertheless, it is evident that breast ultrasound is capable of detecting previously occult cancers in women who had already undergone mammography and clinical examination [8,9,11,12]. However, screening larger collectives with conventional ultrasound is plainly not feasible. With the ABVS, we have a tool that could principally overcome these problems, and the ABVS may make ultrasound available to a larger number of women. Image acquisition with the ABVS can be efficiently performed by a medical assistant. Moreover, the ABVS allows a delayed interpretation of the images at any time, as well as second-readings. On the other hand, it has to be taken into account that we still experience a high number of time-consuming second-look ultrasounds due to the low specificity. This problem may be solved through second-readings by an independent examiner. Our proposed rules are relatively unusual, as, in order to improve the specificity, disagreement between the examiners would be classified as "negative" and only agreement that a scan is suspicious would be classified as "positive". Therefore, further studies should include these concepts. However, we are convinced that the ABVS is a feasible method that can be easily integrated into the workflow of any inpatient or outpatient department.

We can imagine the ABVS being applied in breast cancer screening programs in the future and that additional examinations are offered to women at risk. However, we still have no data focusing on certain subgroups of patients (e.g. high-risk versus low-risk, ACR 1–2 versus ACR 3–4, etc.).

A prospective randomized controlled trial could answer the open questions. This trial should include patients with normal mammograms, some of whom will receive additional ABVS. The primary outcome variables would be the detection rate of breast cancer, the tumor stage and the overall survival of the two groups. Presumably, results could only be obtained if the collectives were sufficiently large, which makes it likewise unrealistic that a corresponding trial will actually be conducted.

Conclusions

In conclusion, the ABVS has demonstrated high sensitivity and a fair inter-observer concordance in the evaluation of breast lesions. However, we have to overcome the problem of the high number of false-positive results in healthy women. Therefore, further prospective validation studies in larger collectives are necessary to define standard procedures in image acquisition and volume interpretation. Nevertheless, the ABVS is a reliable, technically mature and potentially beneficial imaging method. Therefore, we propose that the ABVS can be used in routine diagnostic procedures as an adjunct to mammography and conventional ultrasound, as previously described.

Competing interests
The authors declare that they have no competing interest.

Authors' contributions
SW and SG contributed to the conception and design of the study and SW performed the ultrasound examinations and data collection. SG and AF performed the independent evaluation of the ABVS data sets. SW contributed to the statistical analysis and the interpretation of the data. SW and PS contributed to the writing of the manuscript. FD and PH conducted final reviews of the manuscript and FD provided methodological advice. All authors read and approve the final manuscript.

Acknowledgements

Publication costs were covered by a grant of the DFG (German Research Foundation) within the project "Open Access Publications" at MHH (Hannover Medical School, Germany).

Author details

[1]Department of OB/GYN, Hannover Medical School, OE 6410, Carl-Neuberg-Straße 1, 30625 Hannover, Germany. [2]Department of OB/GYN, Franziskus Hospital, Bielefeld, Germany.

References

1. Parkin DM, Bray F, Ferlay J, Pisani P: **Global cancer statistics, 2002.** *CA Cancer J Clin* 2005, **55**(2):74–108.
2. IARC: *World cancer report 2008.* Lyon: International Agency for Research on Cancer, WHO Press; 2008.
3. IARC: *Globocan database.* Lyon: International Agency for Research on Cancer; 2008.
4. Parkin DM, Fernandez LM: **Use of statistics to assess the global burden of breast cancer.** *Breast J* 2006, **12**(1):S70–80.
5. Duijm LE, Louwman MW, Groenewoud JH, van de Poll-Franse LV, Fracheboud J, Coebergh JW: **Inter-observer variability in mammography screening and effect of type and number of readers on screening outcome.** *Br J Cancer* 2009, **100**(6):901–907.
6. Independent UK Panel on Breast Cancer Screening: **The benefits and harms of breast cancer screening: an independent review.** *Lancet* 2012, **380**(9855):1778–1786.
7. Zonderland HM, Coerkamp EG, Hermans J, van de Vijver MJ, van Voorthuisen AE: **Diagnosis of breast cancer: contribution of US as an adjunct to mammography.** *Radiology* 1999, **213**(2):413–422.
8. Buchberger W, Niehoff A, Obrist P, DeKoekkoek-Doll P, Dunser M: **Clinically and mammographically occult breast lesions: detection and classification with high-resolution sonography.** *Semin Ultrasound CT MR* 2000, **21**(4):325–336.
9. Corsetti V, Ferrari A, Ghirardi M, Bergonzini R, Bellarosa S, Angelini O, Bani C, Ciatto S: **Role of ultrasonography in detecting mammographically occult breast carcinoma in women with dense breasts.** *Radiol Med* 2006, **111**(3):440–448.
10. Gordon PB, Goldenberg SL: **Malignant breast masses detected only by ultrasound: a retrospective review.** *Cancer* 1995, **76**(4):626–630.
11. Kolb TM, Lichy J, Newhouse JH: **Occult cancer in women with dense breasts: detection with screening US–diagnostic yield and tumor characteristics.** *Radiology* 1998, **207**(1):191–199.
12. Nothacker M, Duda V, Hahn M, Warm M, Degenhardt F, Madjar H, Weinbrenner S, Albert US: **Early detection of breast cancer: benefits and risks of supplemental breast ultrasound in asymptomatic women with mammographically dense breast tissue: a systematic review.** *BMC Cancer* 2009, **9**:335.
13. Maturo VG, Zusmer NR, Gilson AJ, Smoak WM, Janowitz WR, Bear BE, Goddard J, Dick DE: **Ultrasound of the whole breast utilizing a dedicated automated breast scanner.** *Radiology* 1980, **137**(2):457–463.
14. Mendelson EB, Baum JK, Berg WA, Merritt CR, Rubin E: **BI-RADS: ultrasound.** In *Breast imaging reporting and data system: ACR BI-RADS - breast imaging atlas.* Edited by D'Orsi CJ, Mendelson EB, Ikeda DM. Reston, VA: American College of Radiology; 2002.
15. Wojcinski S, Farrokh A, Hille U, Wiskirchen J, Gyapong S, Soliman AA, Degenhardt F, Hillemanns P: **The automated breast volume scanner (ABVS): initial experiences in lesion detection compared with conventional handheld B-mode ultrasound: a pilot study of 50 cases.** *International journal of women's health* 2011, **3**:337–346.
16. Tozaki M, Isobe S, Yamaguchi M, Ogawa Y, Kohara M, Joo C, Fukuma E: **Optimal scanning technique to cover the whole breast using an automated breast volume scanner.** *Jpn J Radiol* 2010, **28**(4):325–328.
17. DEGUM (deutsche gesellschaft für ultraschall in der medizin, german association for ultrasound in medicine) - mehrstufenkonzept mammasonographie. http://www.degum.de/Mehrstufenkonzept_Mammasonogra.634.0.html.
18. KBV (kassenaerztliche bundesvereinigung, German federal association of fund doctors) -ultraschallvereinbarung, ultrasound regulations. http://www.kbv.de/2488.html.
19. Zhou XH, Obuchowski NA, McClish DK: *Statistical methods in diagnostic medicine: 2nd ed.* New York: Wiley; 2011.
20. Newcombe RG: **Interval estimation for the difference between independent proportions: comparison of eleven methods.** *Stat Med* 1998, **17**(8):873–890.
21. Landis JR, Koch GG: **The measurement of observer agreement for categorical data.** *Biometrics* 1977, **33**(1):159–174.
22. Hahn M, Roessner L, Krainick-Strobel U, Gruber IV, Kramer B, Gall C, Siegmann KC, Wallwiener D, Kagan KO: **Sonographic criteria for the differentiation of benign and malignant breast lesions using real-time spatial compound imaging in combination with XRES adaptive image processing.** *Ultraschall Med* 2012, **33**(3):270–274.
23. Farrokh A, Wojcinski S, Degenhardt F: **Diagnostic value of strain ratio measurement in the differentiation of malignant and benign breast lesions.** *Ultraschall Med* 2011, **32**(4):400–405.
24. Wojcinski S, Farrokh A, Peisker U, Thomas A, Degenhardt F, Hahn M: **Neue diagnostische verfahren - sono-elastografie der mamma.** *Senologie - Zeitschrift für Mammadiagnostik und -therapie* 2011, **7**:15–18.
25. Smith CM: **Origin and uses of primum non nocere–above all, do no harm!** *J Clin Pharmacol* 2005, **45**(4):371–377.
26. Shin HJ, Kim HH, Cha JH, Park JH, Lee KE, Kim JH: **Automated ultrasound of the breast for diagnosis: interobserver agreement on lesion detection and characterization.** *AJR Am J Roentgenol* 2011, **197**(3):747–754.
27. Golatta M, Franz D, Harcos A, Junkermann H, Rauch G, Scharf A, Schuetz F, Sohn C, Heil J: **Interobserver reliability of automated breast volume scanner (ABVS) interpretation and agreement of ABVS findings with hand held breast ultrasound (HHUS), mammography and pathology results.** *Eur J Radiol* 2013, **82**(8):332–336.
28. Lin X, Wang J, Han F, Fu J, Li A: **Analysis of eighty-one cases with breast lesions using automated breast volume scanner and comparison with handheld ultrasound.** *Eur J Radiol* 2012, **81**(5):873–878.
29. Wang HY, Jiang YX, Zhu QL, Zhang J, Dai Q, Liu H, Lai XJ, Sun Q: **Differentiation of benign and malignant breast lesions: a comparison between automatically generated breast volume scans and handheld ultrasound examinations.** *Eur J Radiol* 2012, **81**(11):3190–3200.
30. Wang ZL, Xu JH, Li JL, Huang Y, Tang J: **Erratum to: comparison of automated breast volume scanning to hand-held ultrasound and mammography.** *Radiol Med* 2012, **117**(8):1443.
31. Wang ZL, Xw JH, Li JL, Huang Y, Tang J: **Comparison of automated breast volume scanning to hand-held ultrasound and mammography.** *Radiol Med* 2012, **117**(8):1287–1293.
32. Zhang J, Lai XJ, Zhu QL, Wang HY, Jiang YX, Liu H, Dai Q, You SS, Xiao MS, Sun Q: **Interobserver agreement for sonograms of breast lesions obtained by an automated breast volume scanner.** *Eur J Radiol* 2012, **81**(9):2179–2183.
33. Tozaki M, Fukuma E: **Accuracy of determining preoperative cancer extent measured by automated breast ultrasonography.** *Jpn J Radiol* 2010, **28**(10):771–773.
34. Isobe S, Tozaki M, Yamaguchi M, Ogawa Y, Homma K, Satomi R, Saito M, Joo C, Fukuma E: **Detectability of breast lesions under the nipple using an automated breast volume scanner: comparison with handheld ultrasonography.** *Jpn J Radiol* 2011, **29**(5):361–365.
35. Kuehn T, Bembenek A, Decker T, Munz DL, Sautter-Bihl ML, Untch M, Wallwiener D: **Consensus committee of the german society of, senology: a concept for the clinical implementation of sentinel lymph node biopsy in patients with breast carcinoma with special regard to quality assurance.** *Cancer* 2005, **103**(3):451–461.
36. de Bresser J, de Vos B, van der Ent F, Hulsewe K: **Breast MRI in clinically and mammographically occult breast cancer presenting with an axillary metastasis: a systematic review.** *Eur J Surg Oncol* 2010, **36**(2):114–119.
37. Schwab FD, Burger H, Isenschmid M, Kuhn A, Mueller MD, Gunthert AR: **Suspicious axillary lymph nodes in patients with unremarkable imaging of the breast.** *Eur J Obstet Gynecol Reprod Biol* 2010, **150**(1):88–91.

11

Mammographic images segmentation based on chaotic map clustering algorithm

Marius Iacomi[1,2], Donato Cascio[1*], Francesco Fauci[1] and Giuseppe Raso[1]

Abstract

Background: This work investigates the applicability of a novel clustering approach to the segmentation of mammographic digital images. The chaotic map clustering algorithm is used to group together similar subsets of image pixels resulting in a medically meaningful partition of the mammography.

Methods: The image is divided into pixels subsets characterized by a set of conveniently chosen features and each of the corresponding points in the feature space is associated to a map. A mutual coupling strength between the maps depending on the associated distance between feature space points is subsequently introduced. On the system of maps, the simulated evolution through chaotic dynamics leads to its natural partitioning, which corresponds to a particular segmentation scheme of the initial mammographic image.

Results: The system provides a high recognition rate for small mass lesions (about 94% correctly segmented inside the breast) and the reproduction of the shape of regions with denser micro-calcifications in about 2/3 of the cases, while being less effective on identification of larger mass lesions.

Conclusions: We can summarize our analysis by asserting that due to the particularities of the mammographic images, the chaotic map clustering algorithm should not be used as the sole method of segmentation. It is rather the joint use of this method along with other segmentation techniques that could be successfully used for increasing the segmentation performance and for providing extra information for the subsequent analysis stages such as the classification of the segmented ROI.

Keywords: Chaotic maps, Clustering algorithms, Cooperative behavior, Segmentation, Mammography, Features, Mass lesions, Microcalcifications, Breast cancer

Background

At present, breast cancer is the most common cancer among women, after cancers of the skin, and the second leading cause of cancer death in women after lung cancer [1-3]. The most widely used method for detecting breast cancer in its early stages is the mammography, a technique which has lately taken advantage of the supplementary features offered by the digital format [1]. During the last decades, the automatic detection of pathologies in the mammographic images has became a widespread auxiliary technique in radiology and the CAD (Computer Aided Detection) systems have proven their effectiveness mostly as a "second reader" (see [4-6]). The partitioning of the image in medically meaningful components (homogeneous with respect to one or several appropriately chosen characteristics) is a compulsory step in the process of automatic searching of pathologies in the images [7-11]. This phase plays a crucial role [12]: any non segmented lesion at this stage will be irremediably lost for any further analysis. While a wide variety of segmentation approaches have been proposed, there is no standard algorithm that can ensure high levels of accuracy for all imaging applications [13-15]. Furthermore, many segmentation methods rely on specific testing on an actual database [16] and the performance depends on database specificities. In particular, the segmentation of mass lesions in mammographies remains a challenging task since the masses are usually embedded and obscured by surrounding normal breast parenchyma [1,17]. The segmentation methods proposed in mammography and more generally in medical imaging span a broad range of techniques, see e.g. [18] for a recent

* Correspondence: donato.cascio@unipa.it
[1]Dipartimento di Fisica e Chimica, Università Degli Studi di Palermo, Palermo, Italy
Full list of author information is available at the end of the article

review and [19,20] for particular examples. One of the generic segmentation approaches proposed more than three decades ago is the feature-based clustering method [21], which associates to each pixel or group of pixels from the image a set of appropriately chosen numerical parameters and transforms the primary segmentation task in a derived clustering problem in the associated feature space. Within this approach, the process of feature clustering becomes the crucial part of the segmentation algorithm. The main advantage of this approach is that the method does not require the use of a training set [15]. Towards the end of the last century, a new promising nonparametric method of clustering relying on the physical properties of the inhomogeneous Potts model has been proposed by Blatt, Wiseman and Domany [22]; a similar approach was proposed in terms of coupled chaotic dynamical networks by Manrubia and Mikhalkov [23] and has been further refined and restated with coupled chaotic maps by L. Angelini et al. [24]. During the last decade, a series of successful applications of this clustering method has emerged in the literature, such as landmine detection [25], EEG signals analysis in medicine [26] or financial analysis (stock markets [27], financial time series [28]). On the other hand, the chaotic map based algorithms have been proposed in many other contexts such as analysis of matrix metalloproteinases [29] or the medical image encryption technology [30]. The wide applicability of the feature clustering with coupled chaotic maps inspired us to investigate its effectiveness in the case of mammographic images with their specific characteristics. This paper focuses on the application of the chaotic maps clustering method for the segmentation of digital mammographic medical images. The results of this application are subsequently presented.

Methods

The chaotic map clustering method has been thoroughly described in several references ([24-27]); the reader is therefore invited to consult them for more details concerning the method. For completeness, we present here a sketch of the method we have used, following the general flowchart in reference [26]. The proposed method consists of three major phases (see the flowchart in Figure 1).

In the initialization phase, the mammographic image to be analyzed is divided into elementary units of pixels (squares) and a feature vector is computed for each elementary unit. A dynamical variable is also associated with each unit and initialized at random. Finally, an "interaction coefficient" is computed for each pair of units.

The second phase is the core of the method as it features the basic idea of chaotic map clustering: the integration of a dynamical system in the feature space. For each point in the feature space, the associated dynamical variable is allowed to iteratively evolve according to a

functional law corresponding to the distance matrix. In mathematical terms, for each point in the feature space $\{r_i\}$, one defines a real dynamical variable $x_i \in [-1,1]$ (i labels the data points). For two points i and j, the "interaction" matrix element is defined as

$$J_{ij} = \exp\left[-(r_i-r_j)^2/2a^2\right]$$

where a is a local scale parameter. The iterative evolution law is given by

$$x_i(t+1) = \left(\sum_{j\neq i} J_{ij} f(x_j(t))\right)/C_i$$

where

$$C_i = \sum_{j\neq i} J_{ij}$$

and

$$f(x) = 1-2x^2$$

is the usual logistic map which is at the origin of the chaotic dynamics of the system. The local length scale a is estimated as average distance of the K-nearest neighbors (KNN), where K is the only free parameter of the algorithm.

The third phase is the analysis of the time evolution of the coupled chaotic map system. The trajectories of the associated maps exhibit a more or less synchronized behavior depending on how close are the corresponding points in the feature space irrespective of the randomly chosen initial state of the maps: the closer are the representative points, the more similar are the trajectories. Since the maps are chaotic, there is no final stationary regime. Hence, to evaluate mutual correlations one has to operate a cut-off after a large enough number of iterations [24]. In order to define a meaningful measure for the actual synchronism of pairs of maps, one extracts the time sequence $S_i(t)$ of the sign bits corresponding to the map $x_i(t)$ as $S_i(t) = 1$ if $x_i(t) > 0$ and $S_i(t) = 0$ otherwise, and one computes on this basis the value of the mutual information as:

$$I_{ij} = H_i + H_j - H_{ij}$$

where H_i is the Boltzmann entropy for the i-th map sequence and H_{ij} is the joint entropy of the maps i and j. The mutual information provides a good measure of the synchronism [31], and it ranges between 0 for completely non-correlated maps and $ln\ 2$ for exactly synchronized maps. All the pairs of maps for which the mutual information exceeds a threshold θ are considered connected and the corresponding points in the feature space are assumed to belong to a same cluster. Thus, each value of the threshold θ defines a clustering of the data points. The number of clusters monotonically increases with the

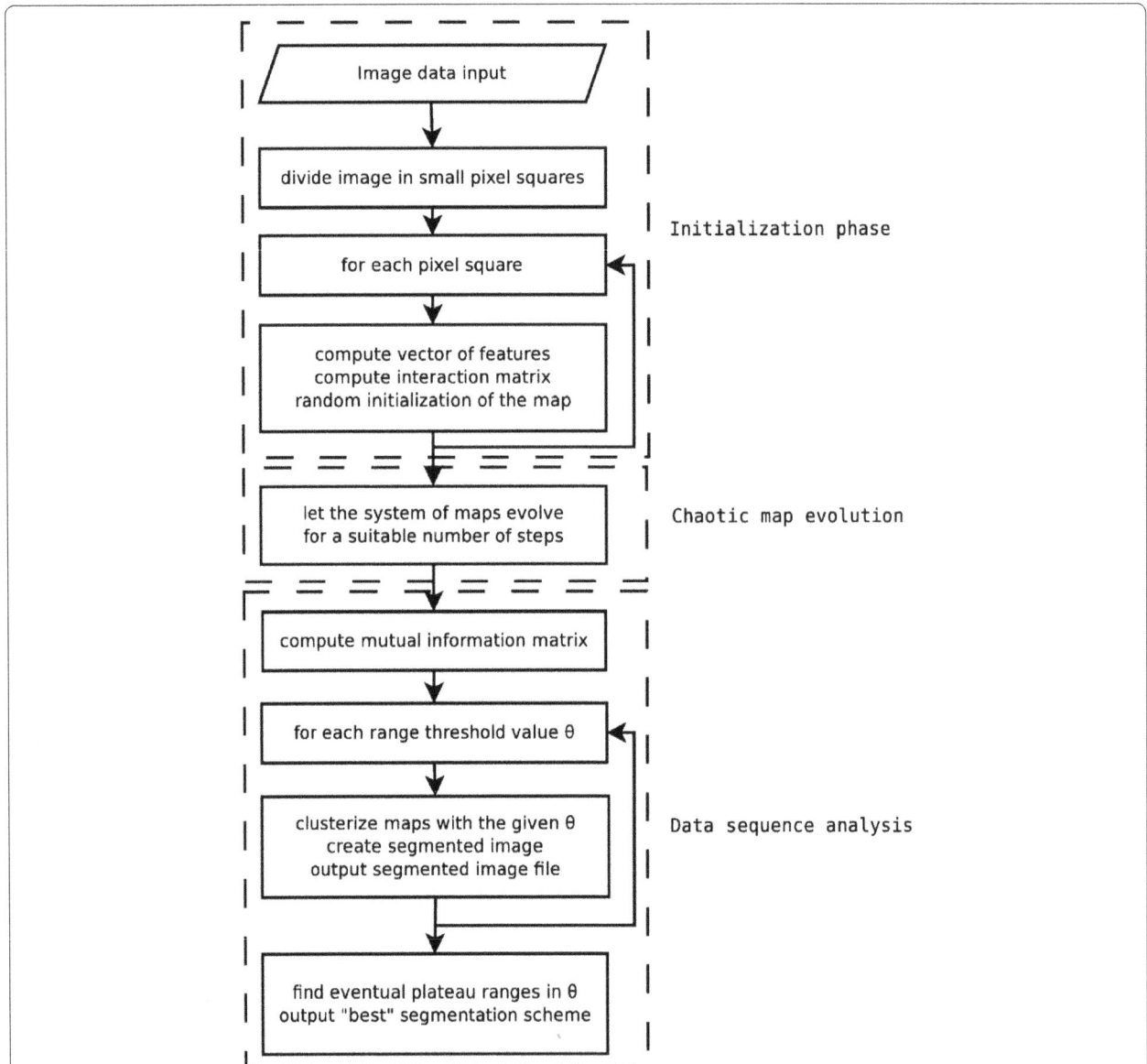

Figure 1 Flowchart of the chaotic map segmentation algorithm. The flowchart of the chaotic map segmentation algoritm used within this work. Its three phases are delimited by dashed lines.

threshold and their hierarchy is naturally obtained from the graph's increasing connectivity. For $\theta = 0$ all data points belong to a single cluster while for $\theta = ln\ 2$ the partitioning will consist in one cluster for each point. Between these extreme values lays the "best" partitioning scheme whose optimality is identified by its maximal stability when varying θ. The stability conditions can be imposed on the number of clusters and on the size of the biggest clusters. These conditions are strong indications that the clustering scheme obtained through application of the algorithm is not a spurious artifact of meaningless numerical output but it rather reflects some deeper similarity property of the input data.

The method has been implemented in order to take as input the data points corresponding to the digital mammographic images to be segmented. The computation begins with the partition of the image into squares small enough to match the typical dimensionality of the smallest objects of interest for the radiologist and rich enough in pixels in order to enable the computation of relevant associated features. In our experiments the side of the square usually ranged around 20 pixels. For each square a vector of features is computed leading to an associated data point in the feature space. Due to the fixed geometry of the initial partitioning, no geometrical or form-based feature can be taken into account at this stage. The position of the square in the image has a definite importance: any segmented lesion should be a contiguous region composed of one or several groups of pixels, therefore any medically meaningful clusters of points in the feature space have to correspond to spatially connected groups of neighbor squares in the image. Hence, it results necessary to treat separately the positional feature (the x and y of a data point) as a compulsory check. Other features used are the usual statistical central moments (mean pixel gray value, variance, kurtosis, skewness) and several autocorrelation values (such as energy, entropy, contrast) accounting for the texture (see [32-34] for other generic texture features and [35-38] for mammographic specific features).

The values of features have been linearly normalized to zero mean and unit variance over the whole image set of points as in [39]. Furthermore, a Karhunen-Loève transformation has been subsequently used in order to eliminate redundancies and focus the analysis on the main independent components of the feature vectors.

In order to make a more meaningful evaluation of the eventual gains of applying the chaotic maps method, the clusters have been also obtained in an alternative manner, by using the simple Euclidean distance in the feature space between the pairs of squares rather than the mutual information.

The clusters obtained on this basis are visualized as different gray-level regions on the image. Due to the border effects, the contour of the breast usually introduces a series of spurious clusters with no real meaning. In our analysis, we have chosen to cut-off these artifacts by default assigning a strip of border pixel squares to the unique border cluster; the choice has the advantage that the breast shape contour is immediately visible on the segmented image (in white), while exhibiting low probability to cut-off also eventual pathologies, usually found more in depth.

The mammographic image database used for this study consists of a group of 149 selected cases for a total of 298 images. More specifically, we operated on three distinct datasets: a first set of 24 digitally acquired cases on a GE Senograph 2000D containing 98 images (characteristics: size 1914×2294 pixels, pixel size 0.094 mm, spatial resolution ~5 lp/mm, log pixel-intensity relationship), a second set of 22 digitalized cases on a Lorad Selenia Full Field Digital Mammograph containing 97 images (characteristics: size 3328×4096 pixels, pixel size 0.070 mm, spatial resolution ~7 lp/mm, linear pixel-intensity relationship); and a third set of 103 anonymized individual images containing micro-calcifications clusters digitally acquired on a Fuji CR mammograph (characteristics: size 1770×2370 pixels, pixel size 0.101 mm, spatial resolution ~5 lp/mm, linear pixel-intensity relationship). The combined first two sets contained a number of 10 cases with small (typical dimension ≤ 2 mm) mass lesions showing up in 20 images (10

images for each set) and 28 cases with large sized (typical dimension > 2 mm) mass lesions showing up in 56 images (30 images for the first set and 26 images for the second). The third set contained 73 cases/images with micro-calcifications clusters and 30 reference healthy images. The digital images were all intended for presentation and had a 12-bit greyscale depth. All the digitally acquired images were subsequently stored on a PACS system. The pathologies have been diagnosed and classified by two expeThe mammographic image database used for this study consists of a group of 149 selected cases for a total of 298 images. More specifically, we operated on three distinct datasets: a first set of 24 digitally acquired cases on a GE Senograph 2000D containing 98 images (characteristics: size 1914×2294 pixels, pixel size 0.094 mm, spatial resolution ~5 lp/mm, log pixel-intensity relationship), a second set of 22 digitalized cases on a Lorad Selenia Full Field Digital Mammograph containing 97 images (characteristics: size 3328×4096 pixels, pixel size 0.070 mm, spatial resolution ~7 lp/mm, linear pixel-intensity relationship) ; and a third set of 103 anonymized individual images containing micro-calcifications clusters digitally acquired on a Fuji CR mammograph (characteristics: size 1770×2370 pixels, pixel size 0.101 mm, spatial resolution ~5 lp/mm, linear pixel-intensity relationship). The combined first two sets contained a number of 10 cases with small (typical dimension ≤ 2 mm) mass lesions showing up in 20 images (10 images for each set) and 28 cases with large sized (typical dimension > 2 mm) mass lesions showing up in 56 images (30 images for the first set and 26 images for the second). The third set contained 73 cases/images with micro-calcifications clusters and 30 reference healthy images. The digital images were all intended for presentation and had a 12-bit greyscale depth. rt senior radiologists; all diagnosed pathologies have been further confirmed by histological examination.

The procedure was tested on images belonging to a private anonymous database collected in the Policlinic Hospital of Palermo. Policlinic Hospital is a hospital firm of University of Palermo in which formation, scientific research and health service are well integrated. Policlinic Hospital attests that all research involving humans is carried out in compliance with the Helsinki Declaration and involves appropriate patient consent.

Results and discussion

The application of this clustering method yielded a series of interesting results. The most striking consideration is that for a wide range of values of the defining parameters k (from the KNN) and a (the scale parameter), there appears to be no automatic "best clustering" criterion since the number of clusters exhibits no obvious stationarity when varying θ. The typical dependence of the number of clusters as a function of the threshold θ is depicted

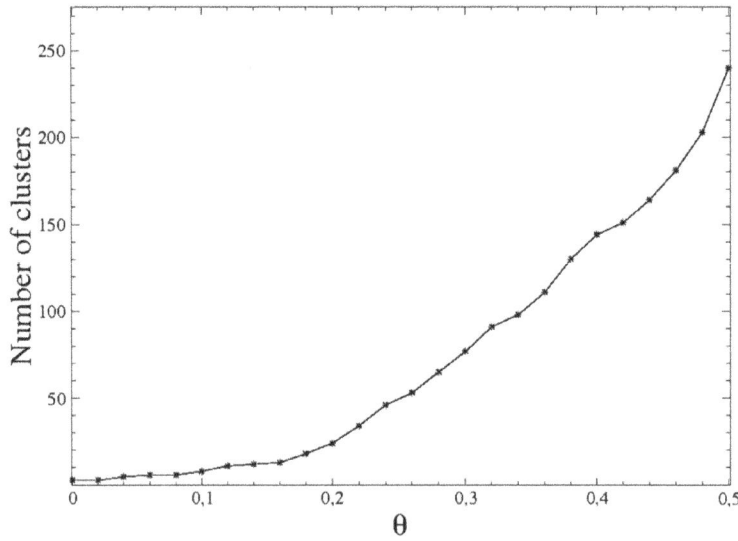

Figure 2 Short title: typical behavior of the number of clusters as a function of the threshold. The figure illustrates the increase in the number of clusters for a given image when increasing the threshold parameter θ. The same behavior is displayed by the number of clusters in all the images, with some slight variations of the actual values not affecting the generic shape of the curve. The upper bound has been set θ = 0.5 rather than θ = ln 2 due to the software limitation of the number of clusters.

in Figure 2. If the clustering is to identify one or a few medically significant regions in the image, it is expected that the corresponding clusters present a minimum of stability also in the number of internal points. The most important clusters in the image actually do exhibit some stability at the varying of the threshold (the internal number of points remains approximately constant on several θ ranges, see e.g. also [26]), but this behavior remains less typical since in a large number of cases, there is no

obvious stability subrange or there is no meaningful cluster in the image. In Figure 3 we have represented a typical behavior of the number of points (pixel squares) contained in the two biggest meaningful clusters (other than the three default ones – image background, border pixels and normal internal breast points).

The segmentation algorithm described above displays a fair number of findings in the images containing mass lesions. The "cluster noise" is very large: in fact, at higher

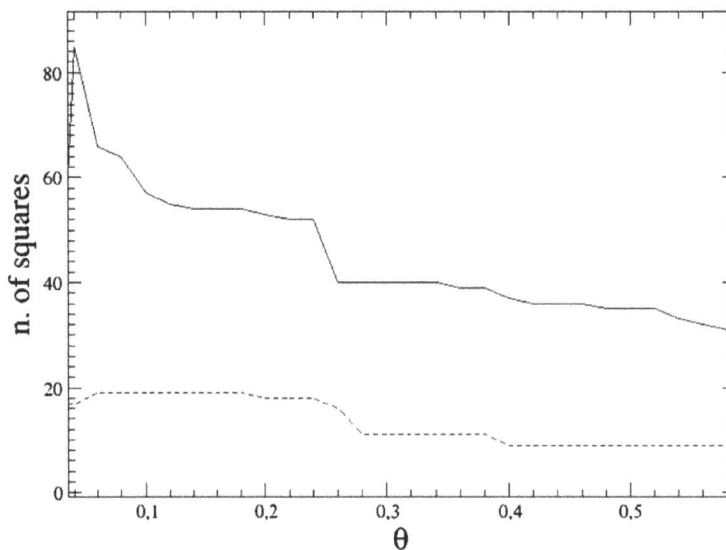

Figure 3 Size of the two largest clusters as a function of the threshold. The number of squares contained in the two largest clusters displayed as a function of the threshold parameter θ for a given image. The solid line refers to the first cluster, the dashed line to the second one. The stability ranges are an indicator of meaningfulness for the clusters.

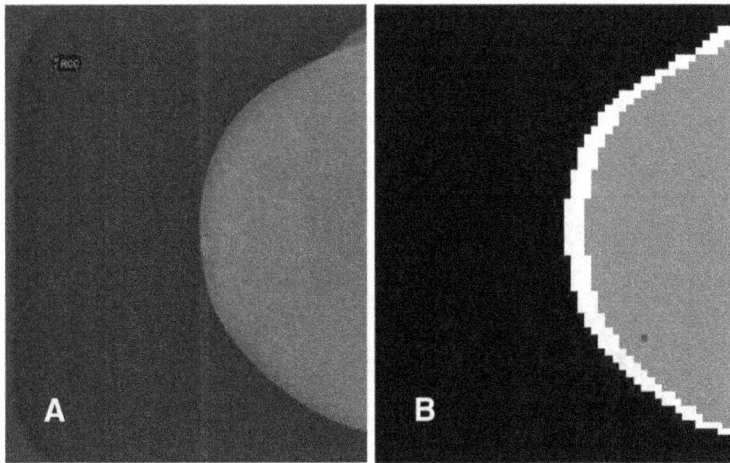

Figure 4 A small mass lesion showing up in the segmented image for most values of θ. Panel **A**. The original image. Panel **B**. The segmented image displaying the small mass lesion for a given threshold value θ = 0.1. An essentially similar segmentation shows up for most values of θ.

threshold levels, most clusters contain actually just one pixel square and show up in internal breast areas characterized by rapid variation of luminosity, typically not far from the breast contour.

Since there is no clear stability range in the threshold θ, assigning these findings to real ROI for a physician (potential mass lesions) remains a hard task, at least for an automatic system such as a CAD. Basically similar segmented images can be obtained with less effort if clustering only the distance features, which means that the chaotic map clustering algorithm brings little (if any) improvement with respect to the more orthodox and less resource consuming distance-based methods. This result is certainly not surprising since if one excludes their geometrical characteristics, mass lesions usually do not share a mathematically well-defined set of features and the identification of mass ROI is a challenge. In the figures below,

some samples illustrating the results of the segmentation algorithm are displayed. Figure 4 exhibits a basic segmentation pattern showing up at most of the threshold values in the case of a small and well-defined mass opacity. Two less satisfactory (according to the physicians opinion) segmentation patterns are shown in the Figures 5 and 6: the first illustrates the occurrence of a potential mass lesion loss within the process, while the second emphasizes the lack of correspondence between the segmented clusters and the shape and size of the actual opacity in the image.

As a general characteristic, the small mass lesions with dimensions of the same order as the size of the pixel square (that is between 1–2 mm), are well identified by the algorithm: practically all of them (15 out of 16, about 94% within this category) show up as isolated point clusters in the segmented image for all but the first threshold

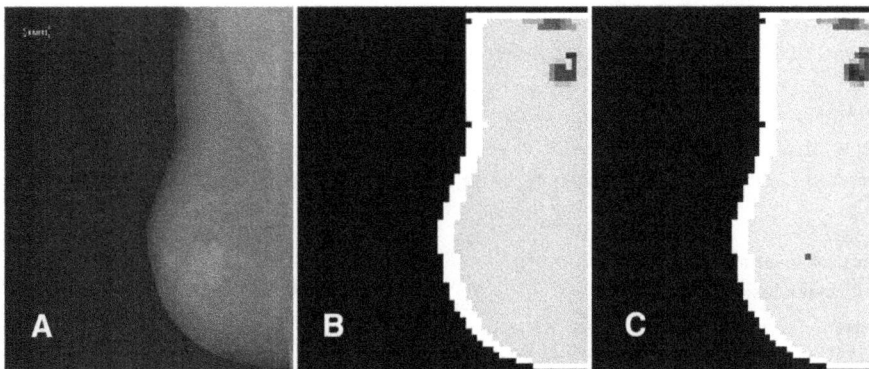

Figure 5 Large-sized mass objects segmentation. Large-sized mass objects in a mammography. Panel **A**. The original image. Panel **B**. The image segmented with θ = 0.04. Panel **C**. The image segmented with θ = 0.36. Note the spurious pixel squares near the upper cluster and the lonely pixel square cluster showing up at higher θ.

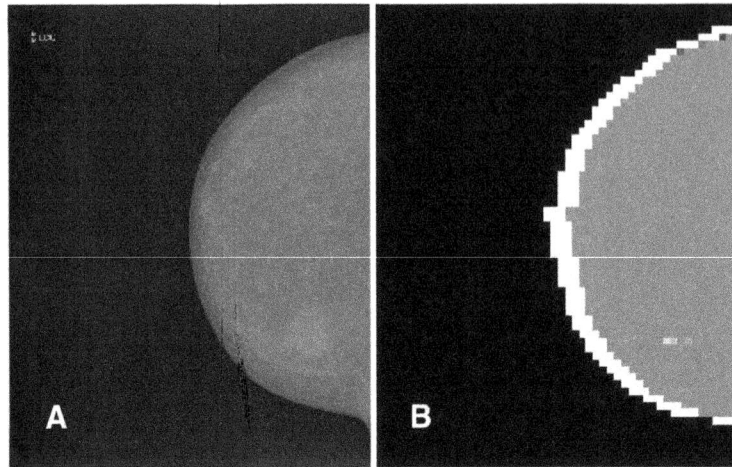

Figure 6 Large-sized massive opacity segmentation. Segmentation of a large-sized massive opacity. Panel **A**. The original image. Panel **B**. The image segmented with θ = 0.24. Note the weak correspondence between the segmented internal areas and the actual shape and size of the ROI.

values. This behavior may be linked with the important differences in the feature characterization of healthy tissue and small lesions. The meaningfulness of the segmented ROI clusters is ensured by their lack of suspicious clusterized neighboring pixel squares rather than by the variational technique used in the original form of the algorithm's implementation: the isolation criterion shows no false positive for cluster groups up to four pixel squares immersed in an uniform (healthy tissue) background, not too close to the border of the breast. If one includes also those small clusters connected with the breast border, the correct recognition rate diminishes accordingly and some false positives show up near the border; it's worthwhile mentioning that in this case the isolation criterion is less operational since all the interesting points cannot be satisfactorily resolved from the spurious pixel squares near the border. No isolated small cluster appears in healthy images.

The results for small mass lesions are summarized in Table 1. In this table, the "Non-Pathologic" label refers to small mass-like objects diagnosed as normal/benign by the physician (4 internal ROI and 4 ROI close to the border). The first row of results contains those ROI segmented as small isolated clusters by the algorithm, while

the second row counts the ROI not identified by the algorithm. These results show that the proposed method might be considered as a potential alternative for finding small mass lesions far from the breast border.

For large-sized mass lesions extending over an area corresponding to more pixel squares (with typical linear diameters ranging from 3 mm up to about 30 mm), the corresponding segmentation clusters rarely match the shape of the lesion due to the usual non-uniformity of the features over ROI area. About 10% of these lesions (5 out of 56) are matched with an overlap of about 80% by the corresponding segmented clusters; the other large lesions either exhibit overlaps under 30% with their segmented cluster counterparts (33 out of 56), or have no meaningful corresponding cluster associated with them (18 out of 56). On the other hand, in the segmented images, the algorithm introduces often bigger-sized cluster artifacts associated with breast borders or non-pathological denser areas in 32 of the cases, and it is difficult to establish an unambiguous automatic decisional criterion for the degree of meaningfulness of these clusters.

Table 2 summarizes the results for large mass lesions. Overall, these results show that the proposed method is

Table 1 Segmentation of images with pathologic and non-pathologic small mass lesions

Only internal isolated ROI, actual diagnosis		Including breast border isolated ROI, actual diagnosis	
Pathologic	Non-pathologic	Pathologic	Non-pathologic
15 TP	0 (FP)	16 TP	3 (FP)
1 FN	4 (TN)	4 FN	5 (TN)

Table 2 Segmentation of large-sized mass lesions (negative images included)

Large mass lesions	
Pathologic	Non-pathologic/absent
38 (= 5 + 33) TP (partial match)	32 (FP)
18 FN	87 (TN)

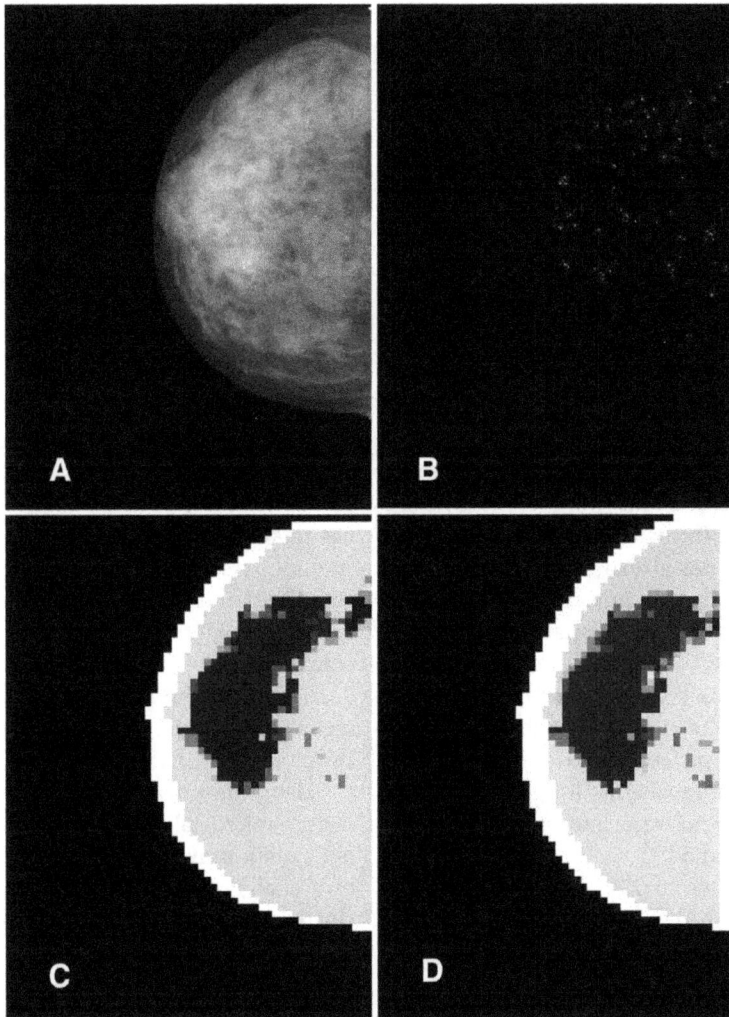

Figure 7 Segmentation of an image with micro-calcifications. Segmentation of an image with micro-calcifications. Panel **A**. The original image containing micro-calcifications clusters. Panel **B**. Actual distribution of micro-calcifications as given by the CAD tool. Panel **C**. The segmented image displaying a big cluster for the ROI. Panel **D**. The image segmented with a feature-based scheme.

not a good potential alternative for finding large mass lesions.

An interesting behavior is displayed by the images containing micro-calcifications. The parts of the image containing micro-calcifications naturally group in a cluster. The feature analysis thus displays the whole ROI rather than finding individual calcifications, as is visible from Figure 7 above[a]. This result is not surprising due to the well-known reliability of the micro-calcifications characterization through the local features on the image. The overlap of the segmented cluster with the micro-calcifications area varies in the range 10-90% with the peak in the range 30-50%. The agreement is better for denser distributed micro-calcifications.

Due to the distinction naturally arising between small and large/sized mass lesions, one can define an accuracy for each class as $acc_i = (TP_i + TN_i)/(TP_i + TN_i + FP_i + FN_i)$ where i labels the mass lesion class and the "true/false" are given with respect to the small or large mass lesions. We find thus for small mass lesions an accuracy $acc_{SMALL\ MASS} = (195\text{-}3\text{-}4)/195 \sim 96\%$ (considering also the isolated clusters near the border) and for large mass lesions an accuracy $acc_{LARGE\ MASS} = (87 + 38)/195 \sim 64\%$, in agreement with our previous observations. Of some

Table 3 Overlap of the cluster with the ROI for micro-calcifications images

Overlap range	0-5%	5-15%	15-25%	25-35%	35-45%	45-55%	55-65%	65-75%	75-85%	85-95%
# of images	11	4	8	12	12	9	2	4	6	5

interest is also the overall accuracy $acc_{MASS} = 118/195 \sim 60.5\%$ for discriminating between images with generic mass lesions and non-pathological/healthy.

The performance of the method doesn't exhibit a significant dependence on the database: the accuracy results restricted to the first set are $acc_{SMALL\ MASS} = 95/98 \sim 97\%$ and $acc_{LARGE\ MASS} = 61/98 \sim 62\%$, while on the second set one has $acc_{SMALL\ MASS} = 93/97 \sim 96\%$ and $acc_{LARGE\ MASS} = 64/97 \sim 66\%$.

Concerning the 103 images in the micro-calcifications dataset, 3 of the healthy images present an internal contiguous cluster similar to the one underlying a part of the positives. The remaining 73 positive ones do exhibit internal "big" clusters distributed according to the following overlaps:

If the overlap in the segmented image with micro-calcifications is enough consistent (our tests show that an overlap of at least 30% with the denser micro-calcification area constitutes already a safe indication) to trigger a further analysis in an automatic system, the internal segmentation cluster will contain most of the micro-calcifications and may be used as a relevant investigation starting point. It should be mentioned at this point that the feature-only based approach produces an essentially similar segmentation pattern. Therefore, the chaotic map clustering of the mammographic images containing micro-calcifications brings no extra information with respect to this alternative method.

Assuming that overlaps up to 25% are not pathology-conclusive, the number of false negatives is essentially given by the sum of the first three terms in Table 3. On the other hand, the false positives are the 3 healthy images segmented with the internal big cluster, therefore one may estimate an accuracy $acc_{MICRO} = (103-23-3)/103 \sim 75\%$.

Conclusion

The non-parametric chaotic map clustering of the mammographic images has been considered here as stand-alone segmentation approach, mainly from an applicability point of view. The ultimate goal of applying such a segmentation method to the medical mammographic images is the potential performance improvement of an automatic detection system based on it. As discussed, the specific aspect of mammographic segmentation which remains a non-trivial challenge is the segmentation of mass lesions, while the identification of micro-calcifications with this new algorithm hardly could lead to any spectacular breakthrough advance (micro-calcifications detection rates of about 94% with 6.25% of false positives and 2% false negatives were already reported more than a decade ago, see [40]).

At this stage of the analysis, the results obtained do allow some general conclusions concerning the valuable applicability of the chaotic map algorithm for the segmentation of mammographic images, in an efficient automatic work-flow, in comparison with the results obtained by alternative methods as those used by present day commercial CAD systems. While many (about 90%) of the mass lesions are either lost or appear with wrong sizes, shapes and as neighboring independent clusters (see Figures 5 & 6 above), most of the smaller ones show up conveniently as internal clusters in the segmented images. Indeed, about 94% of the small lesions more than 6 mm away from the border were correctly segmented by the algorithm; the true positive rate decreases to 80% if the smaller mass lesions near the breast border are included. This fact looks especially important when considering that the small lesions are usually less easily identifiepathologic cases cod than the extended ones, and the support of an automatic CAD system is more useful in their case. On the other hand, one has to keep in mind that the important number of "parasite" clusters with no medical significance adds a further complication in correctly evaluating the output of the segmentation algorithm which the stability analysis cannot eliminate.

Concerning the micro-calcifications, the chaotic maps segmentation process gives interesting and peculiar results. In about 2/3 of the pathologic cases considered here, the algorithm provides an useful shape of the region with denser micro-calcifications. While these results are still not significantly edging the ones derived from simple feature analysis, the algorithm may be used as alternative check in a more complex workflow.

Due to the particularities of the mammographic images, we conclude that the chaotic map clustering algorithm should not be used as unique stand-alone method of segmentation. It is rather the joint use of this method along with other segmentation techniques that could be successfully used for increasing segmentation performance and providing extra information for subsequent analysis stages such as the classification of the segmented ROI.

Endnote

[a]The CAD tool used for computing the position of micro-calcifications is CyclopusCAD Mammo® produced by CyclopusCAD srl.

Competing interests
• We have not received in the past five years reimbursements, fees, funding, or salary from an organization that may in any way gain or lose financially from the publication of this manuscript, either now or in the future.
• We do not hold any stocks or shares in an organization that may in a ny way gain or lose financially from the publication of this manuscript, either now or in the future.
• We do not hold or we are not currently applying for any patents relating to the content of the manuscript. We have not received reimbursements, fees, funding, or salary from an organization that holds or has applied for patents relating to the content of the manuscript.

• We have not any other financial competing interests. Biltawi, M.; Al-Najdawi, N.; Tedmori, S.; Mammogram enhancement and segmentation methods: classification, analysis, and evaluation. The 13th international Arab Conference on Information Technology, December 2012.
• There are not any non-financial competing interests (political, personal, religious, ideological, academic, intellectual, commercial or any other) to declare in relation to this manuscript.

Authors' contributions
MI and DC conceived of the study, carried out the Clustering algorithm implementation and performed the statistical analysis and drafted the manuscript. FF and GR conceived of the study, participated in the design and coordination of the manuscript, and helped to its draft. All authors read and approved the final manuscript.

Acknowledgements
Authors thank Policlinic Hospital of Palermo and in particular Dr. Raffaele Ienzi for providing the images.

Author details
[1]Dipartimento di Fisica e Chimica, Università Degli Studi di Palermo, Palermo, Italy. [2]Institutul de Ştiinţe Spaţiale, Bucharest, Măgurele, Romania.

References
1. Meyer-Bäse A: *Pattern Recognition for Medical Imaging.* San Diego, CA, USA: Elsevier Academic Press; 2003:346–359.
2. American Cancer Society: *Cancer Facts & Figures 2012*; 2012. http://www.cancer.org/acs/groups/content/@epidemiologysurveilance/documents/document/acspc-031941.pdf.
3. Shi J, Sahiner B, Chan HP, Ge J, Hadjiiski L, Helvie MA, Nees A, Wu YT, Wei J, Zhou C, Zhang Y, Cui J: **Characterization of mammographic masses based on level set segmentation with New image features and patient information.** *Med Phys* 2008, **35**:280–290.
4. Azavedo E, Zackrisson S, Mejàre I, Heibert Arnlind M: **Is single reading with computer-aided detection (CAD) as good as double reading in mammography screening? A systematic review.** *BMC Med Imaging* 2012, **12**: art. no. 22.
5. Ciatto S, Cascio D, Fauci F, Magro R, Raso G, Ienzi R, Martinelli F, Simone MV: **Computer assisted diagnosis (CAD) in mammography. Comparison of diagnostic accuracy of a new algorithm (Cyclopus®, Medicad) with two commercial systems.** *Radiol Med* 2009, **114**:626–635.
6. Cascio D, Fauci F, Iacomi M, Raso G, Magro R, Castrogiovanni D, Filosto G, Ienzi R, Vasile MS: **Computer-aided diagnosis in digital mammography: comparison of two commercial systems.** *Imaging in Medicine* 2014, **6**(1):13–30.
7. Nazem-Zadeh M-R, Saksena S, Babajani-Fermi A, Jiang Q, Soltanian-Zadeh H, Rosenblum M, Mikkelsen T, Jain R: **Segmentation of corpus callosum using diffusion tensor imaging: validation in patients with glioblastoma.** *BMC Med Imaging* 2012, **12**: art. no. 10.
8. Montelius M, Ljungberg M, Horn M, Forssell-Aronsson E: **Tumour size measurement in a mouse model using high resolution MRI.** *BMC Med Imaging* 2012, **12**: art. no. 12.
9. Wong KP: **Medical Image Segmentation: Methods and Applications in Functional Imaging.** In *Handbook of Biomedical Image Analysis: Segmentation models Part B.* Edited by Suri JS, Wilson DL, Laxminarayan S. New York, NY, USA: Kluwer Academic/Planum Publishers; 2005:111–115.
10. Cascio D, Fauci F, Magro R, Raso G, Bellotti R, De Carlo F, Tangaro S, De Nunzio G, Quarta M, Forni G, Lauria A, Fantacci ME, Retico A, Masala GL, Oliva P, Bagnasco S, Cheran SC, Torres EL: **Mammogram segmentation by contour searching and massive lesions classification with Neural Network.** *IEEE Trans Nucl Sci* 2006, **53**:2827–2833.
11. Bellotti R, De Carlo F, Tangaro S, Gargano G, Maggipinto G, Castellano M, Massafra R, Cascio D, Fauci F, Magro R, Raso G, Lauria A, Forni G, Bagnasco S, Cerello P, Zanon E, Cheran SC, Lopez Torres E, Bottigli U, Masala GL, Oliva P, Retico A, Fantacci ME, Cataldo R, De Mitri I, De Nunzio G: **A completely automated CAD system for mass detection in a large mammographic database.** *Med Phys* 2006, **33**:3066–3075.
12. Claudia C, Farida C, Guy G, Marie-Claude M, Carl-Eric A: **Quantitative evaluation of an automatic segmentation method for 3D reconstruction of intervertebral scoliotic disks from MR images.** *BMC Med Imaging* 2012, **12**: art. no. 26.
13. Farag AA, Ahmed MN, El-Baz A, Hassan H: **Advanced segmentation techniques.** In *Handbook of Biomedical Image Analysis: Segmentation models Part A.* Edited by Suri JS, Wilson DL, Laxminarayan S. New York, NY, USA: Kluwer Academic/Planum Publishers; 2005:479.
14. Pratt WK: *Digital Image Processing: PIKS Scientific Inside.* 4th edition. Hoboken, NJ, USA: John Wiley & Sons, Inc; 2007:579.
15. Yang S, Sunanda M: **Statistical and adaptive approaches for optimal segmentation in medical images.** In *Handbook of Biomedical Image Analysis: Segmentation models Part B.* Edited by Suri JS, Wilson DL, Laxminarayan S. New York, NY, USA: Kluwer Academic/Planum Publishers; 2005:267–271.
16. Tangaro S, Bellotti R, De Carlo F, Gargano G, Lattanzio E, Monno P, Massacra R, Delogu P, Fantacci ME, Retico A, Mazzocchi M, Bagnasco S, Cerello P, Cheran SC, Lopez Torres E, Zanon E, Lauria A, Sodano A, Cascio D, Fauci F, Magro R, Raso G, Ienzi R, Bottigli U, Masala GL, Oliva P, Meloni G, Caricato AP, Cataldo R: **MAGIC-5: an Italian mammographic database of digitized images for research.** *Radiol Med* 2008, **113**:477–485.
17. Liu J, Chen J, Liu X, Chun L, Tang J, Deng Y: **Mass segmentation using a combined method for cancer detection.** *BMC Syst Biol* 2011, **5**(SUPPL. 3): art. no. S6.
18. Biltawi M, Al-Najdawi N, Tedmori S: **Mammogram enhancement and segmentation methods: classification, analysis, and evaluation. The 13th international Arab conference on information technology.** 2012.
19. Fauci F, Cascio D, La Manna A, Magro R, Raso G, Vasile M, Iacomi M: *A Fourier Based Algorithm for Microcalcifications Enhancement in Mammographic Images,* IEEE Nuclear Science Symposium and Medical Imaging Conference; 2012:4388–4391. art. No. 4774254.
20. Vivona L, Cascio D, Magro R, Fauci F, Raso G: *A Fuzzy Logic Cmeans Clustering Algorithm to Enhance Microcalcifications Clusters in Digital Mammograms,* IEEE Nuclear Science Symposium and Medical Imaging Conference; 2012:3048–3050. art. No. 6152551.
21. Coleman GB, Andrews HC: **Image segmentation by clustering.** *Proc IEEE Inst Electr Electron Eng* 1979, **67**:773–785.
22. Blatt M, Wiseman S, Domany E: **Super-paramagnetic clustering of data.** *Phys Rev Lett* 1996, **76**:3251–3254.
23. Manrubia SC, Mikhalkov AS: **Mutual synchronization and clustering in randomly coupled chaotic dynamical networks.** *Phys Rev E Stat Phys Plasmas Fluids Relat Interdiscip Topics* 1999, **60**:1579–1589.
24. Angelini L, De Carlo F, Marangi C, Pellicoro M, Stramaglia S: **Clustering data by inhomogeneous chaotic map lattices.** *Phys Rev Lett* 2000, **85**:554–557.
25. Marangi C, Angelini L, De Carlo F, Nardulli G, Pellicoro M, Stramaglia S: **Clustering by inhomogeneous chaotic maps in landmine detection.** *Proc SPIE* 2001, **4170**:122–132.
26. Bellotti R, De Carlo F, Stramaglia S: **Chaotic map clustering algorithm for EEG analysis.** *Physica A* 2004, **334**:222–232.
27. Basalto N, Bellotti R, De Carlo F, Facchi P, Pascazio S: **Clustering stock market companies via chaotic map synchronization.** *Physica A* 2005, **345**:196–206.
28. Basalto N, De Carlo F: **Clustering financial time series.** In *Practical Fruits of Econophysics: Proceedings of The Third Nikkei Econophysics Symposium.* Edited by Takayasu H. Tokio, Japan: Springer Verlag; 2006:252–256.
29. Giangreco I, Nicolotti O, Carotti A, De Carlo F, Gargano G, Bellotti R: **Analysis of x-ray structures of matrix metalloproteinases via chaotic map clustering.** *BMC Bioinforma* 2010, **11**:. art. no. 500.
30. Fu C, Meng WH, Zhan YF, Zhu ZL, Lau FCM, Tse CK, Ma HF: **An efficient and secure medical image protection scheme based on chaotic maps.** *Comput Biol Med* 2013, **43**(8):1000–1010.
31. Solé RV, Manrubia SC, Bascompte J, Delgado J, Luque B: **Phase transitions and complex systems.** *Complexity* 1996, **4**:13–26.
32. Haralick R, Shanmugam K, Dinstein I: **Textural features for image classification.** *IEEE Trans Syst Man Cybern C Appl Rev* 1973, **6**:610–621.
33. Haralick R: **Statistical and structural approaches to texture.** *Proc IEEE Inst Electr Electron Eng* 1979, **67**:786–803.
34. Cascio D, Magro R, Fauci F, Iacomi M, Raso G: **Automatic detection of lung nodules in CT datasets based on stable 3D mass-spring models.** *Comput Biol Med* 2012, **42**(11):1098–1109.

35.   Masala GL, Golosio B, Oliva P, Cascio D, Fauci F, Tangaro S, Quarta M, Cheran SC, Lopez Torres E: **Classifiers trained on dissimilarity representation of medical pattern: a comparative study.** *Nuovo Cimento C* 2005, **28:**905–912.

36.   Masala GL, Tangaro S, Golosio B, Oliva P, Stumbo S, Bellotti R, De Carlo F, Gargano G, Cascio D, Fauci F, Magro R, Raso G, Bottigli U, Cgincarini A, De Mitri I, De Nunzio G, Gori I, Retico A, Cerello P, Cheran SC, Fulcheri C, Lopez Torres E: **Comparative study of feature classification methods for mass lesion recognition in digitized mammograms.** *Nuovo Cimento C* 2007, **30:**305–316.

37.   Fauci F, Raso G, Magro R, Forni G, Lauria A, Bagnasco S, Cerello P, Cheran SC, Lopez Torres E, Bellotti R, De Carlo F, Gargano G, Tangaro S, De Mitri I, De Nunzio G, Cataldo R: **A massive lesion detection algorithm in mammography.** *Phys Med* 2005, **21**(1):23–30.

38.   Cascio D, Cheran SC, Chincarini A, De Nunzio G, Delogu P, Fantacci ME, Gargano G, Gori I, Masala GL, Preite Martinez A, Retico A, Santoro M, Spinelli C, Tarantino T: **Automated detection of lung nodules in low-dose computed tomography.** *Int J Comput Assist Radiol Surg* 2007, **2:**357–359.

39.   Angelini L, De Carlo F, Mannarelli M, Marangi C, Nardulli G, Pellicoro M, Satalino G, Stramaglia S: **Chaotic neural networks clustering: an application to landmine detection by dynamic infrared imaging.** *Opt Eng* 2001, **40:**2878–2884. http://www.ba.infn.it/~angelini/minefields.pdf.

40.   Melloul M, Joskowicz L: **Segmentation of microcalcification in X-ray mammograms using entropy thresholding.** *CARS 2002 Computer Assisted Radiology and Surgery* 2002:**671–676.

12

Fractal dimension analysis of malignant and benign endobronchial ultrasound nodes

José Antonio Fiz[1,2]*, Enrique Monte-Moreno[2], Felipe Andreo[1,5], Santiago José Auteri[3], José Sanz-Santos[1], Pere Serra[1], Gloria Bonet[1], Eva Castellà[4] and Juan Ruiz Manzano[1]

Abstract

Background: Endobronchial ultrasonography (EBUS) has been applied as a routine procedure for the diagnostic of hiliar and mediastinal nodes. The authors assessed the relationship between the echographic appearance of mediastinal nodes, based on endobronchial ultrasound images, and the likelihood of malignancy.

Methods: The images of twelve malignant and eleven benign nodes were evaluated. A previous processing method was applied to improve the quality of the images and to enhance the details. Texture and morphology parameters analyzed were: the image texture of the echographies and a fractal dimension that expressed the relationship between area and perimeter of the structures that appear in the image, and characterizes the convoluted inner structure of the hiliar and mediastinal nodes.

Results: Processed images showed that relationship between log perimeter and log area of hilar nodes was lineal (i.e. perimeter vs. area follow a power law). Fractal dimension was lower in the malignant nodes compared with non-malignant nodes (1.47(0.09), 1.53(0.10) mean(SD), Mann–Whitney U test $p < 0.05$)).

Conclusion: Fractal dimension of ultrasonographic images of mediastinal nodes obtained through endobronchial ultrasound differ in malignant nodes from non-malignant. This parameter could differentiate malignat and non-malignat mediastinic and hiliar nodes.

Background

The ultrasound technique (US) applies sound waves (1 MHz up to 100 MHz.) that collide with tissues and thus provide energy as images. US has had a wide-ranging impact in medicine due to its low cost and by offering high resolution images.

Ultrasonography endobronchial (EBUS) has been applied as a routine procedure [1]. Three types of EBUS are currently used: EBUS radial ultra-miniature, radial and the convex or curvilinear (CP EBUS). Radial EBUS allows the evaluation of small outlying lung nodules [2]. CP USEB is the most extensively used technique because it allows to carry out mediastinal lymph node puncture (TBNA) [3,4]. Recently, several studies have demonstrated the relation between macroscopic ultrasonographic appearance and vascular patterns [5] and the likelihood of malignancy [6,7]. Although these studies have shown that some features are associated with malignancy, the evaluation of the ultrasonographic appearance depends on the observer subjectivity, and recently one study demonstrated intraobserver and interobserver disagreement [8]. Because the images contain noises mainly as a result of the reflection among adjacent surfaces, it is necessary to process them to be able to separate the real images from the noise.

The present study describes a method that improves the quality of the image, and in consequence the effectiveness of TBNA. The proposed method consists of two sections: one of having the processed image adapted to the specificities of the ultrasonography obtained by means of EBUS that eliminates the devices and specific noise of the application, and a second that characterizes the morphology of the images with the purpose of distinguishing between normal and pathological nodes.

* Correspondence: jafiz@msn.com
[1]Pulmonology Department, Hospital Universitari Germans Trias Pujol, Planta 8, Carretera del Canyet s/n. 08916, Badalona, Spain
[2]TALP Research Center, UPC, Barcelona, Spain
Full list of author information is available at the end of the article

Material and methods

The study was developed in the Bronchoscopy Dept. of the Hospital University Germans Trias i Pujol and approved by The Human Research and Ethics Committee.

EBUS-TBNA was performed in an outpatient setting using a flexible bronchoscope (BF-UC180F-OL8, Olympus Optical Co Ltd., Tokyo, Japan) with a distal probe capable of producing linear parallel scans of the mediastinal and peribronchial tissues and a working channel suited to the performance of TBNA under direct ultrasound guidance. Local anesthesia and conscious sedation were achieved using topical lidocaine spray and intravenous midazolam, respectively [BTS guidelines]. Mediastinal and lobar nodes with a short-axis diameter of ≥ 5 mm identified during the procedure were sampled under direct ultrasound visualization with a 22-gauge cytology needle specially designed for EBUS-TBNA (NA-201SX-4022, Olympus Optical Co Ltd.). The aspirates were recovered and placed on slides, fixed with 95% ethanol and stained with haematoxylin for rapid on-site evaluation by a cytopathologist. An immediate assessment was given after each pass. Nodes were classified as "normal tissue negative for malignancy" when the sample contained 40 lymphocytes per high-power field in cellular areas of the smear and/or clusters of pigmented macrophages and contained no neoplastic cells or as "metastatic" when recognizable groups of malignant cells were present. Aspirates containing only isolated dysplastic, bronchial or blood cells were considered as inadequate. In these cases the node was punctured as many times as needed to obtain adequate material.

Normal nodes were confirmed to be non-malignant by surgical procedures (patients who underwent mediastinoscopy or thoracotomy with extended nodal dissection) or by clinical and radiological follow-up for at least 18 months. In case of malignant nodes, no further confirmation was performed because the likelihood of false positive EBUS-TBNA results is very low.

Image processing

To improve the quality, we processed the image by means of the following step sequences. The steps are standard image processing procedures that improve the quality of the image [9]. The image was first segmented to select the area of interest. A median filter was applied to remove possible spikes. Afterwards the noise of the image was reduced by a linear average 3×3 low pass filter. Local equalization with structure preserving was applied by means of a histogram 15×15. This last image will be called I1. Then I1 is filtered by means of with two orthogonal Sobel filters, which had the impulsion response (H) of:

$$H = \begin{bmatrix} 1 & 2 & 1 \\ 0 & 0 & 0 \\ -1 & -2 & -1 \end{bmatrix}$$

which yielded images I2 and I3. The Sobel filter was used for enhancing the inner structures of the ganglia.

The final step consisted on combining linearly the filtered images I1, I2 and I3.

Image analysis

The analysis of the images was done by means of two methods: texture and fractal dimension analysis. Texture analysis provides information of the pixels' intensity variability. In areas with soft texture, the range of values around the pixel is small, and when the texture is rough the range is bigger. The texture parameters to analyze are the following: a- Contrast, variance or inertia gives a measure of the intensity between a pixel and its surrounding. For a constant image the contrast is 0. b- Correlation is the relation of a pixel with its surrounding. A constant image has a correlation around 1. c- Homogeneity indicates the degree of vicinity of the elements as well as for intensity of gray. The biggest homogeneity has the value 1.

The fractal dimension of the image was computed by treating the image as a 3D object, and taking horizontal slices of it at different intensity levels. Therefore for each intensity level we created a binary image, where we assigned the value white to the intersection of the surface with the slice and to the inner pixels. In other words, for each gray level we created and image and assigned the white value to the set of pixels with that gray level and the pixels inside the regions. The black value was assigned to the other pixels. The result was that for low values of gray level most of the figure was white, and as the gray level increased, the images begun to take shapes like fiords, as the gray level continued to increase, islands appear, and finally, the whole image finally is black. The algorithm computed the inner area (white space) and its perimeter. We assumed a perimeter model of the node inner structure as follows: Log (Perimeter[n]) = k + α Log(Area[n]). Parameters k and α were computed after a least squares linear regression was applied. The fractal dimension is the α value that models the increase of the perimeter as the area of the figure increases.

A possible characterization of the structures in the images could be done by means of the box counting dimension [10]. We decided not to use it in this problem due to various difficulties.

a) The box counting dimension assumes a binary image with two different zones. The box counting method consists of computing the fractal dimension by counting the boxes that overlap the border between regions at different scales (sizes) of the boxes. This assumes that there is a specific threshold that characterizes the different areas of interest, and the gray level information of the image is lost. In our case, as the different structures of the tissue are reflected in the intensity (or gray level) of the image, we computed the regression of the log perimeter vs log area, not on the different scales of the boxes, but on the variation of the log area/log perimeter relationship at different gray scale levels.

b) The second difficulty was that the size of the areas of interest in the ultrasonography was small (of the order of less than 100x100, depending on the selected area) and therefore the estimate of the fractal dimension by means of the box counting method would have been unreliable, due to the lack of points.

Statistical analysis of differences in image parameters between independent groups were performed with a Mann_Whitney U test. In addition, a receiver-operator characteristic (ROC) curve was applied to measure the capacity of the method to discriminate between neoplasic and non neoplasic nodes.

The Image processing part of the study was made using the Matlab programming language. The texture parameters were computed by means of the subroutines of the same name (i.e. Contrast, variance or inertia) in the 'Image processing Toolbox', and the fractal dimension part was programmed in Matlab. Statistic analysis was developed with Statistica v.12 (StatSoft, Inc 2013. Tulsa.USA).

Results

Table 1 shows the histological results of 23 biopsied mediastinal nodes. Twelve nodes were malignant.

The ultrasound images were processed in order to improve the quality of EBUS image and to enhance the details, as can be seen in Figure 1 (1-A non processed image, 1-B processed image).

Table 2 shows morphologic parameters and fractal dimension of 23 biopsied lymph nodes. Processed images showed that fractal dimension was lower in neoplasic with respect to non neoplasic nodes. There were no differences between both groups in the morphological parameters.

Figure 2 shows the relationship between the log area and the log perimeter. The slope of the straight line would give us the form in that the log-perimeter grows linearly with the log-area. In this example the relationship agrees with a lineal model. Except for fractal dimension, there were no differences in morphological parameters between images (Table 2). On the other hand, the fractal dimension was smaller in malignant lymph nodes (Mann–Whitney U test for independent groups, $p < 0.05$).

Figure 3 shows the ROC curve of fractal dimension parameter. The area under the curve quantifies the overall ability of the fractal dimension measure to discriminate between neoplasic and non neoplasic nodes. The area under the curve was 0.76 with Std Error of 0.11 ($p < 0.03$).

Table 1 Characteristics and results of lymph nodes

ID	Type	Cytological diagnosis	Type	Station	Size (mm)
1	Malignant	Carcinoma	Breast C	7	23.8
2	"	Carcinoma	Breast C	7	28.9
3	"	Squamous		4 L	8.9
4	"	Squamous		11 L	19.1
5	"	Adenocarcinoma	NSCLC	7	13.2
6	"	Squamous	NSCLC	4 L	6.7
7	"	Adenocarcinoma	NSCLC	4R	9.1
8	"	Squamous	NSCLC	4 L	17.1
9	"	SCLC		4R	11.2
10	"	Adenocarcinoma	NSCLC	4R	13.4
11	"	Adenocarcinoma	NSCLC	7	23.0
12	"	Adenocarcinoma	NSCLC	4 L	9.2
13	Benign	Normal		4R	8.2
14	"	Normal		4 L	4.1
15	"	Normal		7	11.8
16	"	Normal		7	14.2
17	"	Normal		4R	5.9
18	"	Normal		4R	8.3
19	"	Normal		4R	8.6
20	"	Normal		11 L	10.6
21	"	Normal		7	10.4
22	"	Normal		4 L	9.8
23	"	Normal		4R	9.1

Histological characteristics of 23 needled lymph nodes.
NSCLC: non-small cell lung cancer.
SCLC: small cell lung cancer.
Breast C: breast cancer.

Discussion

In this work we studied the relationship between parameters that describe the texture and fractal dimension of endobronchial ultrasonographic images of mediastinal nodes and the likehood for malignancy. In both raw images as well as enhanced ones it was found that there is a statistical difference between malignant and non-malignant nodes in terms of fractal dimension.

The introduction of EBUS-TBNA has provided a significant advance in the staging and diagnosis of lung cancer and other malignancies in a safe and minimally invasive procedure [11]. The analysis of the ultrasonographic appearance of the nodes has been applied to predict malignancy. Fujiwara et al. studied morphologic characteristics of lymph nodes by means of a multivariable analysis that included round shape, distinct margin, heterogeneous echogenicity and presence of coagulation necrosis [6]. The authors found that these morphologic characteristics are independent predictive factors for predicting malignancy. Echogenicity was the parameter

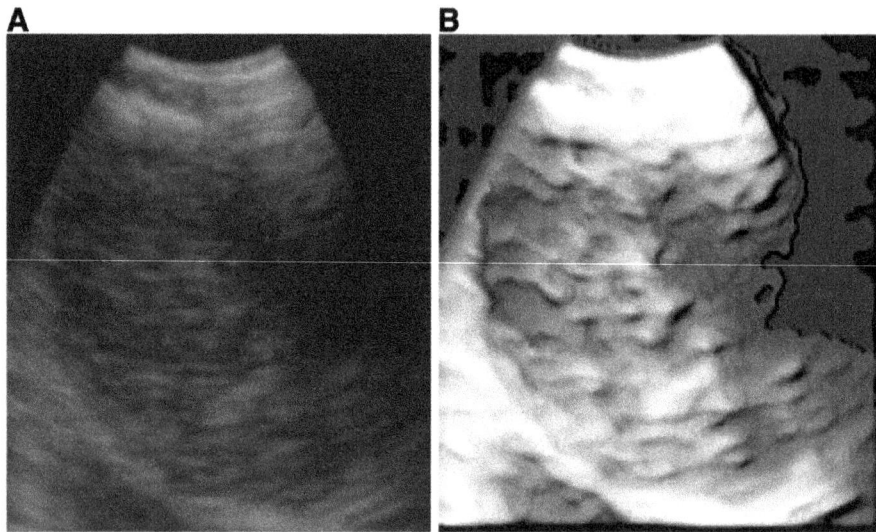

Figure 1 Non processed EBUS image (1-A) and processed image (1-B). Image details are emphasized in image **B** with respect to image **A**.

with the most validated punctuation. The authors did not apply the automatic process of the image, but only qualitative subjective evaluation. Nguyen et al. applied for the first time the second order grayscale texture feature analysis in EBUS [12]. In their study, 52 malignant nodes and 48 benign ones were analyzed. They found that malignant nodes have a higher difference in first and second order texture parameters in relation with benign nodes, using as distinctive features in texture parameters based on first and second order statistics. It should be noted that images were not pre-processed in order to maintain the same real time quality image. On the other hand, the differences in textures after enhancing the image were not significant. This can be attributed to the fact that the processing smoothed the image, eliminated spurious peaks, and enhanced the inner structures of the nodules. This processing that improved the visual appearance of

the details of the nodes, changed the texture of the image.

An interesting aspect of the proposal in this paper of introducing the fractal index α, is that this index is complementary with respect to the texture parameters. This complementariness arises from the fact that the fractal index is adapted to the shape of the internal structures of the nodule, and therefore appears as significant after the enhancement of the image. On the other hand the raw image has too much noise, which gives rise to artifacts when computing the fractal index. The fractal dimension is a real number that generalizes the concept of

Table 2 Morphological image parameters

	Processed image		
	Neoplasic	Non Neoplasic	All
Fractal dimension	1.47(0.09)	1.53(0.10)*	1.50(0.10)
Contrast	0.35(0.09)	0.40(0.14)	0.37(0.12)
Correlation	0.95(0.01)	0.95(0.02)	0.96(0.01)
Homogeneity	0.87(0.03)	0.86(0.04)	0.65(0.03)

Mann–Whitney U test for independent groups.
*P < 0.05. Significant difference between neoplasic and non neoplasic nodes. All values are in mean (SD).
Morphological parameters and fractal dimension of 23 biopsied lymph nodes. The table shows that fractal dimension was lower in neoplasic with respect to non neoplasic nodes. There were no differences in morphology parameters between neoplasic and non neoplasic images.

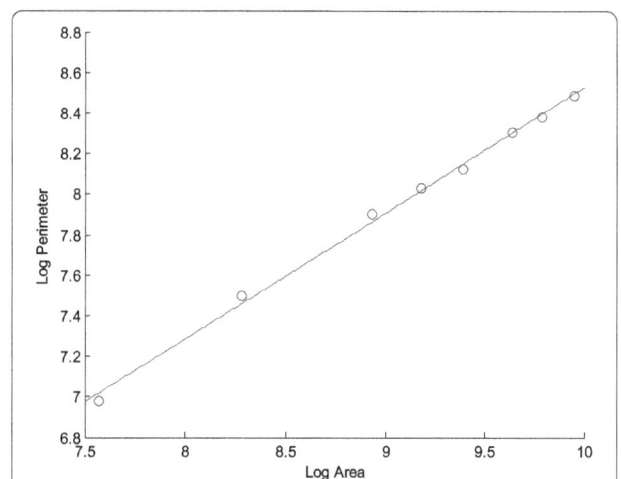

Figure 2 Relationship between the log area and the log perimeter of a node image. The slope of the straight line would give us the form in that the log- perimeter grows linearly with the log-area. In this example the relationship agrees with a lineal model. $Log(Perimeter[n]) = K + aLog(Area[n])$. Coefficients: $a = 0.62$, $K = 2.31$.

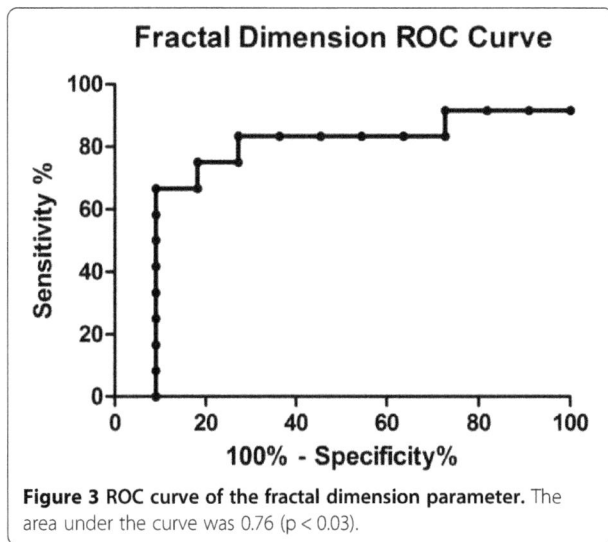

Figure 3 ROC curve of the fractal dimension parameter. The area under the curve was 0.76 (p < 0.03).

ordinary dimension for geometric objects. This process also provides data regarding phenomena like deformation, remodeling, breakup and repair. Cancer in general is associated with a disruption of tissue architecture due to the interaction between cells and stroma [13], and fractal-shape parameters could be descriptors of the cell-stroma system. On the other hand, there is a fractal relationship between the degree of apparent heterogeneity of local tissue and the resolution of the measurement, when heterogeneity provides no uniformity in the cell organs examined.

Fractal dimension has been applied in ultrasound echo signals to detect tissue tumors [14,15]. Texture parameters and fractal Higuchi dimension of the ultrasound series detected prostate cancer in small tissue regions with an accuracy of 91% [15]. Zheng et al. [16] applied fractal Brownian motion and k means cluster analysis to detect breast cancer with a recognition rate of 94.5% for malignant tumors. In the present work, we analyzed 23 nodes (12 of them malignant), and applied an algorithm to compute the inner area (white space) and its perimeter. We assume a power model between the perimeter of the inner structure of the ganglia and the area. Difference of fractal dimension between malignant and non malignant nodes was significant, and less in malignant nodes. A possible cause of this slight reduction in fractal dimension of malignant nodes is that cell membranes spread to take the form of a lower energy structure like a circle, therefore, diminishing the fractal dimension of a neoplasic node [13]. In this way, Kikuchi et al. [17] showed that sonography of solid components in cystic epithelial ovarian cancers had a fractal structure, and the mean fractal dimension decreased from 1.26 for serous intracystic components to 1.18 for clear cell adenocarcinoma. In our study the mean fractal dimension was more than 1, meaning the topological line dimension, and it decreased from 1.53 for benign nodes to 1.47 for malignant nodes, the same proportion of the Kikuchi study.

We believe that the principal limitation of our study is the relatively small number of analyzed nodes, but the objective was to describe the fractal nature of the ultrasonographic images of mediastinal nodes. A future application and validation of the present technique could be developed to distinguish between malignant nodes and other non-malignant pathologies that affect mediastinal nodes (such as tuberculosis and chronic inflammatory diseases like sarcoidosis). We should always try to obtain pathological reference diagnosis from suspicious lymph nodes, but in the future, image analysis could assist the bronchoscopist regarding the likelihood to malignancy of the node, as well as the most suspicious region of the node to sample. In consequence, we believe that fractal dimension can constitute a new EBUS parameter to take into account. To our knowledge, this is the first study that applies fractal dimension analysis to EBUS images.

Conclusion

Fractal dimension of ultrasonographic images of mediastinal nodes obtained through endobronchial ultrasound differ in malignant nodes from non-malignant. This parameter could assist the bronchoscopist to differentiate malignant and non-malignant mediastinic and hiliar nodes.

Competing interest
The authors declare that they have no competing interest.

Authors' contributions
JAF: Participated in the design of study, statistical analysis and manuscript writing. EM: Participated in the study design, statistical analysis and manuscript writing, as well as software programming that computed the fractal dimension of the data and the image processing part. FA: Participated in the study design, manuscript writing and bronchoscopy explorations. SJ: Participated in bronchoscopy explorations and contributed in design and manuscript writing. JS: Participated in bronchoscopy explorations and contributed in design and in the writing and revising of the manuscript. PS: Participated in bronchoscopy explorations and contributed in design and revision of the manuscript. EC: Participated in bronchoscopy explorations and in the design and revising of the manuscript. JR: Participated in the design of study, statistical analysis and manuscript writing. All authors read and approved the final manuscript.

Acknowledgments
The authors thank A. Ruiz and A. Barrios for their technical assistance during the performance of the procedures. This work was partially supported by a grant from the Spanish Society of Pulmonology and Thoracic Surgery (grant SEPAR 2010) and by the grand SpeechTech4All (TEC2012-38939-C03-02).

Author details
[1]Pulmonology Department, Hospital Universitari Germans Trias Pujol, Planta 8, Carretera del Canyet s/n. 08916, Badalona, Spain. [2]TALP Research Center, UPC, Barcelona, Spain. [3]Pulmonology Department Hospital de rehabilitación Respiratoria María Ferrer, Buenos Aires, Argentina. [4]Pathology Department Hospital Universitari Germans Trias Pujol, Badalona, Spain. [5]Ciber de Enfermedades Respiratorias (CiBERES), Bunyola, Balearic Islands, Spain.

References

1. Haas AR, Vachani A, Sterman DH: Advances in diagnostic bronchoscopy. *Am J Respir Crit Care Med* 2010, **182**:589–597.

2. Kurimoto N, Murayama M, Yoshioka S, Nishisaka T: Analysis of the internal structure of peripheral pulmonary lesions using endobronchial ultrasonography. *Chest* 2002, **122**:1887–1894.

3. Herth FJ, Annema JT, Eberhardt R, Yasufuku K, Ernst A, Krasnik M, Rintoul RC: Endobronchial ultrasound with transbronchial needle aspiration for restaging the mediastinum in lung cancer. *J Clin Oncol* 2008, **26**:3346–3350.

4. Wong M, Yasufuku K, Nakajima T, Herth FJ, Sekine Y, Shibuya K, Iizasa T, Hiroshima K, Lam WK, Fujisawa T: Endobronchial ultrasound: new insight for the diagnosis of sarcoidosis. *Eur Respir J* 2007, **29**:1182–1186.

5. Nakajima T, Anayama T, Shingyoji M, Kimura H, Yoshino I, Yasufuku K: Vascular image patterns of lymph nodes for the prediction of metastatic disease during EBUS-TBNA for mediastinal staging of lung cancer. *J Thorac Oncol* 2012, **7**(6):1009–14.

6. Fujiwara T, Yasufuku K, Nakajima T, Chiyo M, Yoshida S, Suzuki M, Shibuya K, Hiroshima K, Nakatani Y, Yoshiro I: The utility of sonographic features during endobronchial ultrasoubd-guided transbronchial needle aspiration for lymph node staging in patients with lung cancer: a Standard endobronchial ultrasound image classification system. *Chest* 2010, **138**:641–647.

7. Tagaya R, Kurimoto N, Osada H, Kobayashi A: Automatic objetive of lymph nodal disease by B-mode images from convex-type echobroncoscopy. *Chest* 2008, **133**:137–142.

8. Garcia-Olivé I, Radua J, Serra P, Andreo F, Sanz-Santos J, Monsó E, Rosell A, Cases-Viedma E, Fernández-Villar A, Nuñez-Delgado M, García-Luján R, Morera J, Ruiz-Manzano: Intra- and interobserver agreement among bronchial endosonographers for the description of intrathoracic lymph nodes. *Ultrasound in Med & Biol* 2012, **38**:1163–1168.

9. Gonzales RC, Woods RE: *Digital Image Processing.* New Jersey: Prentice Hall; 2002.

10. Mandelbrot BB: *The fractal geometry of nature.* San Francisco: Macmillan; 1982.

11. Yasufuku K, Chiyo M, Sekine Y, Chhaied PN, Shibuya K, Lizasa T, Fujisawa T: Real-time endobronchial ultrasound-guided transbronchial needle aspiration of mediastinal and hilar lymph nodes. *Chest* 2004, **126**:122–128.

12. Nguyen P, Bashirzadeh F, Hundloe J, Salvado O, Dowson N, Ware R, Brant I, Bhatt M, Ravi A, Fielding D: Optical differentiation between malignant and benign lymphadenopathy by grayscale texture analysis of endobronchial ultrasound convex probe images. *Chest* 2012, **141**:709–15.

13. Bizarri M, Giuliani A, Cucina A, Anselmi FD, Soto AM, Sonnenschein C: Fractal analysis in a systems biology approach to cancer. *Semin Cancer Biol* 2011, **21**:175–182.

14. Moradi M, Abolmaesumi P, Isotalo PHA, Siemens DR, Sauerbrei EE, Mousavi P: Detection of prostate cancer from RF ultrasound echo signals using fractal analysis. *Conf Proc IEEE Eng Med Biol Soc* 2006, **2006**:2400–2403.

15. Moradi M, Mousavi P, Siemens DR, Sauerbrei EE, Isotalo P, Boag A, Abolmaesumi P: Discrete fourier analysis of ultrasound RF time series for detection of prostate cancer. *Conf Proc IEEE Eng Med Biol Soc* 2007, **2007**:1339–1342.

16. Zheng K, Wang T, Lin JL, Li D: Recognition of breast ultrasound images using a hybrid method. In *IEE/ICME International Conference on Complex Medical Engineering*; 2007:640–643.

17. Kikuchi A, Kozuma S, Kakamaki K, Saito M, Marumo G, Yasugi T, Taketani Y: Fractal tumor growth of ovarian cancer: sono graphic evaluation. *Gynecol Oncol* 2002, **87**:295–302.

13

Malignancy rates of B3-lesions in breast magnetic resonance imaging – do all lesions have to be excised?

H. Preibsch[1], L. K. Wanner[1*], A. Staebler[2], M. Hahn[3] and K. C. Siegmann-Luz[4]

Abstract

Background: Approximately 10% of all MRI-guided vacuum-assisted breast biopsies (MR-VAB) are histologically classified as B3 lesions. In most of these cases surgical excision is recommended. The aim of our study was to evaluate the malignancy rates of different B3 lesions which are visible on MRI to allow a lesion-adapted recommendation of further procedure.

Methods: Retrospective analysis of 572 consecutive MR-VAB was performed. Inclusion criteria were a representative (=successful) MR-VAB, histologic diagnosis of a B3 lesion and either the existence of a definite histology after surgical excision or proof of stability or regression of the lesion on follow-up MRI. Malignancy rates were evaluated for different histologies of B3 lesions. Lesion size and lesion morphology (mass/non-mass enhancement) on MRI were correlated with malignancy.

Results: Of all MR-VAB 43 lesions fulfilled the inclusion criteria. The malignancy rate of those B3 lesions was 23.3% (10/43). The highest malignancy rate was found in atypical ductal hyperplasia (ADH) lesions (50.0%; 4/8), 33.3% (2/6) in flat epithelial atypia (FEA), 28.6% (2/7) in lobular intraepithelial neoplasia (LIN) and 12.5% (2/16) in papillary lesions (PL). All 6 complex sclerosing lesions were benign. Mass findings were significantly more frequently malignant (31.3%, 10/32; $p < 0.05$) than non-mass findings (0/11). Small lesions measuring 5–10 mm were most often malignant (35.0%; 7/20). All large lesions (> 20 mm) were not malignant (0/10). Intermediate sized lesions (11–20 mm) turned out to be malignant in 23.1% (3/13).

Conclusions: The malignancy rate of B3 lesions which were diagnosed after MR-VAB was 23.3%. ADH, FEA and LIN showed considerable malignancy rates (50%, 33% and 29%) and should therefore undergo surgical excision. None of the cases, which were diagnosed as radial scars, non-mass enhancement or larger lesions (> 20 mm) were malignant. Here, a follow-up MRI seems to be advisable to avoid unnecessary operations.

Trial registration: Retrospective study design, waived by the IRB.

Keywords: B3 lesions, Vacuum-assisted biopsy, Breast MRI, MRI-guided breast biopsy

Background

Magnetic resonance imaging (MRI) of the breast is the most sensitive breast imaging modality. It is especially useful in patients with newly diagnosed breast cancer and high breast density on mammography, recurrent breast cancer and screening of high-risk patients. The increasing use of breast MRI results in an increasing number of suspicious findings categorised as category 4 or category 5 according to the Breast Imaging Reporting and Data System (BI-RADS®) [1]. Those lesions demand histologic clarification. If no correlating lesion can be found on second-look breast ultrasound or mammography, MRI-guided vacuum-assisted biopsy (MR-VAB) is necessary. Biopsy specimens of the breast are classified into five histologic categories according to current european guidelines [2] which are based on the international WHO classification of tumours of the breast. Breast lesions which are benign but have an uncertain malignant

---

* Correspondence: heikepreibsch@gmx.de
[1]Department of Diagnostic and Interventional Radiology, University Hospital Tuebingen, Hoppe-Seyler-Str. 3, 72076 Tuebingen, Germany
Full list of author information is available at the end of the article

potential are categorised as B3. This heterogenous group of different histologies is accompanied by an increased risk of associated malignancy. The rate of malignancy in surgical excision of mammographic B3 lesions varies between 0 and 30%, with the highest malignancy rate in ADH (20–30%) [3, 4]. Therefore a surgical biopsy is mostly recommended [5–7]. Approximately 10% of all MRI-BI-RADS® 4 and BI-RADS® 5 lesions clarified by MR-VAB turn out to be B3 lesions [8, 9]. To reduce the rate of benign surgical biopsies of MRI detected B3 lesions it would be desirable to identify low-risk and high-risk lesions before surgery. Until now there is very limited data about the malignancy rate of MRI-only B3 lesions. Therefore the clinical management of these cases is basically derived from the management of mammographic B3 lesions. Hence, the decision on the clinical management of MRI detected B3 lesions is made intuitively in each individual case and varies between different institutions.

The aim of our study was to evaluate the malignancy rate of different MRI-detected and biopsy-proven B3 lesions to optimise clinical management of these lesions due to a reduction of benign surgical excisions. Furthermore we wanded to evaluate the influence of different factors (lesion size, lesion type, patient age, history of breast cancer) on the malignancy rate to derive a management algorithm for clinical routine.

Methods
Patiens and lesions

We retrospectively reviewed the data of 572 consecutive MR-VAB which were carried out during a 100-month period at our institution. Written informed consent was waived by the Institutional Review Board (No. 372/2017BO2). Inclusion criteria were a histologically diagnosed B3 lesion by MR-VAB and either performed excisional biopsy or follow-up breast MRI at our institution. The success of MRI-guided biopsy had to be confirmed by a complete or partial lesion removal on dynamic contrast enhanced breast MRI short term after intervention, usually on the next day. Further MRI follow-up data over a time period of at least 1.5 years had to be available if the targeted B3-lesion was not completely removed or if it did not decrease in size on first follow-up MRI.

Altogether 9.4% (54/572) of the reviewed MRI-guided biopsies revealed a B3 lesion. Four of them had to be excluded because excisional biopsy or follow-up breast MRI was carried out in an external institution or not done at all. Five other patients were lost on follow-up MRI. In 2 patients, the histology of excisional biopsy could not be correlated with the previously diagnosed B3 lesion because the lesion localisation was unclear and no marker clip was set after MR-VAB.

Hence, 43 patients with 43 lesions met the inclusion criteria and could be taken for final analysis. The majority of patients underwent breast MRI due to newly diagnosed breast cancer (28/43; 65.1%). Ten of them presented with ipsilateral breast cancer, 17 patients had contralateral breast cancer and one patient had bilateral breast cancer. Five patients were followed-up after excisional biopsy (5/43; 11.6%) and another five patients had equivocal findings on mammography and ultrasound (5/43; 11.6%). Three patients had a history of breast cancer of the contralateral breast (3/43; 7.0%). In 4.7% (2/43) breast MRI was performed for the clarification of clinical symptoms ($n = 1$ nipple retraction, $n = 1$ nipple discharge).

Mean patient age was 52.0 years (30–81 years). All of them received a diagnostic contrast enhanced breast MRI 2 to 53 days (mean 12 days) before MRI-guided biopsy. Second-look breast ultrasound was performed in all cases without proof of any correlating lesion. The biopsied lesions were visible on MRI only, so MR-guided biopsy was indicated. Thirty-four of them were categorised as BI-RADS® 4 (79.5%) and 9 were categorised as BI-RADS® 5 (20.5%) on MRI.

MRI protocols

Breast MR Imaging in the diagnostic as well as in the follow-up setting was performed at 1.5 T (Achieva, Philips Healthcare, Amsterdam, Netherlands) with a dedicated double breast coil (SENSE breast coil, Philips Healthcare, Amsterdam, Netherlands). After a T2 weighted (T2w) short tau inversion recovery (STIR) sequence in transversal plane (repetition time, 3200 ms; echo time, 50 ms; inversion time, 160 ms; matrix, 512 × 512 pixels; field of view, 360 mm; slice thickness, 3.5 mm), T1w gradient echo sequences (repetition time, 7.5 ms; echo time, 3.7 ms; matrix, 512 × 512 pixels; field of view, 400 mm; flip angle, 20°; slice thickness, 1.5 mm) were acquired before and after i.v. injection of gadolinium contrast agent (0.1 mmol/kg body weight Gadobutrol, Gadovist®, Bayer HealthCare AG, Berlin, Germany). The dynamic series consisted of one unenhanced and seven series after contrast agent injection. Subtraction images of each series were calculated.

MR-guided VAB was performed using the 1.5 T MR machine described above using a dedicated breast surface coil. No T2w sequence was acquired, but a T1w dynamic series in the transversal plane (parameters and contrast agent: see above). Unenhanced, non fat-suppressed T1w sequences in the transveral plane were used as control imaging and an additional sagittal plane after the clip placement. Two different vacuum-assisted breast biopsy systems were used (11G Mammotome®, Devicor, Medical Products, Cincinnati, OH, USA; 10G Vacora®, BARD Biopsy Systems, Karlsruhe, Germany). Partial or total removal of the suspicious lesion was confirmed by a short-interval follow-up MRI one or two days after the MR-guided intervention.

Excisional biopsy and follow-up MRI

In the majority of B3 lesions (33/43; 76.7%) a surgical excision was performed. Thereby the lesions were either removed by a single excisional biopsy (20/33; 60.6%) or during breast conserving therapy or mastectomy because of synchronous ipsilateral breast cancer (13/33 = 39.4%). In 10 patients (23.3%) no surgical resection but MRI follow-up was performed. Reasons for follow-up instead of surgical excision were: a complete lesion removal on short-interval follow-up MRI, a very small lesion which was verifiable histologically only in one biopsy specimen, and the complete disappearance of the lesion on follow-up MRI after the start of neoadjuvant chemotherapy of a contralateral breast cancer. The time interval between MR-VAB and latest MRI follow-up was mean 26.5 months (range 6 to 66 months). The last control MRI showed a disappearance of the B3 lesion in 6 cases (60%), a lesion which was stable in size and contrast enhancement in 2 cases (20%), and a decreased lesion size in 2 cases (20%). In 2 lesions control intervals were shorter than 1.5 years – and showed either disappearance or a decreasing size of the lesion during MRI follow-up. Therefore all lesions with MRI follow-up (n = 10) were classified as benign.

Histopathology – Categories of B3 lesions

All histopathologic diagnoses were made by experienced breast pathologists according to current guidelines [2]. The diagnosed B3 lesions were categorised in 5 groups: Papillary lesions (PL) with or without epithelial atypia, flat epithelial atypia (FEA), radial scar respectively complex sclerosing lesions with or without epithelial atypia (RS), lobular intraepithelial neoplasia (LIN), atypical ductal hyperplasia (ADH). Lobular intraepithelial neoplasia lesions were subdivided into LIN 1, LIN 1–2 and LIN 2. There were no LIN 3 findings because they are considered as malignant lesions and therefore classified as B5a.

Data analysis

All hospital related data like medical history, clinical management, surgery, histopathology and imaging findings were taken from the Hospital Information System (KIS) and the Radiology Information System (RIS) of our institution.

Breast MR images were reviewed by two radiologists in consensus who had one and 14 years experience in reading breast MRI (L. K. W., K. C. S.-L.). MR images were analysed using a dedicated workstation (EWS, Philips Healthcare, Hamburg, Germany). Contrast kinetics were analysed by manually drawn regions of interest (ROI) on the subtraction images.

According to MRI-BI-RADS and lesion morphology all lesions were classified either as non-mass (n = 11; 25.6%; see Figs. 1 and 2) or mass lesions (n = 32; 72.7% see Figs. 3, 4, 5 and 6). The lesion size was measured manually by means of a dedicated workstation and categorised corresponding to the TNM-classification: ≤5 mm: n = 0; > 5 mm and ≤ 10 mm: n = 20; > 10 and ≤ 20 mm: n = 13; > 20 mm: n = 10. Due to the small numbers large lesions of more than 50 mm were not seperately analysed.

The malignancy rate of MRI-only B3 lesions was evaluated. To evaluate the influence of histopathologic type, MRI lesion type, MRI lesion size, and patients' history of breast cancer on the malignancy rate a correlation analysis of those variables with histology (malignant or benign) was performed.

Statistics

Statistical analysis was performed using the chi-squared test to test for stochastic independency. Correlation of the different variables (patient age, risk anamnesis, lesion size, lesion morphology and histology) with the malignancy rate was determined by using a cross table with calculation of 95% confidence intervals. Significant correlation was considered in case of $p \leq 0.05$. Analysis was made using statistical programmes (SPSS 16.0; SPSS, Chicago, IL; JMP 12, SAS, Cary, NC).

Results

Malignancy rate of different B3 lesions

The malignancy rates of each subgroup of B3 histologies are shown in Tables 1 and 2. Papillary lesions were the most frequent B3 lesions (16/43; 37.2%). Two of those

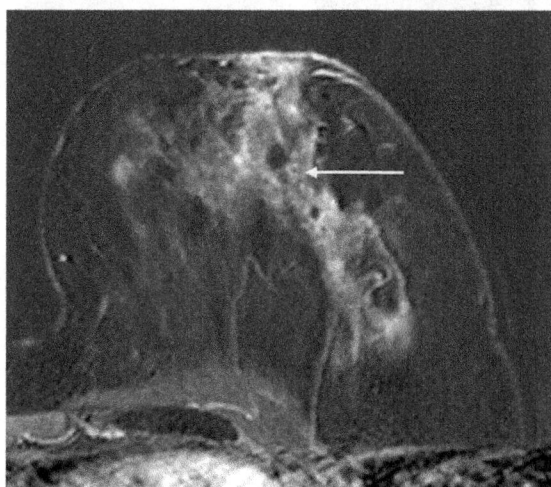

Fig. 1 Non-mass enhancement of 90 mm (subtraction images) in the upper outer quadrant of the left breast. MR-guided VAB (in 40 mm nipple distance, arrow) revealed benign histology (radial scar)

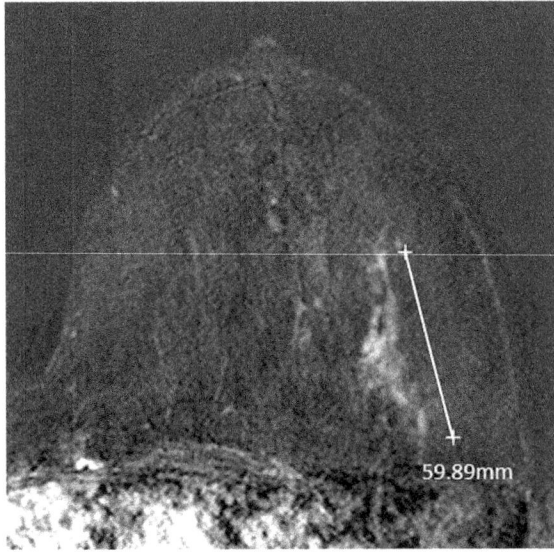

Fig. 2 Non-mass enhencement measuring 60 mm (subtraction images) in the lower outer quadrant of the left breast. MR-VAB had benign histology (papillary lesions and FEA) as a result

lesions (12.5%) turned out to be malignant in excisional biopsy (DIN 1c and DIN 2). Four of the benign lesions were only followed up (see column "no excision histology", Table 1) and appeared constant or disappeared after at least 1.5 years. The final histology of surgical excision was a papillary lesion ($n = 5$), a papillary lesion in combination with FEA ($n = 2$), ADH ($n = 1$), LIN 1 ($n = 1$) and only normal breast parenchyma (B1, $n = 1$) due to complete removal of the B3 lesion through MR-VAB.

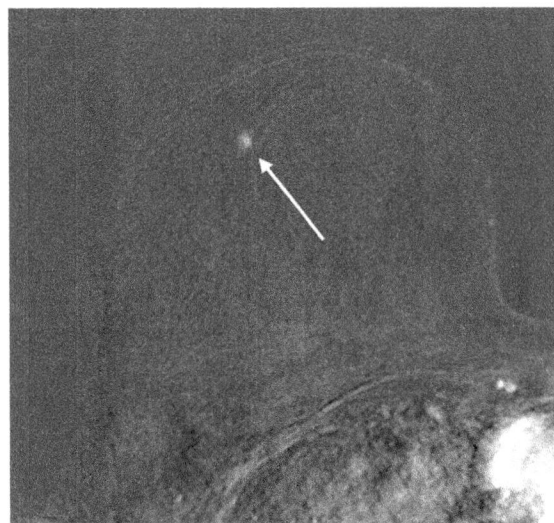

Fig. 4 Irregular shaped mass lesion (subtraction images) in the upper outer quadrant of the right breast with a size of 13 mm. MR-guided VAB showed papillary lesion and ADH on histopathology, but final histology confirmed low grade DCIS

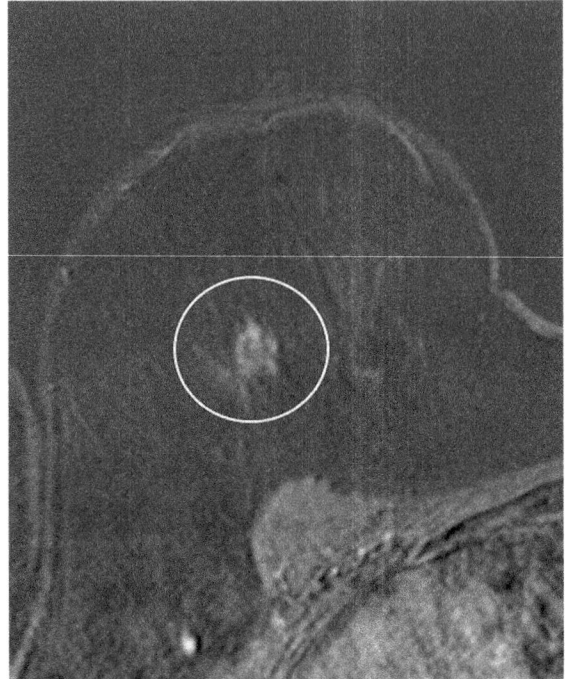

Fig. 3 Subtraction images with contrast-enhancing mass lesion of 7 mm (arrow) in the upper outer quadrant of the right breast, which showed atypical epithelial proliferation of ductal type (B3) on MR-guided biopsy, but proved to be invasive ductal carcinoma (grade 2) on final histology

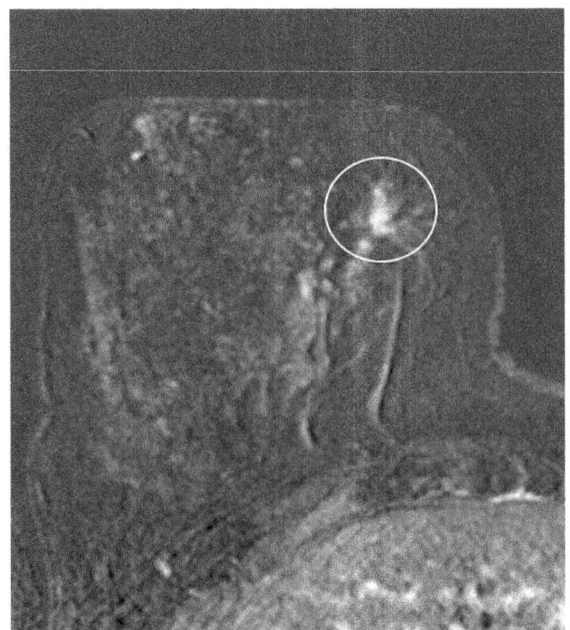

Fig. 5 MR-guided VAB of this 15 mm measuring mass lesion (subtraction images) in the lower inner quadrant of the right breast showed benign histology (radial scar in association with lobular intraepithelial neoplasia)

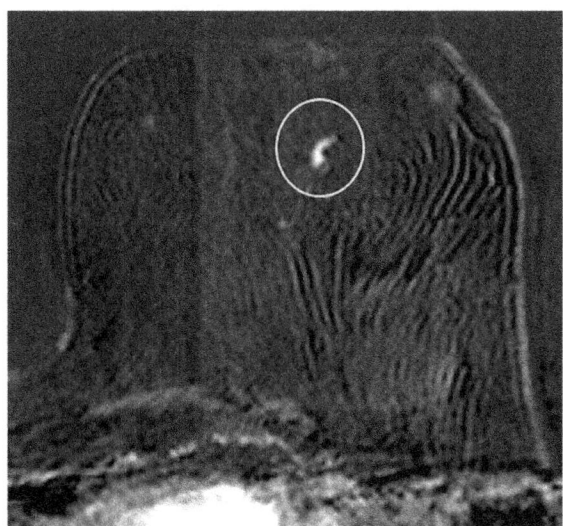

Fig. 6 This 8 mm measuring mass lesion (subtraction images) in the center of the left breast had benign histology (radial scar)

Average age of patients with PL was 52.2 years.

Six of the 43 B3 lesions (14.0%) were classified as radial scar complexes. All 6 turned out to be benign: two of the lesions were controlled by follow-up MRI, both decreasing in size after 9 months or more than 3 years, respectively. Mean patient age in this group was 48.7 years.

In 6 patients (14.0%) a FEA could be identified in MR-VAB. Two of the lesions turned out to be invasive carcinoma in excisional biopsy (33.3%). The benign lesions were associated with another B3 lesion in excisional biopsy in two cases (papillary lesion and radial scar complex, respectively). Mean age of patients with this entity was 50.5 years.

LIN was identified in 7 patients. Here, two lesions (28.6%) turned out to be malignant in final histology: one invasive carcinoma and one DIN 2 lesion. More detailed, the two malignant lesions were reported as LIN

1–2 and LIN 2 in MR-VAB, the benign lesions were LIN 1 ($n = 2$) and LIN 2 ($n = 3$) (see Table 1). Patients with LIN lesions had a mean age of 57.1 years.

Eight of the 43 B3 lesions (18.6%) were classified as ADH, of which 4 lesions turned out to be malignant (50%). Three lesions turned out to be invasive carcinomas, one was classified as DIN 1c. Mean age of patients with ADH was 50.5 years.

The respective positive predictive values (PPV) are 50% for ADH, 33% for FEA, 29% for LIN, 13% for papillary lesions and 0% for radial scars. In total, the PPV for B3 lesions was 24% in our study (also shown in Table 1).

Risk anamnesis and age of patient

Considering risk anamnesis of the patients, in 5 of 10 women (50%) with recently diagnosed carcinoma of the ipsilateral breast, the suspicious B3 lesion turned out to be malignant. In case of contralateral breast cancer, only 17.6% (3/17) of the B3 lesions had a malignant outcome (Table 2). In 25% of the patients with a history of breast cancer and in 11% of the patients without history of breast cancer the outcome was malignant. Risk anamnesis was a factor significantly influencing the malignancy rate ($p = 0.016$).

Considering the age of the patients worst outcome was detected in patients from 46 to 50 years: 6 out of 14 B3 lesions were malignant (42.9%). In the groups from 51 to 55 and older than 55 years, 20% of the lesions had a malignant final histology (2/10 each). Lesions in patients ≤45 years were in no case malignant (0/9) (see Table 3).

Age range of patients with malignant final histology was 46 to 77 years (mean 53.4 years). Patients with benign outcome had a mean age of 52.0 years (30 to 81 years). Patient age was no significant factor influencing the malignancy rate acoording to cross tabulation ($p = 0.530$).

Table 1 Outcome stratified into the different histologic entities classified as B3

Type of B3 lesion	Final histology				PPV (%)	Total
	Benign	DCIS	Malignant invasive	No excision histology		
PL	10	2	0	4	13	16
Radial scar	4	0	0	2	0	6
FEA	3	0	2	1	33	6
LIN 1	1	0	0	1	0	2
LIN 1–2	0	1	0	0	100	1
LIN 2	3	0	1	0	25	4
LIN total	4	1	1	1	29	7
ADH	2	1	3	2	50	8
Total	23	4	6	10	24	43

Papillary lesion (PL); LIN lesions are listed subdivided into LIN 1, LIN 1–2 and LIN 2 lesions (italic), and in total

Table 2 Outcome dependent on individual risk anamnesis of the patients

Risk anamnesis			
	Total	Malignant	% Malignant
Proven ipsilateral Ca	10	5	50
Proven contralateral Ca	17	3	18
Proven bilateral Ca	1	0	0
No present or history of Ca (partly familiar high risk situation)	9	1	11
Mamillary retraction/ secretion	2	0	0
History of Ca	4	1	25

Lesion size and morphology

B3 lesions measured between 5 and 90 mm (mean 18.1 mm) in largest diameter. Non-mass lesions were significantly greater than mass lesions with a mean size of 40.3 mm (7–90 mm) and 10.5 mm (5–24 mm), respectively. Seven out of 20 B3 lesions ≤10 mm had a malignant final histology (35.0%). Lesions from 11 to 20 mm were malignant in only 23.1% (3/13). Lesions taller than 20 mm were in none of the cases malignant (0/10) (see Table 4). Hence, lesions > 20 mm were significantly less likely to be malignant ($p = 0.045$).

Thirteen of the 16 papillary lesions (81.3%) had a mass aspect (including the two malignant lesions) and three (18.7%) were classified as non-mass lesions. Two of the radial scar complexes presented as mass (33.3%), 4 (66.7%) as non-mass lesions. Four of the 6 FEA lesions (66.7%) presented as masses on MRI, including both malignant lesions. All LIN lesions had mass appearance. Six of the 8 ADH lesions (75%) had mass appearance (including all 4 malignant lesions).

Hence, all malignant lesions had a mass aspect on diagnostic MRI (10/10). Non-mass lesions were benign in all cases ($p = 0.031$). Out of 33 lesions with benign outcome (final histology or follow-up MRI), 22 (66.7%) had mass morphology (see Table 5).

Discussion

Some B3 lesions have the potential of malignant degeneration in terms of precancerous lesions, such as ADH [5] and possibly papillary lesions. Some B3 lesions are so-called "indicator lesions", which are frequently associated with coexistent higher grade transformations, i.e.

Table 3 Outcome dependent on patient age

Age				
	≤ 45	46–50	51–55	> 55
n	9	14	10	10
Benign	9	8	8	8
Malignant	0	6	2	2
% Malignant	0	43	20	20

Table 4 Outcome dependent on lesion size

Lesion size	≤ 10 mm	11–20 mm	> 20 mm
n	20	13	10
Benign	13	10	10
Malignant	7	3	0
% Malignant	35	23	0

lobular neoplasia [6]. Analysing actual management of these lesions, practice is varying greatly among surgeons [6]. Because of several surveys reporting high rates of malignancy, routine excision is often recommended [5, 6]. More recent publications suggest vacuum-assisted excision instead of surgical excision in several B3 lesions [10].

As with the term B3 lesions a heterogenous group of lesions with different potential of malignany is summarised, some authors suggest a subclassification according to the presence of atypia into B3a and B3b [11]. This suggestion has not entered guidelines so far.

Most studies evaluating the frequency of malignancy of B3 lesions in excision histology focus on screening-detected mammographic lesions [12–14]. The influence of presentation of the B3 lesion in core biopsies (screen-detected vs. symptomatic) under ultrasound or stereotactic guidance has also been investigated [15]. In a study of 31 patients with high-risk lesions on breast MRI no significant differences considering patient age, indications for breast MRI, size of lesion or morphological features of biopsied lesions was found [16]. The authors concluded that all high-risk lesions diagnosed at MR-guided vacuum-assisted biopsy require surgical excision. Other authors state that in selected cases, if the suspicious lesion is not associated with epithelial atypia, removal by vacuum-assisted biopsy is a safe alternative to surgical excision [13]. Overall, data concerning the outcome of those lesions is still limited and there is no uniform suggestion of further treatment.

Regarding certain B3 lesions, our findings confirm that operative resection is necessary: Particularly ADH show a malignancy rate of 50%. This result is in agreement with a reported malignancy rate of 32 to 59% in mammographic screening [11, 17–19]. The final diagnosis of ADH cannot be made in minimal-invasive biopsy, because here the determination of extensiveness of the lesion is not possible, which is however one of the three main criteria defining ADH [19, 20]. The European

Table 5 Outcome dependent on lesion morphology

Lesion morphology	non-mass	mass	% masses
n	11	32	74
Benign	11	22	67
Malignant	0	10	100
% Malignant	0	31	

Working Group for Breast Screening Pathology therefore recommends to use the term "atypical epithelial proliferation of ductal type" (AEPDT) instead of ADH in diagnostics of minimal-invasive biopsy [2]. The dimension of the lesion is at the same time the most important criterion in the differentiation to low-grade DCIS. Accordingly, the operative resection of an ADH/ AEPDT lesion cannot be questioned.

FEA and LIN also show relevant malignancy rates of 33% respectively 29% in our study and therefore require surgical excision. Crystal et al. observed even higher malignancy rates of 50% for LIN (4/8) and also 50% for FEA (1/2) [14]. Regarding FEA, the precursor lesion of ADH in the low-grade pathway, only very few clinical outcome-studies exist. In observational studies, an association of FEA with lobular neoplasia, ADH, low-grade DCIS, invasive G1 carcinoma and tubular carcinoma is indicated [21]. In approximately one third of subsequent resections, an additional lesion of the low-grade pathway is found [17, 19, 22]. Though, interpretation of these studies is limited because of lacking radiologic-pathologic correlation in several cases and because of different indications for surgical excision. With a malignancy rate of 33% in FEA lesions, our study supports the findings of these previous studies.

Concerning LIN there is still no guideline for the handling of these lesions. Weigel S et al. suggest diagnostic excision of LN lesions only if the lesion is not a coincidental finding accompanying a focal lesion or microcalcifications and if there is a residual lesion detectable after biopsy – with certain radiologic-pathologic correlation [19, 23]. Otherwise annual control mammography is recommended. Our data, however, with a malignancy rate of 29% for LIN, indicates that operative resection in these cases should not be neglected. Therefore especially regarding LIN, further clarification by means of higher patient numbers is required.

Although some studies observed no malignant final histology after MR-VAB of papillary lesions [16] the malignancy rate of our study of 11% for PL however indicates a quite considerable risk for this entity.

In radial scar complexes a more conservative position regarding surgical excision seems justifiable. In our study, out of 6 radial scars, no malignant outcome occurred, which is in accordance with the study of Crystal et al. [16]. Contrarily, Heller S L et al. published data showing high upgrade rates for radial scar lesions at MRI-guided breast biopsies [24]. Hence, regarding this entity, further studies with larger patient cohorts are also essential.

Regarding imaging features predictive of malignancy some authors observed no significant imaging features of upgrade [24]. Here, our study yields some interesting results: mass lesions seem to have a significantly higher malignancy rate than non-mass lesions (31% compared to 0%). This is in accordance with a large retrospective multi-institutional study showing that upgrades of ADH and DCIS diagnosed at MR-guided VAB are significantly associated with the presence of a mass on MR imaging [25]. Furthermore, our study indicates a higher malignant potential for smaller lesions ≤10 mm (PPV 35%) compared to lesions measuring 11–20 mm (PPV 23%) in case of MR-only lesions. Lesions > 20 mm were benign in 100% (10/10). The additional finding that non-mass enhancement in most cases appears as a taller lesion underlines these results. Further investigations in larger patient cohorts are needed to clarify this subject.

With a malignancy rate of 50% for patients with a recently diagnosed carcinoma of the ipsilateral breast, our study confirms the results of Heller et al. stating a significantly higher risk of an upgrade of high-risk lesions in case of ipsilateral cancer or ipsilateral high-risk lesion [24]. Our results also indicate the relevance of previous carcinoma on risk assessment, whereas here our case numbers are too small to be able to differentiate between history of carcinoma of the ipsi- and contralateral breast.

Considering patient age, our data provide no statistical significance, but give clear indication that the outcome of B3 lesions is most unfavorable in the age cohort from 46 to 50 years.

The study has several limitations. Most important, the limited number of patients with 43 inclosed B3 lesions permits only restricted conclusions concerning significance, especially when divided into subgroups. Second, the retrospective study design does not permit to fully reproduce the reasons for indication of surgical excision in all cases. Third, 72% of the patients were referred for breast MRI due to newly diagnosed ipsilateral breast cancer (65%) or history of contraleteral breast cancer (7%), which influences the PPV for malignancy in final histology.

Summarised, the appropriate management of B3 lesions is still discussed controversially in literature. Our study shows that B3 lesions are a summary of different entities with different malignancy rates and that treatment accordingly should be adapted. Further studies with larger patient cohorts and metaanalyses of existing surveys are necessary.

Conclusions

Our study indicates that management of B3 MR-only lesions of the breast should be adapted to the respective histology. ADH, FEA and LIN should undergo surgical treatment, whereas our data did not show any malignancy in complex sclerosing lesions, non-mass lesions or lesions larger than 2 cm.

Funding

We acknowledge support by Deutsche Forschungsgemeinschaft and Open Access Publishing Fund of University of Tuebingen.

Authors' contributions

All authors (HP, LKW, AS, MH and KCS-L) have made substantial contributions to acquisition of data, or analysis and interpretation of data. They have been involved in drafting the manuscript or revising it critically for important intellectual content. The authors have given final approval of the version to be published and agreed to be accountable for all aspects of the work in ensuring that questions related to the accuracy or integrity of any part of the work are appropriately investigated and resolved. Each author – namely HP, LKW, AS, MH and KCS-L – has participated sufficiently in the work to take public responsibility for appropriate portions of the content.

Competing interests

The authors declare that they have no competing interests.

Author details

[1]Department of Diagnostic and Interventional Radiology, University Hospital Tuebingen, Hoppe-Seyler-Str. 3, 72076 Tuebingen, Germany. [2]Department of Pathology and Neuropathology, University Hospital Tuebingen, Liebermeisterstr. 8, 72076 Tuebingen, Germany. [3]Department of Obstetrics and Gynecology, University Hospital Tuebingen, Calwerstr. 7, 72076 Tuebingen, Germany. [4]Diagnostic Breast Centre and Breast Cancer Screening Brandenburg East, Koepenicker Str. 29, 15711 Koenigs Wusterhausen, Germany.

References

1. Morris EA, Comstock CE, Lee CH, et al. ACR BI-RADS® Magnetic Resonance Imaging. In: ACR BI-RADS® Atlas, Breast Imaging Reporting and Data System. Reston: American College of Radiology; 2013.
2. Wells CAAI, Apostolikas N, Bellocq JP. Quality assurance guidelines for pathology. In: Perry NMBM, de Wolf C, editors. EC working group on breast screening pathology: Quality assurance guidelines for pathology in mammography screening – open biopsy and resection specimens European guidelines for quality assurance in mammography screening. 4th ed. Luxembourg: Office for Official Publications of the Eropean Communities; 2006. p. 219–56.
3. Perry N, Broeders M, de Wolf C, Törnberg S, Holland R, von Karsa L. European guidelines for quality assurance in breast cancer screening and diagnosis. Fourth edition--summary document. Ann Oncol. 2008;19:614–22.
4. Saladin C, Haueisen H, Kampmann G, Oehlschlegel C, Seifert B, Rageth L, et al. Lesions with unclear malignant potential (B3) after minimally invasive breast biopsy: evaluation of vacuum biopsies performed in Switzerland and recommended further management. Acta Radiol. 2016;57:815–21.
5. Jacobs TW, Connolly JL, Schnitt SJ. Nonmalignant lesions in breast core needle biopsies: to excise or not to excise? Am J Surg Pathol. 2002;26:1095–110.
6. Johnson NB, Collins LC. Update on percutaneous needle biopsy of non-malignant breast lesions. Adv Anat Pathol. 2009;16:183–95.
7. Nizri E, Schneebaum S, Klausner JM, Menes TS. Current management practice of breast borderline lesions--need for further research and guidelines. Am J Surg. 2012;203:721–5.
8. Siegmann-Luz KC, Bahrs SD, Preibsch H, Hattermann V, Claussen CD. Management of breast lesions detectable only on MRI. Rofo. 2014;186:30–6.
9. Bahrs SD, Hattermann V, Preibsch H, Hahn M, Staebler A, Claussen CD, Siegmann-Luz KC. MR imaging-guided vacuum-assisted breast biopsy: reduction of false-negative biopsies by short-term control MRI 24-48 h after biopsy. Clin Radiol. 2014;69:695–702.
10. Rageth CJ, O'Flynn EA, Comstock C, Kurtz C, Kubik R, Madjar H, et al. First international consensus conference on lesions of uncertain malignant potential in the breast (B3 lesions). Breast Cancer Res Treat. 2016;159:203–13.
11. de Beça FF, Rasteiro C, Correia A, Costa S, Amendoeira I. Improved malignancy prediction by B3 breast lesions subclassification. Ann Diagn Pathol. 2013;17:434–6.
12. El-Sayed ME, Rakha EA, Reed J, Lee AH, Evans AJ, Ellis IO. Predictive value of needle core biopsy diagnoses of lesions of uncertain malignant potential (B3) in abnormalities detected by mammographic screening. Histopathology. 2008;53:650–7.
13. Rakha EA, Lee AH, Jenkins JA, Murphy AE, Hamilton LJ, Ellis IO. Characterization and outcome of breast needle core biopsy diagnoses of lesions of uncertain malignant potential (B3) in abnormalities detected by mammographic screening. Int J Cancer. 2011;129:1417–24.
14. Hayes BD, O'Doherty A, Quinn CM. Correlation of needle core biopsy with excision histology in screen-detected B3 lesions: the Merrion breast screening unit experience. J Clin Pathol. 2009;62:1136–40.
15. Maclean GM, Courtney SP, Umeh H, Sanjeev S, McCormick C, Smith BM. Is mode of presentation of B3 breast core biopsies (screen-detected or symptomatic) a distinguishing factor in the final histopathologic result or risk of diagnosis of malignancy? World J Surg. 2013;37:2607–12.
16. Crystal P, Sadaf A, Bukhanov K, McCready D, O'Malley F, Helbich TH. High-risk lesions diagnosed at MRI-guided vacuum-assisted breast biopsy: can underestimation be predicted? Eur Radiol. 2011;21:582–9.
17. Flegg KM, Flaherty JJ, Bicknell AM, Jain S. Surgical outcomes of borderline breast lesions detected by needle biopsy in a breast screening program. World J Surg Oncol. 2010;8:78.
18. Lieske B, Ravichandran D, Alvi A, Lawrence DA, Wright DJ. Screen-detected breast lesions with an indeterminate (B3) core needle biopsy should be excised. Eur J Surg Oncol. 2008;34:1293–8.
19. Weigel S, Decker T, Korsching E, Biesheuvel C, Wöstmann A, Böcker W, et al. Minimal invasive biopsy results of "uncertain malignant potential" in digital mammography screening: high prevalence but also high predictive value for malignancy. Rofo. 2011;183:743–8.
20. Page DL, Dupont WD, Rogers LW, Jensen RA, Schuyler PA. Continued local recurrence of carcinoma 15-25 years after a diagnosis of low-grade-ductal carcinoma in situ of the breast treated only by biopsy. Cancer. 1995;76:1197–200.
21. Abdel-Fatah TM, Powe DG, Hodi Z, Reis-Filho JS, Lee AH, Ellis IO. Morphologic and molecular evolutionary pathways of low nuclear grade invasive breast cancers and their putative precursor lesions: further evidence to support the concept of low nuclear grade breast neoplasia family. Am J Surg Pathol. 2008;32:513–23.
22. Kunju LP, Kleer CG. Significance of flat epithelial atypia on mammotome core needle biopsy: should it be excised? Hum Pathol. 2007;38:35–41.
23. Kreienberg R, Albert US, Follmann M, Kopp IB, Kühn T, Wöckel A. Interdisciplinary GoR level III guidelines for the diagnosis, therapy and follow-up Care of Breast Cancer: short version - AWMF registry no.: 032-045OL AWMF-register-Nummer: 032-045OL - Kurzversion 3.0, Juli 2012. Geburtshilfe Frauenheilkd. 2013;73:556–83.
24. Heller SL, Elias K, Gupta A, Greenwood HI, Mercado CL, Moy L. Outcome of high-risk lesions at MRI-guided 9-gauge vacuum- assisted breast biopsy. AJR Am J Roentgenol. 2014;202:237–45.
25. Verheyden C, Pages-Bouic E, Balleyguier C, Cherel P, Lepori D, Laffargue G, et al. Underestimation Rate at MR Imaging-guided Vacuum-assisted Breast Biopsy: A Multi-Institutional Retrospective Study of 1509 Breast Biopsies. Radiology. 2016;281:708–19.

14

Mapping breast tissue types by miniature radio-frequency near-field spectroscopy sensor in ex-vivo freshly excised specimens

Zvi Kaufman[1,7]*, Haim Paran[1], Ilana Haas[1], Patricia Malinger[1], Tania Zehavi[2], Tamar Karni[3], Izhak Pappo[3], Judith Sandbank[4], Judith Diment[5] and Tanir Allweis[6]

Abstract

Background: Receiving real-time information on tissue properties while performing biopsy procedures has the potential of improving biopsy accuracy. The study goal was to test the ability of a miniature flexible Radio-Frequency (RF) sensor (Dune Medical Devices), designed to be mounted on the surface of surgical tools, in measuring and mapping the various breast tissue types and abnormalities in terms of electrical properties.

Methods: Between January and October 2012, 102 patients undergoing lumpectomy, open-biopsy or mastectomy, in 3 medical centers, were enrolled in this study. The device was applied to freshly excised specimens, with registration between device measurements and histology analysis. Based on histology, the dielectric properties of the various tissue types were derived. Additionally, the ability of the device to differentiate between malignant and non-malignant tissue was assessed.

Results: A total of 4322 measurements from 106 specimens from 102 patients were analyzed. The dielectric properties of 10 tissue types in the low RF-frequency range were measured, showing distinct differences between the various types. Based on the dielectric properties, a score variable was derived, which showed a correlation of 90 % between the RF measurements and the tissue types. Differentiation ability between tissue types was characterized using ROC curve analysis, with AUC of 0.96, and sensitivity and specificity of 90 and 91 % respectively, for tissue feature sizes at or above 0.8 mm.

Conclusions: Using a radio-frequency near-field spectroscopy miniature flexible sensor the dielectric properties of multiple breast tissue types, both normal and abnormal, were evaluated. The results show promise in differentiating between various breast tissue types, and specifically for differentiation between cancer and normal tissues.

Keywords: Breast cancer, Lumpectomy, Breast biopsy, Surgical margin, Radio-frequency near-field spectroscopy

Background

The response of matter to electromagnetic fields is characterized by the material's dielectric properties: permittivity and conductivity. The conductivity is a measure of the ease with which free electric charges can migrate through the material; the permittivity reflects the extent to which bound charge distributions can be distorted through polarization by an external field.

Differences in dielectric properties between human tissues and specifically between benign and malignant tissue have been studied and are well established [1–3]. Tissue dielectric properties are determined by concentration and mobility of intra and extracellular components, cell size, structure and arrangement, amongst other characteristics. Specifically, the tissue dielectric properties have been extensively studied in breast tissue [4–7], where differences between tissue types, and specifically between normal and malignant were observed over a broad range of frequencies. These properties have been successfully used to differentiate between normal and malignant breast tissue [8, 9] and for intraoperative

---

* Correspondence: zvikau@netvision.net.il
[1]Breast unit, Meir Medical Center, Kfar Saba, Israel
[7]Department of Surgery, Meir Medical Center, Kfar Sava, Israel
Full list of author information is available at the end of the article

margin assessment during lumpectomies [10]. Normal breast tissue is heterogeneous, being composed of three different types of tissue (Adipose, Glandular, and Connective), In all the studies to date, the evaluated dielectric properties were based on measurements and comparisons performed on scales larger than the intrinsic scale of tissue heterogeneity within breast tissue. Therefore, the differences observed represent average values of the dielectric properties. Results were generally reported on properties of "normal" and "cancer" types. In some reports [5, 7] an attempt has been made to partition between the three intrinsic tissue types of the normal breast. There has been no reporting on the specific properties of glandular and connective tissue types. Also, cancer of the breast has three major types: Ductal Carcinoma *in Situ* (DCIS), Invasive Ductal Cancer (IDC), and Invasive Lobular Cancer (ILC). The dielectric properties of these types, to date, have not been characterized separately. Additionally, specifically of importance in breast biopsy procedures, the dielectric characteristics of abnormalities in the breast that may progress to cancer, such as: non-malignant proliferative, non-malignant proliferative with atypia, and LCIS, have not yet been characterized.

The burden of breast cancer is high. Approximately 230,480 American women are diagnosed annually, and 39,520 women die from this disease [11]. Global cancer statistics show that breast cancer is the most frequently diagnosed cancer and the leading cause of cancer death among females, accounting for 23 % of total cancer cases and 14 % of cancer deaths [12]. The majority of breast cancers are diagnosed as a result of an abnormal mammogram or ultrasound, and in selected populations abnormal MRI findings. Some lesions are found by the patient or her physician as a palpable mass. Not all abnormal findings diagnosed by the methods mentioned represent cancer. To determine whether a mass in the breast is a suspicious mass or not the BI-RADS System was developed [13]. All patients with a BI-RADS category of 4 and 5 should undergo a biopsy. Those with category 3 should be followed more frequently. A clinically suspicious mass should also be biopsied, regardless of imaging findings, as about 15 % of such lesions can be mammographically occult [14].

Screening mammography is the most common way to diagnose early breast cancer but carries a high rate of recalls (16.3 % at first and 9.3 % at subsequent mammography) [15]. Biopsy is further recommended in 0.6–1 % of all screened women [16, 17]. Millions of women are screened each year, therefore these figures represent a high number of breast biopsies performed each year, emphasizing the need for accurate biopsy.

During the breast biopsy procedure part or all of a suspicious breast tissue growth is sampled and examined for the presence of cancer, most often in a minimally invasive procedure. Current biopsy techniques have several limitations: First, patients diagnosed with Atypical Ductal Hyperplasia (ADH) are routinely sent for an open surgical biopsy, following which 10–25 % of these patients' diagnosis will be 'upgraded' DCIS, which requires a further lumpectomy or mastectomy [18–21]. Second, patients with a diagnosis of DCIS in biopsy will undergo lumpectomy, typically without a sentinel lymph node biopsy. Following the Lumpectomy, about 20 % of these patients' diagnosis will be upgraded to invasive cancer, requiring a further surgery for node biopsy. Third, studies have shown that up to 10 % of patients endure repeat biopsies [22, 23]. These repeat biopsies reveal carcinoma in up to 25 % of cases [24]. Forth, published data show a 1–7 % false negative rate with current breast core biopsy techniques [25].

The inaccuracies in the biopsy procedure result mainly from the uncertainty in the exact location from which the biopsy sample is taken relative to the image, and from the fact that the features presented on imaging may not be the most abnormal tissue present. Having an *in-situ*, at the needle tip, tissue characterization ability when performing biopsy procedures has the potential to increase the accuracy of the procedure.

In the presented study, we use a miniature, 0.8 mm in diameter, RF sensor to characterize the dielectric properties of different breast tissue types and abnormities. Based on these characteristics, we tested the potential of this type of sensor in differentiating between normal, abnormal, and malignant breast tissue. The sensor has a coaxial opening that results in a fringing electrical field close to the sensor surface. The sensor is manufactured using flexible printed circuit board technology and can be potentially placed on various devices having different geometries, such as open surgical tools as well as minimally invasive ones, like core biopsy needles. A similar device has been already been used for evaluating freshly excised radical prostatectomy specimens [26].

Material and methods
Ethics, consent and permissions
The study was performed at 3 sites under institutional review board approval and in accordance with the Declaration of Helsinki. All subjects signed an informed consent.

General design
Between January to October 2012, subjects undergoing lumpectomy, open biopsy or mastectomy procedure were enrolled. Inclusion criteria specified subjects over 18 years of age.

Tissue measurements were performed on freshly excised breast specimens. Measurements were compared to histological analysis. All medical staff members were blinded to device output. Specimen handling before and after measurements was performed according to routine procedures. As the device was used on ex-vivo specimens in the pathology lab, safety aspects (adverse effects) of the study and device use were monitored only with regards to specimen handling and analysis.

Device description

The device (Dune Medical Devices Ltd., Israel) used in this study is a near-field Radio-Frequency (RF) spectroscopy-based real-time detection device. It consists of a hand-held, pencil like, probe, connected by cables to a console. The console sends RF waves at several frequencies, transmitted to the tissue through the sensor at the probe's tip. The frequencies (4–30 MHz) were chosen based on design considerations, and on where differences between breast tissue types are expected to be substantial [5, 6]. The frequency range at which the tissue is probed has no ionizing effects. The amplitude of the transmitted RF field across the sensor opening is low. The voltage across the sensor is ~ 0.1 Volts, much lower than the ionization voltage. The transmitted RF power is ~ 0.1 mW per square mm. Each measurement takes ~ 3 msec. The RF signals are reflected from the tissue through the sensor, and are received by the console. The sensor is designed as a multi-layer transmission line structure with a coaxial end opening. It is fabricated from flexible circuit board materials, making the sensor (including the transmission line structure) mechanically flexible and thin. The sensor coaxial end conductive regions are gold–plated. The diameter of the sensor coaxial end is 0.8 mm. The sensor end is attached to the flat tip of the probe. The size of the coaxial sensor is much smaller than the transmitted wavelengths, as the highest frequency of 30Mhz corresponds to a wavelength of 10 m. Under this condition the penetration depth of the field is ~0.078 of the coaxial opening [27]. This translates to a penetration depth of ~0.07 mm.

The sensor has a coaxial opening that results in a fringing electrical field close to the sensors surface, which enables direct calculation of the impedance (dielectric properties - permittivity and conductivity) of the tissue in contact with the sensor. Signals at specific frequencies are transmitted to the sensor. The fringing field interacts with the tissue so that the reflected signals are dependent on the impedance of the tissue close to the sensor. From the reflection amplitude and phase the impedance of the tissue at each frequency measured is extracted using the process described in [28].

Tissue measurements and processing

Following excision, the fresh specimens were directly delivered to the pathology laboratory; the fresh, non-fixed, specimens were then fully inked and sliced into 5–7 transverse sections, approximately 1 cm thick, in a bread-loaf manner.

One or two transverse-cut sections were immediately sampled by the probe. The time between performing the measurements and tissue excision was no longer than 30 min. Specially designed stencils were placed on the slice. These stencils contained a matrix of holes of diameter 3.2 mm, which accommodated the probe's distal end, enabling it to contact the tissue surface (Fig. 1). The grid spacing was 6 mm. The probe was operated manually to measure all measurement sites of the slice through the stencil (Fig. 1). Good contact between the sensor and tissue was achieved by applying mechanical pressure by hand to the tissue in the stencil holes. Each individual measurement took 1–3 s to complete. Designated software utility helped the user to record the location of the measurements within the stencil. Once a slice was fully measured it was fixed (24–48 h) and further processed for histological analysis. The histological analysis of the slices was performed en-face, without any further sectioning, so that the full surface of the measurement locations was available for histological examination. The relative position of the stencil and the slice was maintained, thus the sampling locations remain fully registered. The Histological slides were prepared for each measured slice. As the diameter of the stencil holes is 3.2 mm and the probe tip diameter is 3.0 mm, it is estimated that the potential registration error between the actual measured site and the analyzed tissue sample was less than 0.1 mm.

Data analysis

Tissue

Each measurement site was histologically analyzed. The tissue composition and feature sizes of the various tissue types present were recorded. The sites were then classified according to their most advanced abnormality within the 1 mm central area and divided into 6

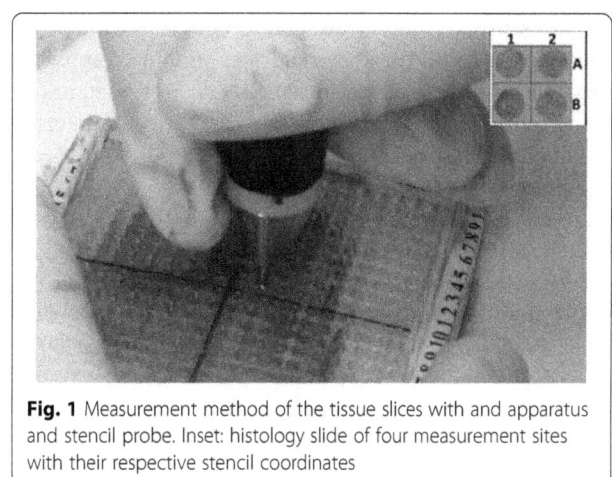

Fig. 1 Measurement method of the tissue slices with and apparatus and stencil probe. Inset: histology slide of four measurement sites with their respective stencil coordinates

categories [29]: 1) normal and non-malignant non-proliferative abnormal tissue; 2) non-malignant proliferative abnormal tissue; 3) non-malignant proliferative tissue with atypia; 4) LCIS; 5) DCIS and 6) invasive cancer.

Measurements

The permittivity and conductivity of each measured tissue site were extracted at all measured frequencies.

Dielectric properties

A subset of measurements in which the size of a given tissue type, the feature size, was larger than 0.7 mm was used for assessment of dielectric properties of various tissue types. As the sensor's size is 0.8 mm, selection of such feature sizes ensures that the sensor came in contact with the specific tissue type being assessed. Analysis was performed by linear regression [30]. Only tissue types presenting in >5 samples were considered. This provided an estimation error of no more than 50 %.

Score variable

The same subset of measurements used to determine the dielectric properties of tissues was used in order to derive a single score variable. The score variable was calculated as a linear combination (using linear discriminant analysis) [31] of the dielectric properties, a linear combination that exhibited differentiation between two selected categories, e.g. normal and malignant tissue. The discriminant analysis was performed for each measurement frequency separately. The analysis presented is based on the results for 10 Mhz. The correlation of the score variable values with tissue type categories was characterized by a linear regression analysis.

ROC curve analysis

A dichotomous device output (positive/negative) for each measurement was derived by placing a threshold for the score variable value. Measurements with a score value lower than the threshold were defined as being negative, and those above the threshold were defined as being positive. Device indication (positive/negative) of qualified measurements was compared to tissue histology. The threshold levels of the score variable were scanned to generate receiver operating characteristics (ROC) curves. Sensitivity and specificity at the optimal cutoff points (points on the ROC curve closest to the upper left corner of the axes) were extracted. This analysis was repeated for normal vs. all abnormal types (malignant and non-malignant). The score variable of normal vs. malignant tissues was also used to estimate the differentiation ability as a function of the malignant tissue feature size.

Results

Out of 104 enrolled subjects, 102 were analyzed (their baseline characteristics are presented in Table 1). Two subjects were excluded from the analysis: one due to neo-adjuvant treatment and one specimen was inserted into formaldehyde prior to device use. Four subjects had bilateral surgery, thus 106 specimens were included in the analysis. Device measurements were found to be non-destructive and had no effect on the specimens or on the ability to inspect them histopathologically.

In the 106 specimens included in the analysis 5262 measurements were performed. Altogether 940 measurements (18 %) were not analyzed. 388 sites were not reproduced during slide preparation, i.e. no histology to compare to measurement, and in 119 sites the exact registration between measurement site and histology could not be verified. The remaining 433 sites were disqualified due to predefined criteria related to poor quality of the histology slides (fragmented tissue, torn tissue, uneven tissue surface, color covering sample). Altogether, 4322 measurements were analyzed. The distribution of tissue histology of all qualified tissue measurements is shown in Table 2. Note that the

Table 1 Patient Cohort

Characteristic	Value
Number of Patients	102
Number of Specimens	106
Age, mean (range)	57 (18–9) years
Procedure	
Lumpectomy	74
Open biopsy	17
Mastectomy	15
Lesion size, mean (range)	1.9 (0.2–13.5) cm
Histology	
IDC	50
ILC	6
DCIS	21
Mixed invasive	6
Other cancer	4
Non-malignant[a]	19
ER/PR[b]	
+/+	64
-/-	7
+/-	9
HER2[c]	
+	24
-	41

[a] 5 ADH, 10 Fibroadenoma, 4 Other
[b] 9 Undetermined
[c] 24 Undetermined

Table 2 Distribution of tissue histology

	Tissue type	Number of samples
Malignant	In- Situ	111
	Invasive	390
Abnormal (Non-Malignant)	Hyperplasia	25
	Cyst	41
	Misc. Non Proliferative	63
	Fibroadenoma	210
	Atypia	19
	Misc. Proliferative	10
	LCIS	2
Normal	Adipose	2435
	Connective	777
	Mixture	239

numbers present the most advanced abnormality, according to the established 6 category scale described earlier, within each tissue site analyzed. This was recorded irrespective of size of the abnormality within the sensed area. For example, in some of the sites categorized as malignant some non-malignant abnormalities may be present, as well.

Dielectric properties

The dielectric properties (conductivity, y-axis, and permittivity, x-axis) of 10 tissue types, as assessed from the data at 4, 10 and 30 MHz, are presented in Fig. 2. The assessment was based on a subset of 1253 tissue measurements which had feature sizes above 0.7 mm of a single tissue type. The dielectric properties were calculated using a linear regression with respect to the relative tissue compositions of these samples. Only tissue types that were present within at least 5 samples were analyzed. The estimation error for each tissue type is also presented. The error depends on the actual spread of values as measured, the feature sizes, and the number of the samples at which a given tissue type is present (e.g. the error for ADH is larger as the number of samples containing ADH was only 7). Additional tissue types present in the breast were either not present in the subset or were very rare, rendering the assessment impractical. The results are similar across the frequency range measured, but the distinction between the various breast tissue types is clearer at 4 and 10 MHz.

Correlation between tissue types and score variable

Figure 3 presents the average (and standard deviation) of the score variable (y-axis), derived based on the tissue dielectric properties, vs. the tissue type categories (x-axis). Although tissue were grouped into 6 categories, in the data used (feature size >0.7 mm) for this analysis only 4 categories were present (after excluding Fibroadenoma).

LCIS and proliferative lesions were not present in these samples. The more severe the tissue abnormality, progressing from left to right, the higher the score variable, starting at -0.4 (+/- 1.2) for normal and non-proliferative abnormal tissue, up to 2.6 (+/- 1.4) for invasive cancer. The linear regression coefficient between the score variable and the tissue type grouping for the dataset was 0.59 [95 % CI: 0.11–1.07, $P = 0.033$]. The need to identify an abnormality such as Fibroadenoma is usually in young women, where these are the majority of the biopsy findings. In these young women the prevalence of cancer (or atypia) is very low. In women who are biopsied with more "suspicion" for cancer, the more relevant differentiation required does not include Fibroademona. Therefore, Fibroademona presents an "isolated" tissue type, with the background tissue being, most always, normal breast tissue.

Differentiation between tissue categories

It is clear from Fig. 2 that various tissue types have different dielectric properties. To further assess whether these differences can serve as a basis for differentiation between various tissue categories, the subset of measurements with feature sizes of >0.7 mm was grouped into binary categories. The resulting ROC curves for two interesting cases, normal vs. malignant (blue line) and normal vs. all abnormal types (red line), are presented in Fig. 4. In both cases the curves follow the left and upper axes, reaching very close to the upper left corner, with the areas under the curve approaching unity; 0.95 (95 % CI: 0.94–0.96) and 0.96 (95 % CI: 0.94–0.97), respectively. The sensitivity and specificity evaluated for each curve at the optimal cut-off point (the point in the curve closest to the upper left corner) are: Sensitivity 90.5 % (95 % CI: 86–94) and Specificity 90.1 (95 % CI: 88–92) for differentiating between normal and malignant tissue, and Sensitivity 88.6 % (95 % CI: 85–92) and Specificity 91.7 (95 % CI: 90–93) for differentiating between normal and all abnormal tissue types, both malignant and non-malignant.

In general, it is expected during a biopsy procedure to encounter lesions of ~1 mm or larger. From analysis of SEER (Surveillance, Epidemiology, and End Results program of the National Cancer Institute) data, more than 97 % of the malignant lesions are larger than 3 mm [32]. Still, it is interesting to analyze the separation ability of the device between normal and malignant tissues for various tissue feature sizes. Figure 5 presents 3 ROC curves for 3 feature size categories - above 0.8 mm (the size of the sensor), 0.5–0.8 mm and below 0.5 mm (including any detectable cancer by pathology, even below 0.1 mm). As seen in the figure, the ability to detect cancer (quantified by the areas under the curves, also presented in Table 3) depends, as expected, on the

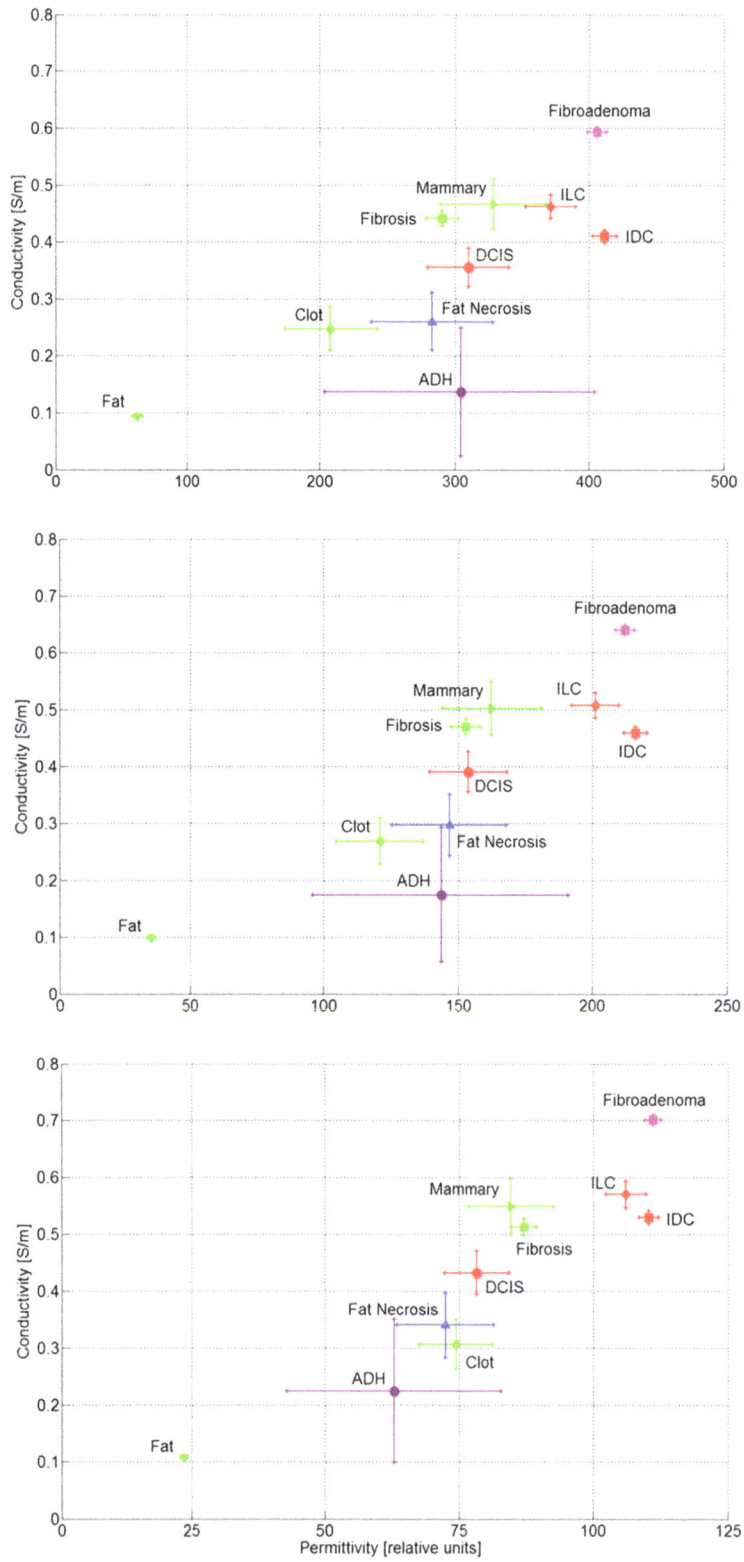

Fig. 2 Dielectric properties, evaluated from measurements performed at 4, 10 and 30 MHz (*top to bottom*), of various tissue types

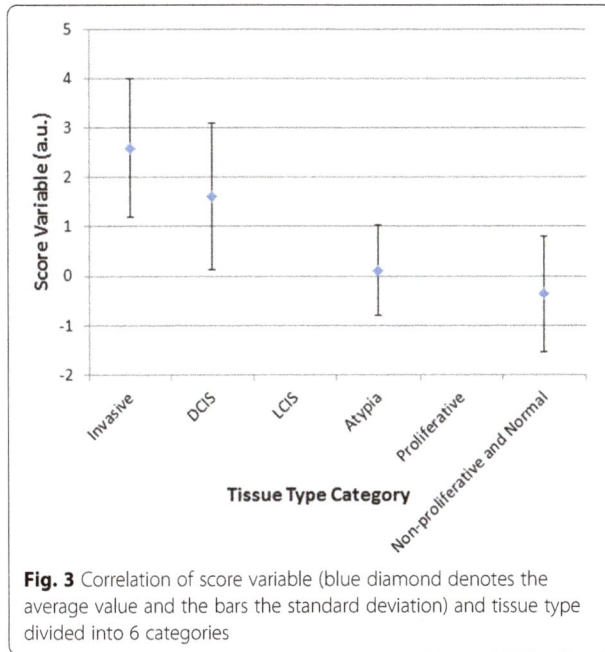

Fig. 3 Correlation of score variable (blue diamond denotes the average value and the bars the standard deviation) and tissue type divided into 6 categories

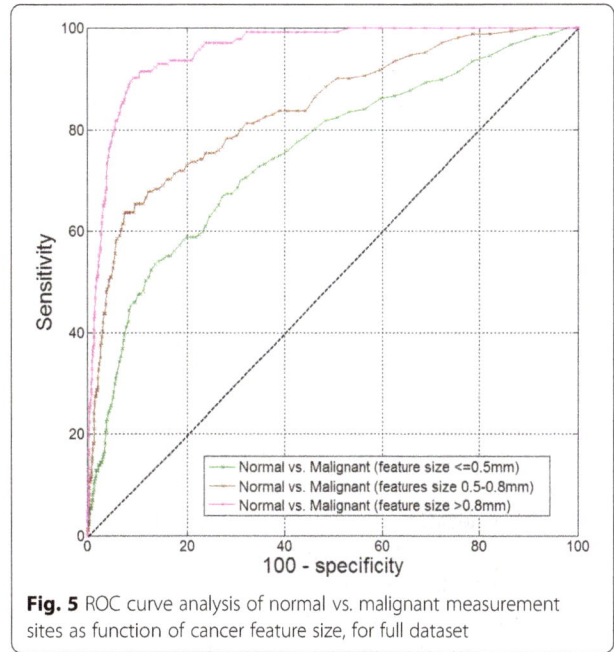

Fig. 5 ROC curve analysis of normal vs. malignant measurement sites as function of cancer feature size, for full dataset

feature size. Table 3 also presents the sensitivity and specificity for each case at the optimal cutoff point of the score variable.

Discussion

Our results quantify dielectric properties of 10 different tissue types present within the breast, and show that they all have different dielectric properties. These includes the types related to normal breast tissue

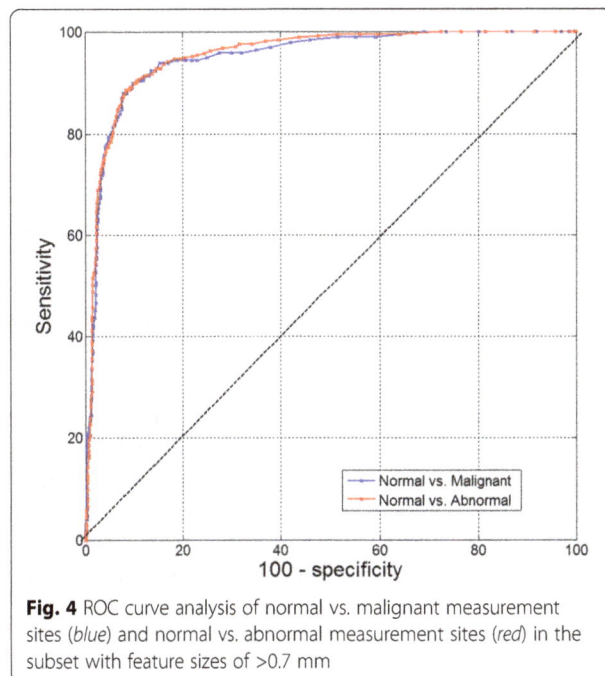

Fig. 4 ROC curve analysis of normal vs. malignant measurement sites (*blue*) and normal vs. abnormal measurement sites (*red*) in the subset with feature sizes of >0.7 mm

(Adipose, Glandular, and Connective), and types associated with various abnormalities, including the differentiation between the dielectric properties of the 3 types of cancer types: IDC, ILC, and DCIS. Prior studies [4–7] have demonstrated that, generally, there are differences between normal and cancer tissue within the breast, but have not provided the level of differentiation presented in this work. Additionally, the data on the dielectric properties of pre-malignant types is new. These identified differences served as a basis for constructing a score variable that demonstrated correlation with the degree of abnormality, including pre-malignant phase, of the breast tissue. Additionally, using the dielectric properties and the score variable good differentiation between normal and malignant, or non-malignant abnormal, tissue was established. The configuration of the sensor as a 0.8 mm circular sensor can be thought of as a basic sensing unit for use in breast biopsy procedures, with an array of sensors aligned along the biopsy needle.

The goal of the initial biopsy is to obtain sufficient diagnostic material using the least invasive approach and to avoid surgical excision of benign lesions. CNB offers a definitive histologic diagnosis, avoids inadequate samples

Table 3 Differentiation ability for various cancer feature sizes

Feature size	Sensitivity	Specificity	AUG
>0.8 mm	90.2 (95 % CI: 84–95)	90.9 (95 % CI: 90–92)	0.957 (95 % CI: 0.95–0.96)
0.5 to 0.8 mm	73.1 (95 % CI: 66–80)	80.4 (95 % CI: 79–82)	0.84 (95 % CI: 0.83–0.85)
<0.5 mm	66.8 (95 % CI: 60–74)	72.8 (95 % CI: 71–74)	0.75 (95 % CI: 0.74–0.77)

and may permit the distinction between invasive versus *in situ* cancer. In most centers, image guided CNB has replaced wire localization and surgical excision as the most common initial biopsy method for nonpalpable abnormalities [33–35]. The accuracy of CNB was shown in a series of 952 consecutive breast CNBs performed at one institution (342 without image guidance, 241 with ultrasound guidance, and 369 using a stereotactic vacuum assisted biopsy (VAB)) [36]. The false-negative rate with 11-gauge VAB was 3 %, compared to 13, 5, and 22 % for non-image guided, surgeon-performed ultrasound-guided, and 14-gauge VAB, respectively. In most of these false negative patients (5–22 %) the reason for the false negative result was due to sampling error, meaning that the biopsy was not taken from the lesion as planned.

The false negative rate can be reduced by using very large needles [37]. An alternative approach could be to keep the needle size relatively small, but add local sensors located at the needle's tissue collection region that provide *in-situ* information on the tissue about to be sampled. The basic units for these sensors can be sub-millimeter, circular near-field radio-frequency sensing units, as those we have used in this work for characterizing breast tissue properties. These sensors may provide real-time measurements of tissue dielectric properties at the locations of tissue to be biopsied. As the power transmitted by the sensor is very low and the RF radiation is non-ionizing, these type of sensors are well suited for in-vivo use.

As per the current standard of care, imaging will be used to direct the needle to the general location of the suspected abnormality. The in-site sensors will provide indication of the tissue type at the immediate vicinity of the needle and in contact with the sensor, as the sensor is effectively a surface characterization sensor. The penetration depth the 0.8 mm sensor in no more than 0.1 mm. By scanning/moving the needle around the suspected region, the most suspicious tissue abnormality can be identified, and biopsied. The spatial resolution of a sensing device designed using the sensors as the basic building blocks is dictated by the sensor size and by the ability to arrange sensors close together. Arranging 0.8 mm sensors in an array will preserve this resolution, as the sensors can share the same ground plane (the outer conductor of the coaxial aperture).

For a potential set-up for use in a biopsy device configuration, approximately 10 0.8 mm circular sensors will be arranged in a 1D array on the biopsy needle, in a location overlapping the biopsy sampling cavity. As each measurement takes approximately 2.5 msec, a reading from all 10 sensors will take ~ 0.025 s. The full measurement cycle, including displaying the results to the user, will take approximately 0.2 s, thus providing real-time

tissue characterization as the needle is progressed through the tissue. Therefore, when the sensors will be integrated with the biopsy needle, it is anticipated that the duration of the biopsy procedure will not be extended.

DCIS is presented mostly as microcalcifications on mammography and diagnosed by stereotactic mammography guided biopsy (mammotomy). The ability of the sensor to distinguish between DCIS and normal breast tissue elements seems promising for using this type of sensor also in mammotomies.

Patients with ADH that were diagnosed on a CNB will be found to have in up to 25 % DCIS or even IDC present at open biopsy. Therefore patients with ADH on CNB are routinely sent for an open surgical biopsy [18–21]. A more accurate CNB can reduce the number of unnecessary open biopsies in these patients. The ability of the sensor to differentiate between normal breast tissue, ADH and DCIS, can potentially improve the accuracy of CNB and reduce the number of open biopsies.

The diagnostic capability of the sensor for differentiating between malignant and normal tissue is high, with a Sensitivity of 90.5 % and Specificity of 90.1 %. This is also reflected by the ROC curves, with an area under the curve of 0.95. The ability of the sensor to differentiate any abnormal tissue from normal tissue is also high, Sensitivity 88.6 % and Specificity 91.7 %. With the current false-negative rates of CNB, this level of sensitivity has the potential of reducing the false negative rates in biopsy procedures to below 1 %.

The detection sensitivity of the sensor is dependent on the feature size of the malignant tissue. A 90.2 % Sensitivity features of at least 0.8 m in size, down to 66.8 % sensitivity for features smaller than 0.5 mm. It is anticipated that most biopsied malignancies will be of at least 1 mm in size, as, based on final pathology, most all of the malignant lesions are found to be larger than 3 mm.

There are some limitations to this type of sensor design. The manufacturing process of the sensor has to account for potential chemical modifications (over time) of the senor face, which can affect the reflected signals. Arranging sensors in a tightly packed array provides an additional challenge in isolating the electrical response of the individual sensors from their neighbors. The tissue has to be in direct contact with the sensor. Therefore, a practical device will need good attachment to substrate, as any (air) voids between the sensor and the tissue will skew the impedance measurement results. The very low penetration depth may limit the scope of applications in which this type of sensor will provide benefit. The sensor is gold-plated, with gold known not to be durable with regards to mechanical abrasion. In a biopsy procedure each sensor would be used for a limited duration, typically no more than a few minutes.

Also, breast tissue is soft, and therefore it is not expected that the sensor structure will be mechanically effected during use.

Conclusion

By use of a miniature flexible radio-frequency near-field spectroscopy sensor the dielectric properties of 10 tissue types present within the breast were quantified, showing distinct differences between the all these types. Using these differences a good differentiating was achieved between breast tissue states, specifically between cancerous and normal tissue. The sensor's dimensions and design may enable the use of such sensors in minimally invasive procedures, including breast biopsy.

Abbreviations

ADH: Atypical Ductal Hyperplasia; CNB: Core Needle Biopsy; DCIS: Ductal Carcinoma *In Situ*; RF: Radio Frequency; ROC: Receiver Operating Characteristics; VAB: Vacuum assisted Biopsy

Acknowledgements

None.

Funding

The study was sponsored by Dune Medical devices.

Authors' contributions

ZK, HP, IH, PM, TK, IP, and TA participated in the design of the study. TZ, JS, and JD performed the pathological evaluation. ZK and TE drafted the manuscript. All authors read and approved the final manuscript.

Competing interests

The authors declare that they have no competing interests.

Author details

[1]Breast unit, Meir Medical Center, Kfar Saba, Israel. [2]Department of pathology, Meir Medical Center, Kfar Saba, Israel. [3]Breast unit, Assaf Harofeh Medical Center, Zrifin, Israel. [4]Department of Pathology, Assaf Harofeh Medical Center, Zrifin, Israel. [5]Department of Pathology, Kaplan Medical Center, Rehovot, Israel. [6]Breast Unit, Kaplan Medical Center, Rehovot, Israel. [7]Department of Surgery, Meir Medical Center, Kfar Sava, Israel.

References

1. Gabriel S, Lau RW, Gabriel C. The dielectric properties of biological tissue II: Measurements in the frequency range 10 Hz to 20 GHz. Phys Med Biol. 1996;41:2251.
2. Foster KR, Schepps JL. Dielectric properties of tumor and normal tissues at radio through microwave frequencies. J Micro Power. 1981;16(2):107–19.
3. Joines WT, Zhang Y, Li C, Jirtle RL. The measured electrical properties of normal and malignant human tissues from 50 to 900 MHz. Med Phys. 1994;21(4):547–50.
4. Sha L, Ward ER, Stroy B. A review of dielectric properties of normal and malignant breast tissue. PIEEE Southeast Con. 2002; 457-462.
5. Surowiec AJ, Stuchly SS, Barr JR, Swarup A. Dielectric properties of breast carcinoma and the surrounding tissue. IEEE Trans Biomed Eng. 1988;35(4):257–63.
6. Zou Y, Guo Z. A review of electrical impedance techniques for breast cancer. Med Eng Phys. 2003;25(2):79–90.
7. Lazebnik M, et al. A large-scale study of the ultrawideband microwave dielectric properties of normal breast tissue obtained from reduction surgeries. Phys Med Biol. 2007;52:6093–115.
8. Pappo I, Spector R, Schindel A, Morgenstern S, Sandbank J, Leider LT, et al. Diagnostic performance of a novel device for real-time margin assessment in lumpectomy specimens. J Surg Res. 2010;160(2):277–81.
9. Karni T, Pappo I, Sandbank J, Lavon O, Kent V, Spector R, et al. A device for real-time, intraoperative margin assessment in breast-conservation surgery. Am J Surg. 2007;194:467–73.
10. Allweis TM, Kaufman Z, Lelcuk S, Pappo I, Karni T, Schneebaum S, et al. A prospective, randomized, controlled, multicenter study of a real-time, intraoperative probe for positive margin detection in breast-conserving surgery. Am J Surg. 2008;196:483.
11. Siegel R, Ward E, Brawley O, Jemal A. Cancer statistics, 2011: The impact of eliminating socioeconomic and racial disparities on premature cancer deaths. CA Cancer J Clin. 2011;61:212.
12. Jemal A, Bray F, Center MM, et al. Global cancer statistics. CA Cancer J Clin. 2011;61:69.
13. Breast Imaging Reporting and Data System (BI-RADS) Atlas, 4th ed, American College of Radiology, Reston, VA 2003.
14. Barlow WE, Lehman CD, Zheng Y, et al. Performance of diagnostic mammography for women with signs or symptoms of breast cancer. J Natl Cancer Inst. 2002;94:1.
15. Hubbard RA, Kerlikowske K, Flowers CI, et al. Cumulative probability of false positive recall or biopsy recommendation after 10 years of screening mammography: a cohort study. Ann Intern Med. 2011;155:481–92.
16. Ghosh K, Melton 3rd LJ, Suman VJ, Grant CS, Steriolf S, et al. Breastbiopsy utilization: a population-based study. Arch Intern Med. 2005;165:1593–8.
17. Nelson HD, et al. Screening for breast cancer: an update for the U.S. Preventive services task force. Ann Intern Med. 2009;151:727–37.
18. Chae BJ, Lee A, Song BJ, Jung SS. Predictive factors for breast cancer in patients diagnosed atypical ductal hyperplasia at core needle biopsy. World J Surg Oncol. 2009;7:77.
19. Elsheikh TM, Silverman JF. Follow-up surgical excision is indicated when breast core needle biopsies show atypical lobular hyperplasia or lobular carcinoma in situ: a correlative study of 33 patients with review of the literature. Am J Surg Pathol. 2005;29:534.
20. Anderson BO, Calhoun KE, Rosen EL. Evolving concepts in the management of lobular neoplasia. J Natl Compr Canc Netw. 2006;4:511.
21. Margenthaler JA, Duke D, Monsees BS, et al. Correlation between core biopsy and excisional biopsy in breast high-risk lesions. Am J Surg. 2006;192:534.
22. Lui, et al. Rebiopsy after stereotactic core-needle breast biopsy: prospective study. J HK Coll Radiol. 2004;7:116–20.
23. Youk JH, et al. Missed breast cancers at US-guided core needle biopsy: How to reduce them, radio graphics, vol. 27. 2007. p. 79–94.
24. Brun del Re R. Minimally invasive breast biopsies, recent results in cancer research 173. Berlin Heidelberg: Springer; 2009. p. 149.
25. Fajardo, et al. Stereotactic and sonographic large-core biopsy of nonpalpable breast lesions: results of the radiologic diagnostic oncology group V study. Acad Radiol. 2004;11(3):293–308.
26. Dotan ZA, Fridman E, Lindner A, Ramon J, Pode D, Bejar J, Kopolovic J, Pizov G, Sandbank J, Katz R, Shapiro A, Shilo Y, Nativ O. Detection of prostate cancer by radio-frequency near-field spectroscopy in radical prostatectomy ex vivo specimens. Prostate Cancer Prostatic Dis. 2013;16(1):73–8.
27. Meaney PM, Williams BB, Geimer SD, Flood AB, Swartz HM. A coaxial dielectric probe technique for distinguishing tooth enamel from dental resin. Adv Biomed Eng Res. 2015;3:8–17.
28. Misra DK. A quasi-static analysis of open-ended coaxial lines. IEEE Trans Microwave Theory Tech. 1987;MTT-35:925–8.
29. Dupont WD, Page DL. Risk factors for breast cancer in women with proliferative breast disease. N Engl J Med. 1985;312:146–51. American Cancer Society, Non-cancerous Breast Conditions.

30. Rawlings JO, Pantula SG, Dickey DA. Applied regression analysis: a research tool. Springer; 1998.

31. Estrela da Silva JE, Marques de Sa JP, Jossinet J. Classification of breast tissue by electrical impedance spectroscopy. J Med Biol Eng Comput. 2000;38:26–30.

32. Ries LAG, Young JL, Keel GE, Eisner MP, Lin YD, Horner M-J, editors. SEER survival monograph: cancer survival among adults: U.S. SEER program, 1988-2001, patient and tumor characteristics. Bethesda: National Cancer Institute; 2007. SEER Program, NIH Pub. No. 07-6215.

33. Gutwein LG, Ang DN, Liu H, et al. Utilization of minimally invasive breast biopsy for the evaluation of suspicious breast lesions. Am J Surg. 2011;202:127.

34. Verkooijen HM, Core Biopsy After Radiological Localisation (COBRA) Study Group. Diagnostic accuracy of stereotactic large-core needle biopsy for nonpalpable breast disease: results of a multicenter prospective study with 95 % surgical confirmation. Int J Cancer. 2002;99:853.

35. Stomper PC, Winston PS, Proulx GM, et al. Mammographic detection and staging of ductal carcinoma in situ: mammographic-pathologic correlation. Semin Breast Dis. 2000;3:1.

36. Shah VI, Raju U, Chitale D, et al. False-negative core needle biopsies of the breast: an analysis of clinical, radiologic, and pathologic findings in 27 consecutive cases of missed breast cancer. Cancer. 2003;97:1824.

37. Jackman RJ, Marzoni Jr FA, Rosenberg J. False-negative diagnoses at stereotactic vacuum-assisted needle breast biopsy: long-term follow-up of 1,280 lesions and review of the literature. AJR Am J Roentgenol. 2009;192:341.

15

Quantification of FDG-PET/CT with delayed imaging in patients with newly diagnosed recurrent breast cancer

Christina Baun[1]* (ID), Kirsten Falch[1], Oke Gerke[1,2], Jeanette Hansen[1], Tram Nguyen[1], Abass Alavi[3], Poul-Flemming Høilund-Carlsen[1] and Malene G. Hildebrandt[1]

Abstract

Background: Several studies have shown the advantage of delayed-time-point imaging with 18F-FDG-PET/CT to distinguish malignant from benign uptake. This may be relevant in cancer diseases with low metabolism, such as breast cancer. We aimed at examining the change in SUV from 1 h (1h) to 3 h (3h) time-point imaging in local and distant lesions in patients with recurrent breast cancer. Furthermore, we investigated the effect of partial volume correction in the different types of metastases, using semi-automatic quantitative software (ROVER™).

Methods: One-hundred and two patients with suspected breast cancer recurrence underwent whole-body PET/CT scans 1h and 3h after FDG injection. Semi-quantitative standardised uptake values (SUVmax, SUVmean) and partial volume corrected SUVmean (cSUVmean), were estimated in malignant lesions, and as reference in healthy liver tissue. The change in quantitative measures from 1h to 3h was calculated, and SUVmean was compared to cSUVmean. Metastases were verified by biopsy.

Results: Of the 102 included patients, 41 had verified recurrent disease with in median 15 lesions (range 1-70) amounting to a total of 337 malignant lesions included in the analysis. SUVmax of malignant lesions increased from 6.4 ± 3.4 [0.9-19.7] (mean $\pm$ SD, min and max) at 1h to 8.1 ± 4.4 [0.7-29.7] at 3h. SUVmax in breast, lung, lymph node and bone lesions increased significantly ($p < 0.0001$) between 1h and 3h by on average 25, 40, 33, and 27%, respectively. A similar pattern was observed with (uncorrected) SUVmean. Partial volume correction increased SUVmean significantly, by 63 and 71% at 1h and 3h imaging, respectively. The highest impact was in breast lesions at 3h, where cSUVmean increased by 87% compared to SUVmean.

Conclusion: SUVs increased from 1h to 3h in malignant lesions, SUVs of distant recurrence were in general about twice as high as those of local recurrence. Partial volume correction caused significant increases in these values. However, it is questionable, if these relatively modest quantitative advances of 3h imaging are sufficient to warrant delayed imaging in this patient group.

Keywords: FDG-PET/CT, Breast cancer, Delayed-time-point, Standardised uptake values, Partial volume correction

* Correspondence: Christina.baun@rsyd.dk
[1]Department of Nuclear Medicine, University Hospital, Sdr. Boulevard 29, 5000 Odense C, Denmark
Full list of author information is available at the end of the article

Background

Breast cancer is the most frequent cancer among women in western countries, and up to 30% of patients are likely to develop recurrence [1, 2]. 18F-fluoro-deoxy-glucose positron emission tomography/computed tomography (FDG-PET/CT) is useful in the diagnosis, staging and therapeutic follow-up of patients with recurrent breast cancer, and is especially better than conventional imaging at detecting distant metastases [3–5].

FDG is not specific for malignancy; however, recent studies have shown the advantage of delayed or dual-time imaging with FDG-PET to distinguish malignant from benign uptake [6–8]. The underlying rationale is that malignant cells have more glucose transporters and hexokinases and less glucose-6-phosphatase (G6Pase), which leads to FDG accumulation over time compared to benign cells [9, 10]. Delayed scan time-points may thus improve the image quality due the greater difference between tumour and background levels [11–14]. This may be relevant in cancer diseases with low metabolism, such as breast cancer.

Only a few studies have examined the use of delayed time-point imaging (DTPI) in whole-body FDG-PET/CT to show the FDG accumulation over time associated with distant metastases [15–17]. The literature suggests that more prospective studies are needed to provide a better understanding of the use of DTPI in detecting recurrent breast cancer [6, 18, 19]. Analysis of PET data is often performed semi-quantitatively by measuring standardised uptake values (SUV) in lesions suspected of malignancy [20–22]. SUV has been referred to correlate well with histological and biological tumour characteristics, and can be an important tool in the diagnostic report for breast cancer patients [23–25]. SUV is strongly affected by the partial volume effect (PVE), however, which can cause a significant underestimation of the lesion uptake level [26–28]. Although methods for partial volume correction (PVC) have been developed to overcome this limitation, no method has yet found its place in daily clinical practice. Further evidence is needed to state the usefulness and feasibility of these software methods [29–32].

We aimed at examining the value of whole-body FDG-PET/CT performed at 3 h (3h) compared to the standard imaging time-point at 1 h (1h), in patients suspected of recurrent breast cancer, using quantitative software that included PVC.

Our objectives were to investigate i) the change in standardised uptake values from early (1h) to delayed (3h) time-point imaging in local and distant lesions, by measuring SUVmax, SUVmean and correcting SUVmean for PVE (cSUVmean), and ii) the effect of PVC by comparing SUVmean and cSUVmean at both time-points.

Methods

One-hundred and two women with suspected breast cancer recurrence or with verified local recurrence and potential distant disease were enrolled in the study. The patients were part of a larger prospective accuracy study comparing FDG-PET/CT to conventional imaging in detecting recurrent breast cancer [33]. The prospective study was conducted at the PET centre, Odense University Hospital, Denmark, from December 2011 to September 2014. Exclusion criteria were history of other malignancies, age < 18 years, pregnancy or breastfeeding, diabetes mellitus, or considered unable to cooperate. For further methodological details we refer to our recent publication [33].

FDG-pet/CT

Patients were required to fast for at least 6 h before the FDG-PET/CT scan. A maximum blood glucose level of 144 mg/dL was allowed prior to intravenous injection of 4 MBq/kg FDG. Whole-body FDG-PET/CT scans were performed 1h and 3h after FDG injection on a General Electric Discovery STE or Discovery RX system (GE Healthcare, Milwaukee, USA). A low-dose CT scan (140 kV, 30-110 mA; Auto- and Smart mA) was performed followed by a 3D PET scan. Acquisition time was of 2.5 min/frame for the 1h scan and 3.5 min/frame for the 3h scan, for patients with a normal body mass index (BMI) between 18.5 kg/m^2 and 24.9 kg/m^2. If BMI was lower or higher, the scan time was adjusted according to BMI and either decreased or increased by ½ min/frame, respectively. Images were reconstructed iteratively using an ordered subset expectation maximization (OSEM) algorithm, with 2 iterations, and 21 or 28 subsets, a slice thickness of 3.3 mm and matrix size of 128 × 128 (pixel size of 5.47mm^2) with CT-based attenuation correction and 5 mm Gaussian post-filtering.

Reference standard

Suspected recurrence was verified by biopsy. If biopsy was not possible, a composite reference standard comprising all available imaging procedures (MRI, CT, PET/CT, bone scan, ultrasound, x-ray and mammography) and/or clinical follow-up data over 6 months was used as gold standard, using the patients' medical files as necessary. In patients with multiple lesions, it was not possible to obtain a biopsy from all lesions for ethical reasons. The patients were categorised into groups of 'local recurrence' or 'distant recurrence' based on reference standard and in accordance with treatment decision.

Image interpretation

The scans were visually interpreted by an experienced nuclear medicine physician using the General Electric acquisition workstation. The 1h and 3h images were read independently. Each lesion was described with anatomic site and exact image number for further semi-quantitative analysis. The lesions were divided into seven subgroups according to lesion site: cerebrum, lung, liver, breast, lymph node, bone and 'other' (subcutaneous and muscle metastasis).

Semi-quantitative analysis

Semi-quantitative analysis of the malignant lesions was retrospectively performed using dedicated image analysis software (ROVER™, ABX, Radeberg, Germany). This software provides semi-automatic image segmentation with a model-free method for PVE correction of SUVmean values. The software performs lesion delineation within a user-defined 3D mask using fixed, peak-based thresholding to delineate the lesion region-of-interest (ROI), which represents the metabolic active tumour volume (MTV). In the following step, ROVER performs PVC using an algorithm that defines a spill-out region of the lesion ROI from which a background corrected estimate of the spill-out region is calculated and used to perform PVC of SUVmean resulting in cSUVmean. Further details regarding software algorithms are explained by Hofheinz et al. [32, 34]. The ROVER software was used in standard mode with a threshold setting of 40% of maximum 3D mask value, including a minimum ROI volume of 1cm^3 and excluding ROI intersection. SUV values were normalised to body weight. Manually placement of 3D masks was performed after visual identification of the lesion by the interpreting physician. Masks were placed 2-4 pixels beyond the visual margin of each lesion, and ROVER automatically delineated the lesion ROI and performed PVC. It automatically calculated ROI values of SUVmax, SUVmean, cSUVmean and MTV. Separate 3D masks were used for the same lesions in the 1h and 3h scans. If a lesion had no discernible FDG uptake in the early images, the 3D mask was placed as close as possible to the assumed origin based on anatomic orientation. A reference measurement in healthy liver tissue was obtained in all patients at both time-points. This was performed by drawing a mask of a proximately 36 cm^3 in the upper right lobe of healthy liver tissue, avoiding malignancies and organ boundaries. Potential metastatic lesions without FDG-uptake would not be registered for analysis. The difference in SUVmax, SUVmean, cSUVmean, and MTV between the two time-points were calculated as ΔSUV=SUV3h - SUV1h, and ΔMTV = MTV3h - MTV1h.

Statistical analysis

Descriptive statistics were performed for demographic variables and scanning parameters. The semi-quantitative analysis parameters from the 1h and 3h scans were expressed as mean ± standard deviation (SD) and range. Boxplots were used for graphical display of the data. The differences in SUVs between the two time-points as well as the difference between SUVmean and cSUVmean measurements at each time-point were estimated together with 95% confidence intervals (CI) and p-values that were derived from univariate linear regression models using robust standard errors to allow for intragroup correlation (i.e. multiple lesions in the same patient). Subgroup analyses were conducted by recurrence category (distant versus local recurrence) and lesion site, where healthy liver tissue was used as the reference category. Analyses were supplemented by relative changes of mean values in groups, e.g. (mean value of 3h measurements – mean value of 1h measurements)/ (mean value of 1h measurements)*100%.

Statistical tests were two-sided with a significance level of 5%. Analyses were conducted with Stata/MP 14.0 (StataCorp LP, College Station, Texas 77845, USA).

Results

Of the 102 patients who initially agreed to participate in the study one patient changed her mind before FDG-PET/CT, another was excluded due to a previous biopsy-verified bone metastasis, and a third patient did not complete the 3h scan, leaving 99 women available for analysis. Forty-one of these (41.4%) were diagnosed with recurrent breast cancer, with a total of 337 malignant lesions (mean 15, range 1-70) available for analysis. The patient and scanning characteristics are given in Table 1.

Nineteen patients had local recurrence comprising 21 lesions, and 22 patients had distant disease with 316 lesions. All patients had at least one biopsy to verify recurrence. Biopsies were primarily taken from breast lesions. For patients with recurrent disease and multiple distant metastases, only one distant lesion was verified by biopsy due to ethical aspect. All remaining metastatic lesions were verified by the composite reference standard, as

Table 1 Patient and scanning characteristics of 1h and 3h FDG-PET/CT, performed in the 41 patients with recurrent breast cancer

Patient characteristics	Mean ± SD, range
Patient age (years)	62 ± 4.2 [57;74]
Body mass index	27 ± 7.1 [22;32]
Blood glucose level (mmol/L)	5.4 ± 1.0 [3.8;7.7]
Years since treatment of primary breast cancer	6 ± 8.2 [0;30]
Scanning characteristics	
Dose (MBq)	281 ± 56.0 [208;401]
Time (min) between injection and early scan (1h)	62 ± 6.0 [53;80]
Time (min) between injection and late scan (3h)	180 ± 6.0 [170;200]

described in the method section. Distribution of lesions and biopsies are shown in Table 2.

Local vs. distant recurrence

The overall SUV measurements for all 41 patients increased, on average, significantly between 1h and 3h, i.e., SUVmax by 1.8 (+ 28% increase), SUVmean by 1.1 (+ 28%), and cSUVmean by 2.3 (+ 35%). Overall, MTV decreased significantly over time, particularly for patients with distant recurrence in whom it decreased by 16%, shown in Table 3.

The values of distant recurrence were in general about twice as high as those of local recurrence, but the relative average increase was the same for the two groups. In both groups, the relative increase in cSUVmean (35-36%) was greater than the increase in SUVmean and SUVmax (25-28%). Despite these average tendencies, some lesions showed reduced SUVmax values at 3h, i.e., 8 lesions (38%) in patients with local recurrence and 31 lesions (10%) in patients with distant recurrence.

Changes by lesion subgroup

Except for and the lesion group 'other', all subgroups showed a significant increase in SUVmax and SUVmean over time, compared to the reference measurements in healthy liver tissue (Fig. 1). Lymph node metastases showed the highest absolute increase in SUVmax by 2.1 [1.4-2.8] (mean, 95% CI) (+ 33%), SUVmean by 1.5 [0.1-0.7] (+ 36%) and cSUVmean by 3.2 [2.6-3.2] (+ 47%). The highest relative increase in SUVmax, SUVmean and cSUVmean over time was seen for lung metastases at 40, 44 and 52%, respectively. Breast lesions showed the smallest absolute increase from 1h to 3h in SUVmax, SUVmean and cSUVmean at 0.7 [0.2-1.1] (+ 25%), 0.4 [0.1-0.7] (+ 24%) and 1.2 [0.4-1.9] (+ 42%). Liver lesions showed the lowest relative increase in SUVmax, SUVmean and, cSUVmean of 18, 16 and 18% respectively. Reference tissue in healthy liver showed a significant average decrease in SUVmax by 11 and 20%, respectively.

Despite the overall increase in SUV for lesion subgroups, some lesions showed reduced SUV over time, i. e., 1 (4%) in the lung, 1 (14%) in liver, 11 (41%) in breast, 3 (6%) in lymph nodes, 22 (7%) in bone and 1 (10%) of the 'other' lesions. The percentages of lesions with decreased values between the two time-points were the same for SUVmax, SUVmean and cSUVmean. Due to only one cerebral metastasis, this lesion group was not considered representative and is not commented upon in the results or discussion sections. MTV decreased, on average, significantly for all lesion subgroups between 1h and 3h; however, for liver lesions and 'other' lesions the decrease was not significant. The greatest decrease (of 43%) in MTV was seen in breast lesions. For details regarding lesion subgroups, see supplementary data given in Additional file 1.

Partial volume correction

For all lesions as a whole, cSUVmean was significantly higher than SUVmean at both 1h (mean difference of 2.5 equal to 63%) and 3h (3.6 equal to 71%) except lesions 'other' and liver metastases at 1h, which was insignificantly higher (Table 4). For patients with local recurrence cSUVmean was 70% higher than SUVmean at 1h and 84% at 3h and for distant recurrence 63% higher at 1h and 71% at 3h, see Table 4.

At lesion site the largest difference was at 3h for breast lesions, where cSUVmean was 87% higher than SUVmean. The smallest difference was at 1h for liver lesions, in which cSUVmean was 39% higher than SUVmean (Table 4). Generally, cSUVmean varied more than SUVmean in all lesion sites (Fig. 2). Further details regarding lesion subgroups, see supplementary data given in Additional file 1.

Discussion

This study of malignant lesions in 41 out of 99 analysed patients with breast cancer recurrence showed significant overall increase in uptake of FDG between 1h and 3h scans. The values of distant recurrence were in general about twice as high as those of local recurrence, but the relative increase was the same for the two groups (Table 3). Lymph node metastases showed the highest absolute increase in SUV between the two time-points, whereas lung metastases displayed the highest relative increase. PVC led to higher uptake estimates, especially for patients with local recurrence and for breast lesions at the 3h scan (Table 4 and Fig. 2). We found decreased SUV over time in reference tissue (healthy liver) as expected and hence an increased tumour-to-background ratio for delayed imaging.

Table 2 Distribution of 337 malignant lesions in 41 recurrent breast cancer patients, according to recurrence status and lesion site. Lesion group 'other' consisted of subcutaneous and muscle metastases

Sites of recurrence	Number of patients	Number of lesions	Number of biopsies
Local recurrence	19	21	19
Distant recurrence	22	316	22
Cerebrum	1	1 (0.3%)	1
Lung	6	25 (7.4%)	1
Liver	4	7 (2.1%)	3
Breast	23	27 (8.0%)	21
Lymph node	13	54 (16.0%)	8
Bone	18	213 (63.2%)	7
Other	2	10 (3.0%)	5

Table 3 Standard uptake values (SUVmax, SUVmean, partial volume corrected SUVmean (cSUVmean) and MTV of malignant lesions at 1h and 3h (mean ± SD, min and max), and the change over time (ΔSUV with 95% CI) by patient recurrence status. **Δ**SUV% and ΔMTV% were calculated by using mean values of 1h and 3h groups. *P*-values refer to the hypothesis test that the mean difference of the paired observations at 1h and 3h is equal to 0

	1h	3h	ΔSUV (3h-1h)	p-value	ΔSUV%
All 41 patients with recurrence (337 lesions)					
SUVmax	6.4 ± 3.4 [0.9-19.7]	8.1 ± 4.4 [0.7-29.7]	1.8 [1.5 to 2.1]	< 0.0001	28
SUVmean	4.0 ± 2.0 [0.5-11.3]	5.1 ± 2.6 [0.4-16.5]	1.1 [1.0 to 1.3]	< 0.0001	28
cSUVmean	6.5 ± 3.5 [0.7-20.8]	8.8 ± 4.7 [0.5-30.9]	2.3 [1.9 to 2.6]	< 0.0001	35
MTV (cc)	12.5 ± 42.4 [0.3-562]	10.4 ± 39.9 [0.2-565.5]	−2.1 [− 3.1 to − 1.0]	< 0.0001	− 17
19 patients with local recurrence (21 lesions)					
SUVmax	3.0 ± 1.9 [0.9-8.7]	3.8 ± 3.0 [0.7-12.3]	0.8 [0.2 to 1.4]	0.006	27
SUVmean	1.9 ± 1.3 [0.5-5.9]	2.4 ± 2.0 [0.4-8.6]	0.5 [0.08 to 0.9]	0.022	25
cSUVmean	3.2 ± 2.4 [0.7-8.9]	4.4 ± 3.9 [0.5-14.4]	1.2 [0.3 to 2.1]	0.014	36
MTV (cc)	8.4 ± 10.3 [0.3-33.3]	5.7 ± 5.5 [0.2-22.3]	−2.8 [−6.2 to 0.7]	0.11	−33
22 patients with distant recurrence (316 lesions)					
SUVmax	6.6 ± 3.3 [1.2-19.7]	8.4 ± 4.4 [1.2-29.7]	1.8 [1.5 to 2.2]	< 0.0001	28
SUVmean	4.1 ± 2.0 [0.8-11.3]	5.3 ± 2.6 [0.6-16.5]	1.2 [1.0 to 1.4]	< 0.0001	28
cSUVmean	6.7 ± 3.5 [0.8-20.8]	9.1 ± 4.6 [0.8-30.9]	2.3 [2.0 to 2.7]	< 0.0001	35
MTV (cc)	12.8 ± 43.7 [0.4-562.0]	10.7 ± 41.1 [0.2-565.5]	−2.1 [−3.2 to −0.9]	0.001	−16

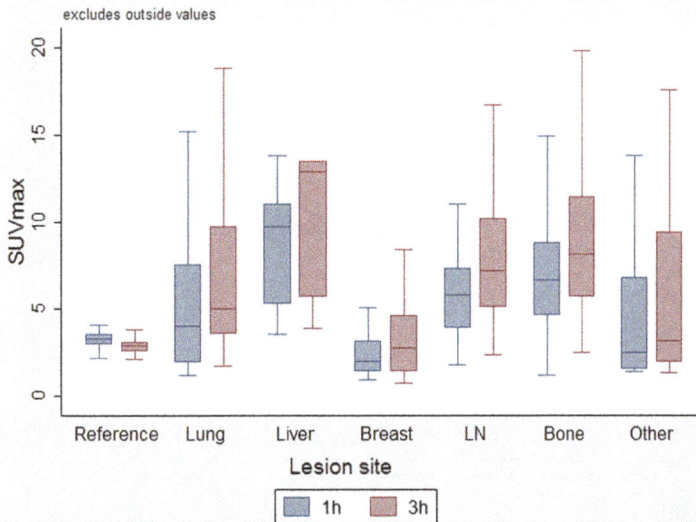

Fig. 1 Boxplots of SUVmax, at 1h and 3h imaging time-point, for the 337 malignant lesions according to the different subgroups and reference tissue (healthy liver) in 41 patients with recurrent breast cancer. Due to only one cerebral lesion, data are not shown for this group

Table 4 Difference between SUVmean and cSUVmean for 1h and 3h measurements for all lesions according to recurrent status and lesion subgroups (mean and 95% CI). Percentage difference was calculated by using mean values of cSUVmean and SUVmean groups for 1h and 3h. P-values refer to the hypothesis test that the mean difference of the paired observations at each time-point for SUVmean and cSUVmean is equal to 0

Group	Difference 1h (cSUVmean-SUVmean)	p-value	% diff	Difference 3h (cSUVmean-SUVmean)	p-value	% diff
All lesions (337 lesions)	2.51 [2.14 – 2.88]	< 0.0001	63	3.64 [3.22 – 4.06]	< 0.0001	71
Local recurrence (21 lesions)	1.32 [0.74 – 1.91]	< 0.0001	70	2.02 [1.07 - 2.98]	< 0.0001	84
Distant recurrence (316 lesions)	2.59 [2.21 - 2.98]	< 0.0001	63	3.75 [3.32 - 4.18]	< 0.0001	71
Lung (25 lesions)	1.88 [0.48 – 3.27]	0.018	60	3.09 [1.28 - 4.91]	0.007	68
Liver (7 lesions)	2.17 [−0.80 – 5.14]	0.103	39	2.67 [0.91 - 4.44]	0.017	41
Breast (27 lesions)	1.09 [0.59 - 1.60]	< 0.0001	63	1.86 [1.06 - 2.66]	< 0.0001	87
Lymph node (54 lesions)	2.77 [1.62 - 3.92]	< 0.0001	69	4.49 [3.16 - 5.82]	< 0.0001	82
Bone (213 lesions)	2.73 [2.43 - 2.92]	< 0.0001	63	3.80 [3.45 - 4.14]	< 0.0001	69
Other (10 lesions)	2.32 [−21.82 – 26.46]	0.437	78	2.73 [−21.54 – 27.00]	0.389	73

Although our study, in line with previous literature, demonstrated an increased tumour-to-background ratio in delayed images, the diagnostic accuracy at patient level did not improve in our overall prospective accuracy study [33]. The clinical usefulness of delayed imaging in this category of patients may thus be limited. Furthermore, it is our experience that DTPI caused planning challenges in daily workflow and patient discomfort due to a longer fasting period.

Change in SUV from early to late time-point imaging
Patients with local recurrence had in general lower SUV-max and SUVmean measurements compared to the group with distant recurrence at both time-points. This

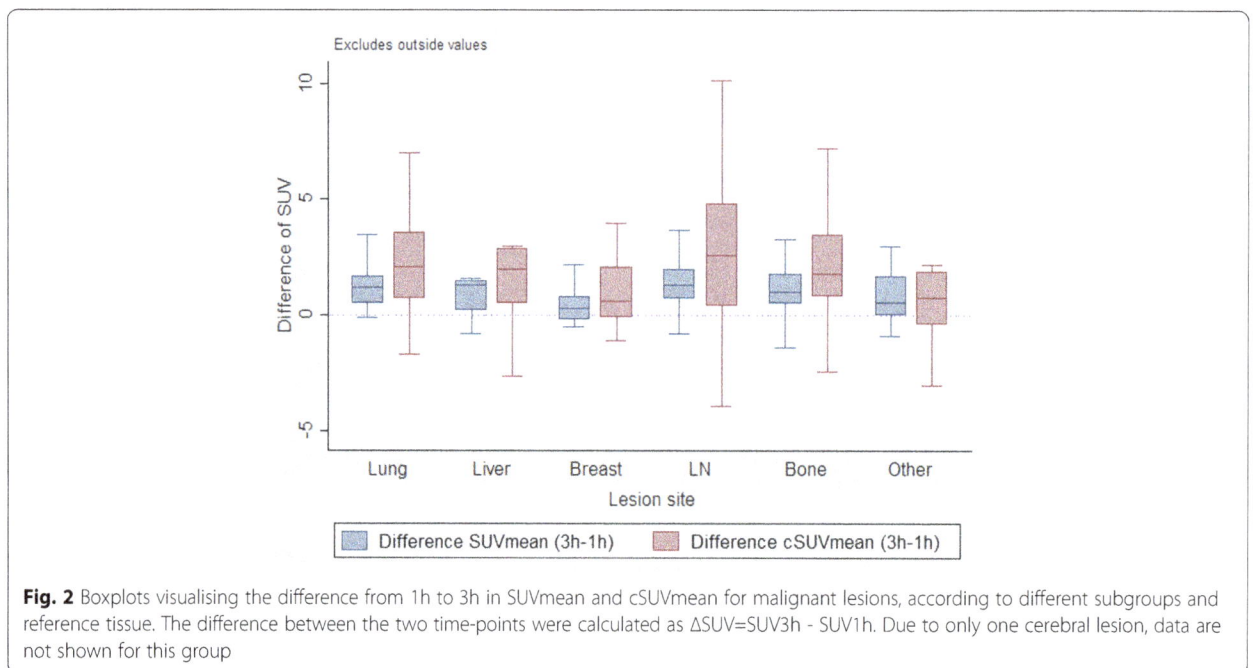

Fig. 2 Boxplots visualising the difference from 1h to 3h in SUVmean and cSUVmean for malignant lesions, according to different subgroups and reference tissue. The difference between the two time-points were calculated as ΔSUV=SUV3h - SUV1h. Due to only one cerebral lesion, data are not shown for this group

could partly be due to the finding that 8 of the 21 lesions (38%) in the group with local recurrence showed decreased SUV from 1h to 3h compared to only 10% in patients with distant recurrence. Suga et al. reported similar results from 52 patients with suspected local recurrence of breast cancer, where SUVmax increased in 84% of the lesions and decreased in 16% of the lesions between 1h and 2h scans, while overall SUVmax increased by 18% [35]. The higher increase in SUVmax in our study could be due to the later imaging point at 3h. Several studies have performed delayed or dual-time imaging in breast cancer but have only shown a small improvement in detecting local recurrence, despite an increased tumour-to-background ratio [11, 12, 36, 37].

Distant metastases in lung, lymph node, liver and bone all increased in SUVmax, SUVmean, and cSUVmean from 1h to 3h, and especially for lymph node metastases. These findings are supported by the literature, where several publications have stated the increased FDG accumulation over time in different malignant lesions [7, 16, 17, 35].

In our study, we used healthy liver tissue for reference measurement, which has previously been demonstrated useful by Chirindel et al. [38]. For bone metastases, we found a significant increase for SUVmax, SUVmean, and cSUVmean between 1h and 3h. These findings are supported by a study of bone metastases in breast cancer patients from Tian et al. [39]. Other diagnostic studies of bone metastases and FDG-PET/CT have found that FDG has a high sensitivity for detecting osteolytic and mixed bone lesions compared to osteoblastic lesions, which can be false-negative due to low metabolic activity [40, 41].

SUV can be influenced by a range of physiological and technical parameters, which should be taken in consideration by quantitative image analysis, to minimize bias [42–44]. SUVmax demonstrates a high inter-observer reproducibility and is often used as a semi-quantitative measure of FDG-uptake. However, SUVmax is more sensitive to image noise, and has been shown to have a lower inter-study repeatability than SUVmean [45, 46]. While SUVmean may be a more reliable measure in heterogeneous tumours, it can be observer-dependent due to lesion delineation dependency with variability in mask placement and sensitivity to PVE, especially in smaller lesions [26, 27, 47].

Impact of PVC performed with ROVER software

PVC of SUVmean had as expected a significant impact in our study, in both the overall lesion group and the various subgroups. However, PVC increased the standard deviation of cSUVmean compared to uncorrected SUVmean, probably due to incorrect lesion delineation caused by segmentation challenges (Fig. 2). The highest impact of PVC was seen for breast lesions which also

had the smallest MTV according to ROVER. Our results agree with the literature, showing that partial volume effects influence measured uptake in all lesions, especially those smaller or of a size close to the limited spatial resolution of the PET scanner, for which it causes a significant underestimation of lesion extent and activity level [26, 27, 47].

Several studies have demonstrated observer-related variability associated with manual delineation of ROI, which can be reduced by the use of automatic or semi-automatic contour drawing [48–50]. Prevalently employed automatic delineation methods employing different threshold and cut-offs, however, are also known to be suboptimal in many cases, leading to segmentation bias [20, 49]. We used ROVER software for PVC, which has previously been shown to be feasibly and clinically useful [31, 34]. ROVER software included background subtraction for each lesion, but despite this we discovered practical challenges due to non-uniformity of lesions and background activity. We experienced against expectation a decrease in MTV defined by ROVER from 1h to 3h, despite the general known tendency of increased FDG accumulation over time in malignant lesions. This issue was probably caused by crucial segmentation challenges associated with the semi-automatic lesion delineation. Thus, by visual inspection of the automatic lesion delineation in our study, the lesion ROI in the 1h image often included background voxels and thereby overestimated lesion size, compared to the same lesion in the 3h image, where the lesion delineation appeared more well-defined (Fig. 3). This indicates that the threshold-based segmentation in ROVER led to overestimated volumes of small lesions, particularly in the early scan, where the lesion-to-background ratio was low, and through that an underestimation of SUVmean. We used a fixed 40% threshold setting to semi-automatically delineate lesions. This approach was based on the current use in the literature and similar to the threshold of 41% recommended by updated European guidelines [48, 51]. A more systematic search of other threshold levels or rather alternative segmentation methods that can provide more accurate lesion delineation could be beneficial [32, 42, 49], but lies outside the scope of this article.

Strengths and limitations of the study

The main strengths of our study are its prospective design and clinically representative patient group with newly diagnosed recurrence – verified by biopsy in all patients – and, hence, yet untreated metastases. The scanning protocol consisted of whole-body scans at both 1h and 3h allowing us to compare SUV measurements over time in all recurrent lesions. A major limitation was that histological proof was not available for all lesions due to ethical and practical reasons, and therefore a composite reference

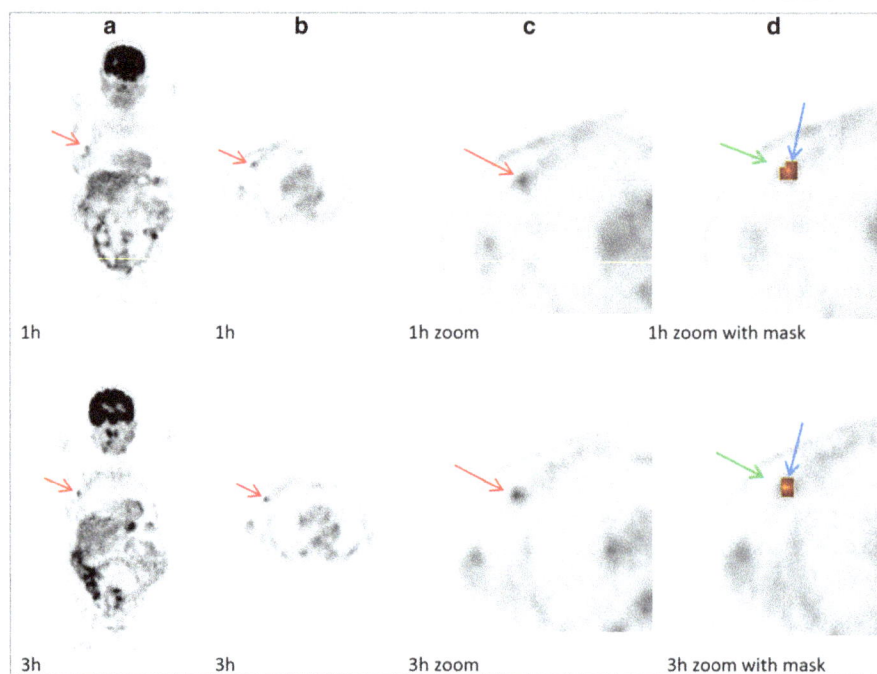

Fig. 3 FDG-PET/CT images of a 73 years old woman with local recurrence in her right breast (red arrow) displayed in ROVER. **a** Maximum intensity projection images 1 h (1h) and 3 h (3h) after injection, **b** Transaxial images of thorax at 1h and 3h, **c** Zoomed transaxial images of the left side of thorax at 1h and 3h, and **d** Zoomed transaxial images with masks at 1h and 3h, where the green arrow shows the user defined 3D mask (equal mask size at 1h and 3h images), and the blue arrow shows the lesion ROI delineated by the ROVER software, which yielded the following values after 1h and 3h, respectively: MTV (cc) 3.8 and 2.1; SUVmax 3.2 and 3.7; SUVmean 1.8 and 2.6; cSUVmean 2.3 and 5.1

standard was the best option. Another limitation was the observed suboptimal segmentation with a fixed 40% of maximum value threshold. Segmentation methods using separate masks for 1h and 3h images in each patient were associated with challenges such as spatial mismatch between 1h and 3h acquisitions. This could contribute to segmentation variability and potentially incorrect comparison of quantitative results from the two time-points. Being the outcome of a single institution study, the generalizability of our results is uncertain.

The overall intention with this study was to consider whether a 3h scan should replace the 1h standard imaging in patients with metastatic breast cancer. Although we found an increased tumour-to-background ratio in 3h compared to 1h scans, this was not associated with improved diagnostic accuracy on a per-patient level as shown in our previous publication [33]. Furthermore, 3h protocols cause challenges regarding planning, patient discomfort and healthcare costs. Based on these experiences, it may not be justified to replace the standard 1h by a delayed imaging protocol.

Conclusion

SUVs of FDG increased significantly from 1h to 3h in malignant lesions of recurrent breast cancer and in all types of lesions, while reference measurements in healthy liver tissue decreased. PVC increased these values significantly as expected, especially in breast metastases. However, the demonstrated modest quantitative advances of 3h imaging can hardly justify delayed PET imaging on a routine basis in this patient group.

Abbreviations

1h: 1 h; 3h: 3 h; BMI: Body mass index; CI: Confidence interval; cSUVmean: Partial volume corrected SUVmean; CT: Computed tomography; DTPI: Delayed time-point imaging; FDG-PET/CT: ^{18}F-fluoro-deoxy-glucose positron emission tomography/computed tomography G6PaseGlucose-6-phosphatase; MBq: Mega Becquerel; MRI: Magnetic resonance imaging; MTV: Metabolic active tumour volume; OSEM: Ordered subset expectation maximization; PVC: Partial volume correction; PVE: Partial volume effect; ROI: Region-of-interest; SD: Standard deviation; SUV: Standard uptake values; SUVmax: Maximum standard uptake value; SUVmean: Mean standard uptake value

Acknowledgements

The authors would like to express their gratitude towards two reviewers whose comments significantly improved former versions of the manuscript. Moreover, the authors acknowledge the support of the staff at the Department of Nuclear Medicine, Odense University Hospital, Denmark. Special thanks to the PET/CT technologists for technical assistance with the imaging studies and to Birgitte B. Olsen for ongoing constructive feedback on the project.

Funding
The project was implemented without the involvement of private organizations or companies.

Authors' contributions
CB, MGH, KF AA and PFC conceptualised and designed the study CB and MGH acquired and analysed data and drafted the manuscript. KF acquired and analysed data. JH and OG analysed and interpreted data. PFHC, AA, OG and TQN enhanced the intellectual content of and reviewed the manuscript. All authors have read and approved the final version of the manuscript.

Competing interests
The authors declare that they have no competing interests.

Author details
[1]Department of Nuclear Medicine, University Hospital, Sdr. Boulevard 29, 5000 Odense C, Denmark. [2]Centre of Health Economics Research, University of Southern Denmark, Odense, Denmark. [3]University of Pennsylvania, Philadelphia, USA.

References
1. Jemal A, Bray F, Center MM, Ferlay J, Ward E, Forman D. Global cancer statistics. CA Cancer J Clin. 2011;61(2):69–90.
2. International Agency for Research on Cancer, Globocan 2012. http://globocan.iarc.fr/Pages/fact_sheets_cancer.aspx. Accessed 11 May 2016.
3. Groheux D, Espie M, Giacchetti S, Hindie E. Performance of FDG PET/CT in the clinical management of breast cancer. Radiology. 2013;266(2):388–405.
4. Pennant M, Takwoingi Y, Pennant L, Davenport C, Fry-Smith A, Eisinga A, Andronis L, Arvanitis T, Deeks J, Hyde C. A systematic review of positron emission tomography (PET) and positron emission tomography/computed tomography (PET/CT) for the diagnosis of breast cancer recurrence. Health Technol Asses. 2010;14(50):1–103.
5. Eubank WB, Mankoff DA, Vesselle HJ, Eary JF, Schubert EK, Dunnwald LK, Lindsley SK, Gralow JR, Austin-Seymour MM, Ellis GK, et al. Detection of locoregional and distant recurrences in breast cancer patients by using FDG PET. Radiographics. 2002;22(1):5–17.
6. Cheng G, Torigian DA, Zhuang H, Alavi A. When should we recommend use of dual time-point and delayed time-point imaging techniques in FDG PET? Eur J Nucl Med Mol I. 2013;40(5):779–87.
7. Matthies A, Hickeson M, Cuchiara A, Alavi A. Dual time point 18F-FDG PET for the evaluation of pulmonary nodules. J Nucl Med. 2002;43(7):871–5.
8. Houshmand S, Salavati A, Segtnan EA, Grupe P, Hoilund-Carlsen PF, Alavi A. Dual-time-point imaging and delayed-time-point Fluorodeoxyglucose-PET/computed tomography imaging in various clinical settings. PET Clin. 2016;11(1):65–84.
9. Cheng G, Alavi A, Lim E, Werner TJ, Del Bello CV, Akers SR. Dynamic changes of FDG uptake and clearance in normal tissues. Mol Imaging Biol. 2013;15(3):345–52.
10. Gillies RJ, Robey I, Gatenby RA. Causes and consequences of increased glucose metabolism of cancers. J Nucl Med. 2008;49(Suppl 2):24s–42s.
11. Boerner AR, Weckesser M, Herzog H, Schmitz T, Audretsch W, Nitz U, Bender HG, Mueller-Gaertner HW. Optimal scan time for fluorine-18 fluorodeoxyglucose positron emission tomography in breast cancer. Eur J Nucl Med. 1999;26(3):226–30.
12. Kumar R, Loving VA, Chauhan A, Zhuang H, Mitchell S, Alavi A. Potential of dual-time-point imaging to improve breast cancer diagnosis with (18)F-FDG PET. J Nucl Med. 2005;46(11):1819–24.
13. Mavi A, Urhan M, Yu JQ, Zhuang H, Houseni M, Cermik TF, Thiruvenkatasamy D, Czerniecki B, Schnall M, Alavi A. Dual time point 18F-FDG PET imaging detects breast cancer with high sensitivity and correlates well with histologic subtypes. J Nucl Med. 2006;47(9):1440–6.
14. Beaulieu S, Kinahan P, Tseng J, Dunnwald LK, Schubert EK, Pham P, Lewellen B, Mankoff DA. SUV varies with time after injection in (18)F-FDG PET of breast cancer: characterization and method to adjust for time differences. J Nucl Med. 2003;44(7):1044–50.
15. Basu S, Mavi A, Cermik T, Houseni M, Alavi A. Implications of standardized uptake value measurements of the primary lesions in proven cases of breast carcinoma with different degree of disease burden at diagnosis: does 2-deoxy-2-[F-18]fluoro-D-glucose-positron emission tomography predict tumor biology? Mol Imaging Biol. 2008;10(1):62–6.
16. Chan WL, Ramsay SC, Szeto ER, Freund J, Pohlen JM, Tarlinton LC, Young A, Hickey A, Dura R. Dual-time-point (18)F-FDG-PET/CT imaging in the assessment of suspected malignancy. J Med Imag Radiat On. 2011;55(4):379–90.
17. Lee JW, Kim SK, Lee SM, Moon SH, Kim TS. Detection of hepatic metastases using dual-time-point FDG PET/CT scans in patients with colorectal cancer. Mol Imaging Biol. 2011;13(3):565–72.
18. Basu S, Alavi A. Partial volume correction of standardized uptake values and the dual time point in FDG-PET imaging: should these be routinely employed in assessing patients with cancer? Eur J Nucl Med Mol I. 2007;34(10):1527–9.
19. Kadoya T, Aogi K, Kiyoto S, Masumoto N, Sugawara Y, Okada M. Role of maximum standardized uptake value in fluorodeoxyglucose positron emission tomography/computed tomography predicts malignancy grade and prognosis of operable breast cancer: a multi-institute study. Breast Cancer Res Tr. 2013;141(2):269–75.
20. Vriens D, Visser EP, de Geus-Oei LF, Oyen WJ. Methodological considerations in quantification of oncological FDG PET studies. Eur J Nucl Med Mol I. 2010;37(7):1408–25.
21. Gamez-Cenzano C, Pino-Sorroche F. Standardization and quantification in FDG-PET/CT imaging for staging and restaging of malignant disease. PET Clin. 2014;9(2):117–27.
22. Basu S, Zaidi H, Houseni M, Bural G, Udupa J, Acton P, Torigian DA, Alavi A. Novel quantitative techniques for assessing regional and global function and structure based on modern imaging modalities: implications for normal variation, aging and diseased states. Semin Nucl Med. 2007;37(3):223–39.
23. Groheux D, Giacchetti S, Moretti JL, Porcher R, Espie M, Lehmann-Che J, de Roquancourt A, Hamy AS, Cuvier C, Vercellino L, et al. Correlation of high 18F-FDG uptake to clinical, pathological and biological prognostic factors in breast cancer. Eur J Nucl Med Mol I. 2011;38(3):426–35.
24. Morris PG, Ulaner GA, Eaton A, Fazio M, Jhaveri K, Patil S, Evangelista L, Park JY, Serna-Tamayo C, Howard J, et al. Standardized uptake value by positron emission tomography/computed tomography as a prognostic variable in metastatic breast cancer. Cancer. 2012;118(22):5454–62.
25. Garcia Vicente AM, Soriano Castrejon A, Leon Martin A, Chacon Lopez-Muniz I, Munoz Madero V. Munoz Sanchez Mdel M, Palomar Munoz a, Espinosa Aunion R, Gonzalez Ageitos a: molecular subtypes of breast cancer: metabolic correlation with (1)(8)F-FDG PET/CT. Eur J Nucl Med Mol I. 2013;40(9):1304–11.
26. Soret M, Bacharach SL, Buvat I. Partial-volume effect in PET tumor imaging. J Nucl Med. 2007;48(6):932–45.
27. Hoetjes NJ, van Velden FH, Hoekstra OS, Hoekstra CJ, Krak NC, Lammertsma AA, Boellaard R. Partial volume correction strategies for quantitative FDG PET in oncology. Eur J Nucl Med Mol I. 2010;37(9):1679–87.
28. Gallivanone F, Canevari C, Sassi I, Zuber V, Marassi A, Gianolli L, Picchio M, Messa C, Gilardi MC, Castiglioni I. Partial volume corrected 18F-FDG PET mean standardized uptake value correlates with prognostic factors in breast cancer. Q J Nucl Med. 2014;58(4):424–39.
29. Aston JA, Cunningham VJ, Asselin MC, Hammers A, Evans AC, Gunn RN. Positron emission tomography partial volume correction: estimation and algorithms. J Cerebr Blood F Met. 2002;22(8):1019–34.
30. Boussion N, Hatt M, Lamare F, Bizais Y, Turzo A, Cheze-Le Rest C, Visvikis D. A multiresolution image based approach for correction of

partial volume effects in emission tomography. Phys Med Biol. 2006; 51(7):1857–76.

31. Torigian DA, Lopez RF, Alapati S, Bodapati G, Hofheinz F, van den Hoff J, Saboury B, Alavi A. Feasibility and performance of novel software to quantify metabolically active volumes and 3D partial volume corrected SUV and metabolic volumetric products of spinal bone marrow metastases on 18F-FDG-PET/CT. Hell J Nuc Med. 2011;14(1):8–14.

32. Hofheinz F, Langner J, Petr J, Beuthien-Baumann B, Oehme L, Steinbach J, Kotzerke J, van den Hoff J. A method for model-free partial volume correction in oncological PET. Eur J Nucl Med Mol I Research. 2012;2(1):16.

33. Hildebrandt MG, Gerke O, Baun C, Falch K, Hansen JA, Farahani ZA, Petersen H, Larsen LB, Duvnjak S, Buskevica I, et al. [18F]Fluorodeoxyglucose (FDG)-positron emission tomography (PET)/computed tomography (CT) in suspected recurrent breast Cancer: a prospective comparative study of dual-time-point FDG-PET/CT, contrast-enhanced CT, and bone scintigraphy. J Clin Oncol. 2016;34:1889–97.

34. Hofheinz F, Potzsch C, Oehme L, Beuthien-Baumann B, Steinbach J, Kotzerke J, van den Hoff J. Automatic volume delineation in oncological PET. Evaluation of a dedicated software tool and comparison with manual delineation in clinical data sets. Nuklearmedizin. 2012;51(1):9–16.

35. Suga K, Kawakami Y, Hiyama A, Matsunaga N. Differentiation of FDG-avid loco-regional recurrent and compromised benign lesions after surgery for breast cancer with dual-time point F-18-fluorodeoxy-glucose PET/CT scan. Ann Nucl Med. 2009;23(4):399–407.

36. Caprio MG, Cangiano A, Imbriaco M, Soscia F, Di Martino G, Farina A, Avitabile G, Pace L, Forestieri P, Salvatore M. Dual-time-point [18F]-FDG PET/CT in the diagnostic evaluation of suspicious breast lesions. Radiol Med. 2010;115:215–24.

37. Choi WH, Yoo IR, JH O, Kim SH, Chung SK. The value of dual-time-point 18F-FDG PET/CT for identifying axillary lymph node metastasis in breast cancer patients. Brit J Rad. 2011;84(1003):593–9.

38. Chirindel A, Alluri KC, Tahari AK, Chaudhry M, Wahl RL, Lodge MA, Subramaniam RM. Liver standardized uptake value corrected for lean body mass at FDG PET/CT: effect of FDG uptake time. Clin Nucl Med. 2015;40(1):e17–22.

39. Tian R, Su M, Tian Y, Li F, Li L, Kuang A, Zeng J. Dual-time point PET/CT with F-18 FDG for the differentiation of malignant and benign bone lesions. Skelet Radiol. 2009;38(5):451–8.

40. Hamaoka T, Madewell JE, Podoloff DA, Hortobagyi GN, Ueno NT. Bone imaging in metastatic breast cancer. J Clin Oncol. 2004;22(14):2942–53.

41. Cook GJ, Houston S, Rubens R, Maisey MN, Fogelman I. Detection of bone metastases in breast cancer by 18FDG PET: differing metabolic activity in osteoblastic and osteolytic lesions. J Clin Oncol. 1998;16(10):3375–9.

42. Boellaard R, Krak NC, Hoekstra OS, Lammertsma AA. Effects of noise, image resolution, and ROI definition on the accuracy of standard uptake values: a simulation study. J Nucl Med. 2004;45(9):1519–27.

43. Huang SC. Anatomy of SUV. Standardized uptake value. Nucl Med Biol. 2000;27(7):643–6.

44. Keyes JW Jr. SUV: standard uptake or silly useless value? J Nucl Med. 1995; 36(10):1836–9.

45. Krak NC, Boellaard R, Hoekstra OS, Twisk JW, Hoekstra CJ, Lammertsma AA. Effects of ROI definition and reconstruction method on quantitative outcome and applicability in a response monitoring trial. Eur J Nucl Med Mol I. 2005;32(3):294–301.

46. Nahmias C, Wahl LM. Reproducibility of standardized uptake value measurements determined by 18F-FDG PET in malignant tumors. J Nucl Med. 2008;49(11):1804–8.

47. Bai B, Bading J, Conti PS. Tumor quantification in clinical positron emission tomography. Theranostics. 2013;3(10):787–801.

48. Boellaard R. Standards for PET image acquisition and quantitative data analysis. J Nucl Med. 2009;50(Suppl 1):11s–20s.

49. Tomasi G, Turkheimer F, Aboagye E. Importance of quantification for the analysis of PET data in oncology: review of current methods and trends for the future. Mol Imaging Biol. 2012;14(2):131–46.

50. Houshmand S, Salavati A, Hess S, Werner TJ, Alavi A, Zaidi H. An update on novel quantitative techniques in the context of evolving whole-body PET imaging. PET Clin. 2015;10(1):45–58.

51. Boellaard R, Delgado-Bolton R, Oyen WJ, Giammarile F, Tatsch K, Eschner W, Verzijlbergen FJ, Barrington SF, Pike LC, Weber WA, et al. FDG PET/CT: EANM procedure guidelines for tumour imaging: version 2.0. Eur J Nucl Med Mol I. 2015;42(2):328–54.

16

Evaluation of dynamic infrared thermography as an alternative to CT angiography for perforator mapping in breast reconstruction: a clinical study

Sven Weum[1,2*], James B. Mercer[1,2] and Louis de Weerd[1,3]

Abstract

Background: The current gold standard for preoperative perforator mapping in breast reconstruction with a DIEP flap is CT angiography (CTA). Dynamic infrared thermography (DIRT) is an imaging method that does not require ionizing radiation or contrast injection. We evaluated if DIRT could be an alternative to CTA in perforator mapping.

Methods: Twenty-five patients scheduled for secondary breast reconstruction with a DIEP flap were included. Preoperatively, the lower abdomen was examined with hand-held Doppler, DIRT and CTA. Arterial Doppler sound locations were marked on the skin. DIRT examination involved rewarming of the abdominal skin after a mild cold challenge. The locations of hot spots on DIRT were compared with the arterial Doppler sound locations. The rate and pattern of rewarming of the hot spots were analyzed. Multiplanar CT reconstructions were used to see if hot spots were related to perforators on CTA. All flaps were based on the perforator selected with DIRT and the surgical outcome was analyzed.

Results: First appearing hot spots were always associated with arterial Doppler sounds and clearly visible perforators on CTA. The hot spots on DIRT images were always slightly laterally located in relation to the exit points of the associated perforators through the rectus abdominis fascia on CTA. Some periumbilical perforators were not associated with hot spots and showed communication with the superficial inferior epigastric vein on CTA. The selected perforators adequately perfused all flaps.

Conclusion: This study confirms that perforators selected with DIRT have arterial Doppler sound, are clearly visible on CTA and provide adequate perfusion for DIEP breast reconstruction.

Trial registration: Retrospectively registered at ClinicalTrials.gov with identifier NCT02806518.

Keywords: Deep Inferior Epigastric Perforator (DIEP), Medical thermography, Perforator flap surgery, Perforator imaging, CT angiography, Radiology, Plastic surgery, Reconstructive surgery, Breast reconstruction

* Correspondence: sven.weum@unn.no
[1]Medical Imaging Research Group, Department of Clinical Medicine, UiT The Arctic University of Norway, 9037 Tromsø, Norway
[2]Department of Radiology, University Hospital of North Norway, Sykehusveien 38, P.O. Box 103, 9038 Tromsø, Norway
Full list of author information is available at the end of the article

Background

Breast reconstruction with a deep inferior epigastric perforator (DIEP) flap utilizing skin and subcutaneous tissue from the patient's lower abdomen has become a popular option for women treated for breast cancer. The DIEP flap receives its blood supply from a perforator consisting of an artery and one or two comitant veins arising from the deep inferior epigastric artery (DIEA) and vein [1, 2]. In DIEP breast reconstruction the blood supply to the DIEP flap is reestablished by anastomosing the perforator to the internal mammary vessels.

The selected perforator is crucial for flap survival as it is the only source of blood supply to the flap. Although intraoperative perforator selection without preoperative perforator mapping is possible, the large variability in the numbers, locations and diameters of perforators makes this rather difficult [3–5]. A multicenter consensus study considered CTA the preferred method for preoperative perforator mapping [6]. CTA allows for precise anatomical description of the origin of perforators, their intramuscular course and point of fascia penetration. The main disadvantages of CTA are exposure to ionizing radiation and the use of intravenous contrast medium. The use of CTA is also associated with high costs. CTA can be time consuming due to delays in obtaining CTA preoperatively leading to delay in surgery, time the patient has to expend to obtain the CTA, and time of the surgeon and radiologist to review the imaging.

In 1993 Itoh and Arai described for the first time in English literature the use of dynamic infrared thermography (DIRT) for perforator mapping in DIEP flaps [7, 8]. Perforators that transport blood to the subdermal plexus cause a local heating at the skin surface that can be visualized as hot spots on infrared images. In DIRT a cold challenge is applied to the skin surface and temperature changes at the hot spots during the rewarming period are registered with an infrared camera. It might be beneficial for patients if DIRT could replace CTA in preoperative perforating mapping as DIRT, unlike CTA, does not involve the exposure to ionizing radiation or the use of intravenous contrast medium. DIRT has been used in the preoperative planning as well as intraoperative and postoperative monitoring of flap perfusion [9–14]. To our knowledge there are no studies that systematically have compared DIRT with other techniques for preoperative perforator mapping.

In this study the results of preoperative perforator mapping in DIEP breast reconstruction with DIRT were compared with those obtained with the most frequently used techniques hand-held Doppler and CTA. As flap sur·:val is dependent on the selected perforator, all breast reconstructions were based on the perforator selected with DIRT and the surgical outcome was evaluated.

Methods

This prospective clinical study was approved by the Regional Committee for Research Ethics. After giving informed consent to participation and publication of data, 25 women with mean age 57 years (range 38–69) and mean body mass index 27.2 kg/m^2 (range 21.6–32.4) scheduled for DIEP breast reconstruction were included. Perforator mapping on the lower abdomen was performed with hand-held Doppler, DIRT and CTA in the same supine position. In all cases the DIEP breast reconstruction was based on the perforator selected with DIRT. The DIRT results were compared to the results obtained with the hand-held Doppler and CTA. Evaluation of the surgical outcome related to flap survival was made.

The flap was marked on the lower abdomen. The lateral border of each rectus abdominis muscle was marked following palpation before and during muscle contraction. To describe the locations of perforators, a quadrant system was used. The flap surface overlying each rectus fascia was divided into 4 quadrants (Fig. 1). The vertical line at the midline between the upper and lower border of the flap is bisected in two equal lengths and defines the horizontal line between upper and lower quadrants. The area between the lateral border of each rectus abdominis muscle and the linea alba is bisected in equal parts by a vertical line.

Hand-held Doppler (8 MHz, Multi Dopplex II, Huntleigh Healthcare, Cardiff, UK) was used to locate arterial Doppler sounds within the quadrants and these were marked as black dots on the skin. DIRT included a 5-min acclimatization of the exposed abdomen at room temperature (22–24 °C).

An infrared camera (FLIR ThermaCAM S65 HS, FLIR Systems, Boston, MA) was used to capture video sequences of thermal images before, during and after exposure of the lower abdomen to a cold challenge. This cold challenge was provided by blowing air at room temperature for 2 min over the abdomen using a desktop fan (Fig. 2). The temperature changes were well within the physiological range. After a recovery period of 3 min, the presence of arterial Doppler sounds at the first appearing hot spots was evaluated with hand-held Doppler. If present at a hot spot, its location was marked with a cross on the skin. A digital photo of the abdomen was taken at the end of the DIRT examination using the same angle as the infrared camera (Fig. 3). Thermal images and photos were stored on the hospital's picture archiving and communication system (PACS).

The thermal images were qualitatively analyzed for the rate and pattern of rewarming of the hot spots. The first appearing hot spots and their associated quadrants were registered and named with increasing identification numbers based on their order of appearance. Hot spots showing the same rate of rewarming were ranked on basis of

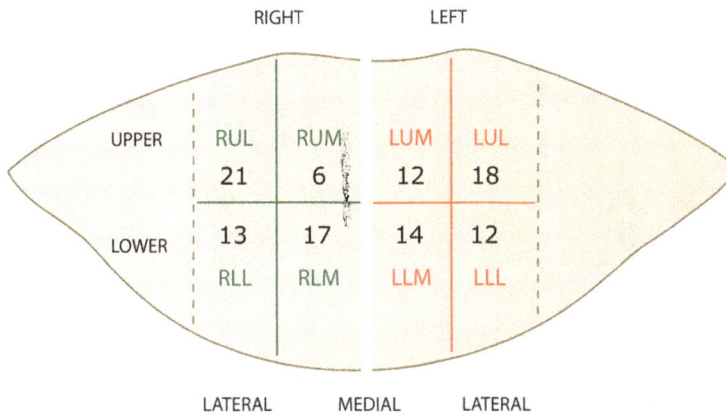

Fig. 1 The quadrant system: The flap surface over each rectus fascia is divided into four quadrants. The abbreviations indicate right/left (R/L), upper/lower (U/L) and lateral/medial (L/M). The numbers indicate the distribution of hot spots in the 25 patients

rewarming of the area around the hot spot. The hot spot with most progressive rewarming was given the lowest number.

CTA was performed (SOMATOM Sensation 16, Siemens Medical Solutions, Erlangen, Germany) after intravenous

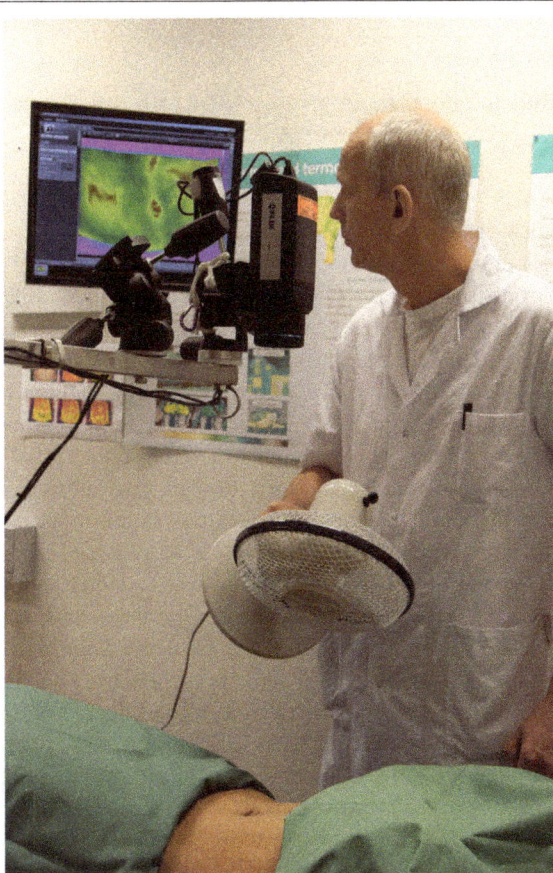

Fig. 2 An infrared camera captures video sequences of thermal images before, during and after a cold challenge delivered by a desktop fan

injection of contrast medium (Ultravist 370, Schering AG, Berlin, Germany or Iomeron 350, Bracco, Milan, Italy) with bolus triggering on the distal aorta. Scan parameters are summarized in Table 1. Three- dimensional (3D) and multiplanar reconstructions (MPR) were used to evaluate the DIEA and its perforators within the flap area (OsiriX version 4.0, OsiriX foundation, Geneva, Switzerland). On coronal thick maximum intensity projection (MIP) images the course and ramifications of the DIEA were evaluated on both sides. Axial thick MIP images were used to evaluate if there was a dominating DIEA system with perforators suitable for a DIEP reconstruction.

CTA images were analyzed by consensus between a radiologist (SW) and plastic surgeon (LdW). MPR images were used to see if the locations of the first appearing hot spots could be related to perforators from the DIEA. Axial images were used to decide if perforators were classified as lateral or medial. Sagittal images were used to decide if perforators were cranially or caudally located to the level midway between the umbilicus and the pubic symphysis.

Results

Preoperative results

DIRT revealed a large variability in location, size, and number of hot spots between patients. This variability was also seen between the left and right side. Hot spots were always associated with arterial Doppler sounds. First appearing hot spots during rewarming were brighter than those appearing later. The hand-held Doppler does not allow for quantitative volume registration but, subjectively, the brightness of hot spots was related to the volume of Doppler sounds. All first appearing hot spots were also associated with clearly visible perforators on CTA and located in the same quadrants (Fig. 4). Hot spots were always slightly laterally located to the exit points of the perforators through the rectus fascia as seen on CTA.

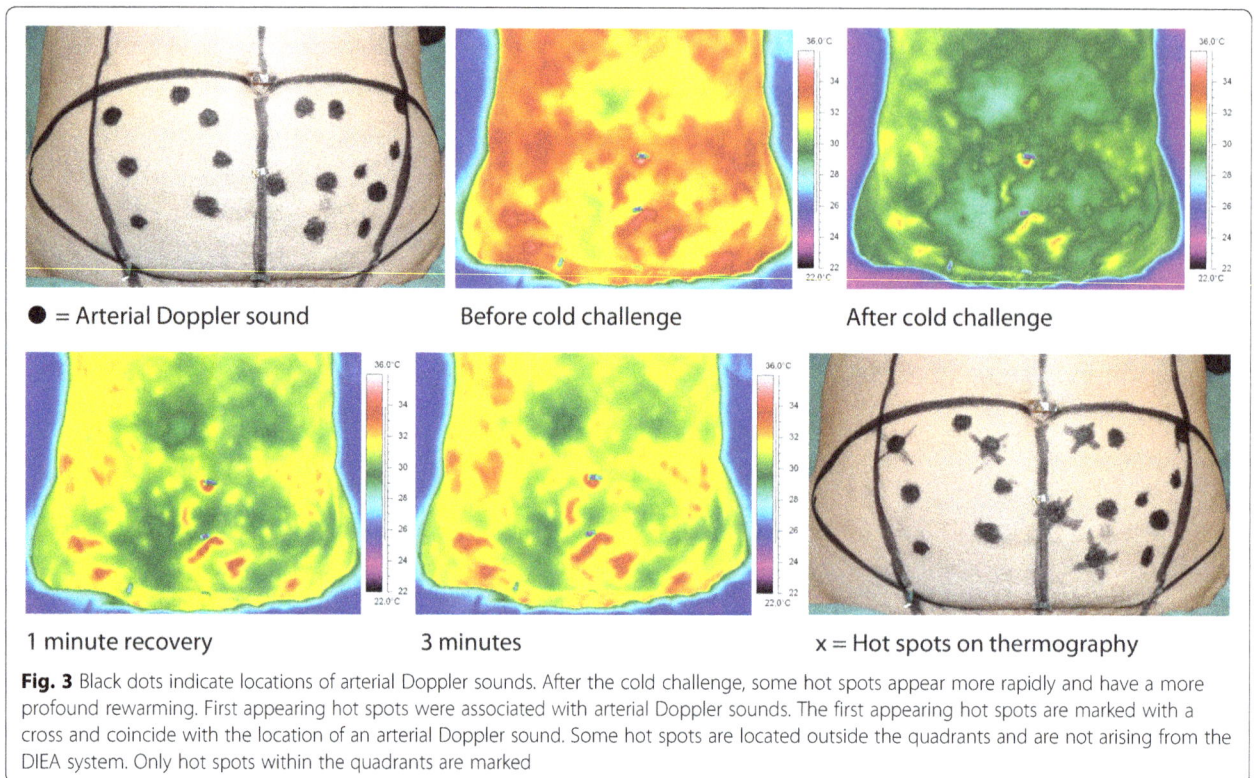

Fig. 3 Black dots indicate locations of arterial Doppler sounds. After the cold challenge, some hot spots appear more rapidly and have a more profound rewarming. First appearing hot spots were associated with arterial Doppler sounds. The first appearing hot spots are marked with a cross and coincide with the location of an arterial Doppler sound. Some hot spots are located outside the quadrants and are not arising from the DIEA system. Only hot spots within the quadrants are marked

In our 25 patients 113 hot spots were registered using DIRT and 108 (95.6 %) corresponded to a perforator in the same quadrant seen on CTA (Fig. 1). The remaining 5 hot spots (4.4 %) were all found in the lower part of the lower quadrants and corresponded to perforators coming from other arteries than the DIEA. The 113 hot spots were evenly distributed between the right and left side (57/56), as well as between the upper and lower quadrants (57/56). In the upper quadrants there were fewer medial than lateral hot spots (18/39).

Some large periumbilical perforators on CTA were associated with arterial Doppler sounds but not with hot spots. In these cases 3D reconstruction revealed a connection between the perforator and the superficial inferior epigastric vein in the periumbilical area. Not all arterial Doppler sounds locations could be associated with a hot spot on DIRT or a perforator on CTA.

Surgical results

In all cases, the selected hot spots could be related to perforators found intraoperatively. Large periumbilical perforators that were not associated with a hot spot consisted of a small artery with one or two large comitant veins. The marked hot spots were always slightly laterally located to the exit points of the perforator through the fascia. While all first appearing hot spots could be related to suitable perforators, not all arterial Doppler sound locations on the skin could be related to suitable perforators intraoperatively. All flaps were based on the selected perforator from DIRT and were adequately perfused. Of the 25 flaps, 24 survived. One flap was lost on the second postoperative day due to a bleeding beneath the flap that was diagnosed too late to save the flap. This complication could not be related to the selected perforator. The mean flap weight was 713 grams (range 302–1270). Twelve flaps were based on one perforator, nine flaps on two perforators, two flaps on three perforators and two flaps on four perforators. In all cases the selected perforator visualized with DIRT was the most suitable perforator, additional perforators were added in cases with large volume flaps to guarantee adequate flap perfusion.

Table 1 CT scan parameters

Patient position: Head first supine
Range: 3 cm cranial of umbilicus to symphysis
Bolus tracking: Abdominal aorta 2 cm cranial to bifurcation
Contrast medium: 120 mL Ultravist 370 or Iomeron 350, 4.0 mL/s
Voltage: 120 kV
Current: 150–200 mA
Slice collimation: 0.75 mm
Kernel: B20f medium
Slice width/increment: 1.0 mm/0.7 mm reconstruction

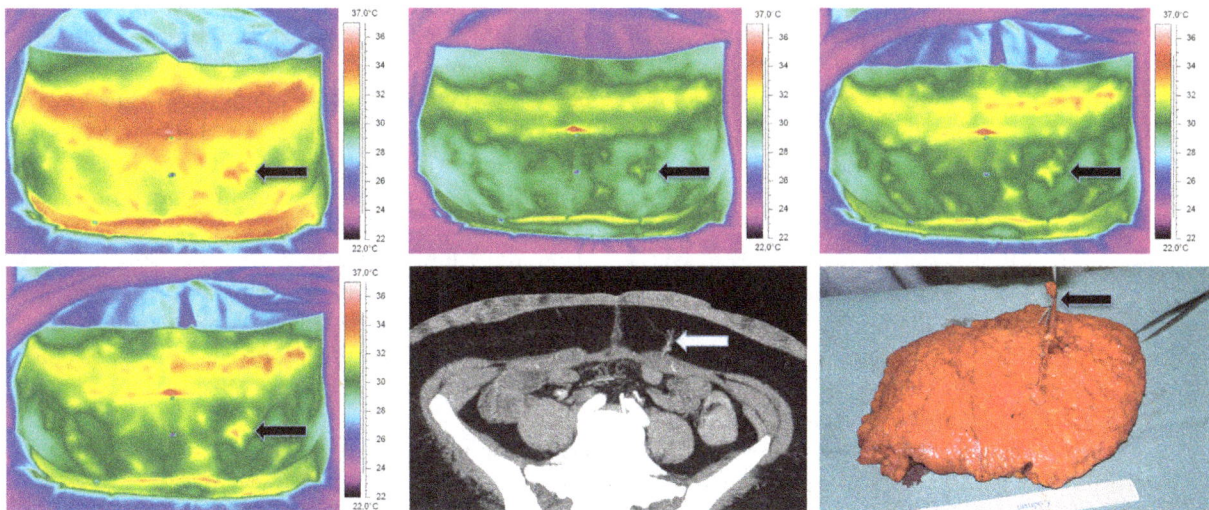

Fig. 4 The selected hot spot (*arrow* on IR images) is associated with a perforator on CTA (arrow on CTA image) and intraoperatively (*arrow* on intraoperative flap image)

Discussion

The main finding of this study is that the first appearing hot spots on DIRT were always associated with arterial Doppler sounds as well as clearly visible perforators on CTA and intraoperatively. The use of DIRT in preoperative perforator mapping provided a suitable perforator for DIEP breast reconstruction in all 25 cases.

Surgeons want information on the hemodynamic properties of a perforator as well as its location. Hand-held Doppler is frequently used for preoperative perforator mapping. Giunta et al. attributed the high number of false-positive results in their study to the relative high sensitivity of the hand-held Doppler [15]. Very small perforating vessels were also located, unsuitable for perforator flaps because of their narrow caliber. Others have abandoned hand-held Doppler because the results often proved to be aberrant from the intraoperative observations [16]. Similar to Giunta we found arterial Doppler sounds that could not be associated with hot spots, nor with suitable perforators intraoperatively.

CTA has become the current gold standard for perforator mapping and is based on the perfusion of the perforators with contrast medium during the arterial phase. It provides information on the caliber of each perforator, its intramuscular course and its exit point through the anterior rectus fascia [6]. However, a recent study by Cina et al. revealed that the sum of the diameter of the perforating artery and vein with color Doppler was in agreement with the diameter of the presumed artery on CTA [2]. However, there was a significant disagreement between the measured diameters of the arteries measured with color Doppler and CTA, as well as for CTA and intraoperative findings. Thus, measurement of the assumed perforating artery on CTA may in fact constitute the sum of the diameters of the perforating artery and vein(s). Mathes et al. warned against sole reliance on CTA perforator mapping as they had to make a significant number of changes intraoperatively [17]. Important disadvantages of CTA are exposure to ionizing radiation and the use of intravenous contrast medium. A method without these disadvantages would be beneficial.

In our study, the rate and pattern of rewarming of the hot spots were analyzed. There was a large variability in the number of hot spots and in the rate and pattern of rewarming. As first appearing hot spots were associated with perforators on CTA and arterial Doppler sounds, the rewarming at the hot spot is a result of blood perfusion through the perforator to the skin surface.

During the rewarming period all perforators compete with each other in skin rewarming. A rapid rewarming indicates that the associated perforator transports more blood to the skin surface than a perforator that produces a slower rewarming. Progressive rewarming around the hot spot indicates a well-developed vascular network around this hot spot. A well-developed branching pattern is also considered an important criterion when selecting a perforator on CTA [18, 19]. By analyzing the rate and pattern of rewarming, the surgeon obtains information on the perforator's hemodynamic properties.

Information on the location where the suitable perforator can be found is of great value to the surgeon. Chubb et al. reported their preliminary results with DIRT and reported that this technique matched the accuracy of CTA for perforator location [20]. We found, however, that the hot spot on the skin was always slightly laterally located in relation to the perforator's exit point through the rectus abdominis fascia. Using CTA, Rozen et al. found in their perforator angiosome study that lateral row perforators have a long and laterally directed course, whereas the medial perforators show a straighter course from the rectus sheath towards the skin [21]. An explanation for this lateral orientation of vessels was given by the eminent anatomist John Hunter (1728–1793), who saw it as a product of growth that occurs from the stage of fetus to adulthood [22]. In contrast to CTA, DIRT does not provide information on the intramuscular course of the perforator. Although the main goal of perforator mapping is to find a perforator that can provide adequate blood perfusion of the flap, a perforator with a short intramuscular course is preferred to a perforator with the same caliber and a longer intramuscular course. Interestingly, de Weerd et al. found in a DIRT study that first appearing hot spots were often associated with perforators passing through the tendineous intersection [19]. These perforators have a very short intramuscular course. A further advantage of CTA over DIRT is that CTA can provide information on the continuity of the deep inferior epigastric system in patients that have been previously operated in that area. In cases with large flap volumes, additional perforators were added to the selected perforator to optimize flap perfusion, as also reported by Gill et al. in their retrospective study [23].

Our results showed cases in which large periumbilical perforators on CTA could not be associated with hot spots. This indicates that these perforators do not transport much blood the skin surface. We postulate that such perforators consist of a small caliber artery and one or two large caliber comitant veins and that these large veins communicate with the superficial inferior epigastric vein. This postulation is supported by our intraoperative findings and CTA. The existence of these communications was already described by Carramenha e Costa et al. in an anatomic study and nicely illustrated with the use of CTA by Rozen at al. in a study on the venous anatomy of the abdominal wall [24, 25].

One of the disadvantages of DIRT is that only perforators that transport blood to the skin surface are detected. It is possible that a perforator that ends in the subcutaneous tissue might be a suitable perforator for DIEP breast reconstruction. Such a perforator can be detected with CTA but not with DIRT. From earlier studies it is known that the subdermal plexus contributes to the perfusion of the underlying subcutaneous tissue. In their cross sectional radiographic study, Taylor et al. revealed blood supply to the subcutaneous layer caused by "raining down" from the subdermal plexus, a result confirmed by Schaverien et al. [26, 27]. Initially, the perfusion of the DIEP flap depends on this mechanism. During the first postoperative week, the interconnections between the vascular structures within the flap increase in size and, as a result, tissue perfusion improves [28]. The main limitation of this study is the small number of 25 patients. Because of the small study size our results are indicative and should be

interpreted within the context of this limitation. One limitation in this study is that we were unable to objectively measure perfusion of subcutaneous tissue. Such is possible using indocyanine green angiography intraoperatively [29]. Inadequate perfusion of subcutaneous tissue fat may cause fat necrosis or wound-healing problems. None of our patients had a wound-healing problem at the reconstructed site or required a reoperation for fat necrosis. Another limitation is that DIRT was used in relatively healthy patients. The mean BMI was 27.2 kg/m^2 (range 21.6–32.4). Further studies are required to evaluate the usefulness of DIRT in preoperative perforator mapping in patients with co-morbidities and obesity.

Conclusions

We conclude that the locations of first appearing hot spots on DIRT are associated with arterial Doppler sounds and with perforators on CTA. In addition, the surgical results revealed that DIEP breast reconstruction could reliably be performed using DIRT for perforator selection. DIRT provides information on the location of the perforator and its hemodynamic properties. DIRT is easy to interpret and it does not involve exposure to ionizing radiation or the use of intravenous contrast medium. Based on our results we conclude that DIRT is a promising alternative to CTA for preoperative perforator mapping in DIEP breast reconstruction.

Abbreviations
3D, Three-dimensional; CT, Computed tomography; CTA, Computed tomographic angiography; DIEA, Deep inferior epigastric artery; DIEP, Deep inferior epigastric artery perforator; DIRT, Dynamic infrared thermography; MIP, Maximum intensity projection; MPR, Multiplanar reconstruction; PACS, Picture archiving and communication system

Acknowledgements
Not applicable.

Funding
The corresponding author has received research grants provided by the Norwegian Research School in Medical Imaging (MedIm) and Northern Norway Regional Health Authority (Helse Nord RHF). The other authors have not received any funding.

Authors' contributions
All three authors have participated in the planning of the study, the collection of data, interpretation of data and writing of the manuscript. All authors read and approved the final manuscript.

Authors' information
SW is a Consultant Radiologist and Associate Professor at the University Hospital of North Norway and Head of Medical Imaging Research Group at UiT the Arctic University of Norway. JM is a Professor at UiT the Arctic University of Norway and the University Hospital of North Norway where he is responsible for the thermography laboratory. JM was the President of European Association of Thermology from 2009 to 2015. LdW is a Plastic Surgeon and Professor at the University Hospital of North Norway. LdW specializes in reconstructive surgery and the development of new surgical techniques in plastic surgery.

Competing interests
The authors declare that they have no competing interests.

Author details
[1]Medical Imaging Research Group, Department of Clinical Medicine, UiT The Arctic University of Norway, 9037 Tromsø, Norway. [2]Department of Radiology, University Hospital of North Norway, Sykehusveien 38, P.O. Box 103, 9038 Tromsø, Norway. [3]Department of Plastic Surgery and Hand Surgery, University Hospital of North Norway, P.O. Box 66, 9038 Tromsø, Norway.

References
1. El-Mrakby HH, Milner RH. The vascular anatomy of the lower anterior abdominal wall: a microdissection study on the deep inferior epigastric vessels and the perforator branches. Plast Reconstr Surg. 2002;109(2):539–43. discussion 544–537.
2. Cina A, Salgarello M, Barone-Adesi L, Rinaldi P, Bonomo L. Planning breast reconstruction with deep inferior epigastric artery perforating vessels: multidetector CT angiography versus color Doppler US. Radiology. 2010; 255(3):979–87.
3. Blondeel PN. One hundred free DIEP flap breast reconstructions: a personal experience. Br J Plast Surg. 1999;52(2):104–11.
4. Mathes DW, Neligan PC. Current techniques in preoperative imaging for abdomen-based perforator flap microsurgical breast reconstruction. J Reconstr Microsurg. 2010;26(1):3–10.
5. Blondeel PN, Beyens G, Verhaeghe R, Van Landuyt K, Tonnard P, Monstrey SJ, Matton G. Doppler flowmetry in the planning of perforator flaps. Br J Plast Surg. 1998;51(3):202–9.
6. Rozen WM, Garcia-Tutor E, Alonso-Burgos A, Acosta R, Stillaert F, Zubieta JL, Hamdi M, Whitaker IS, Ashton MW. Planning and optimising DIEP flaps with virtual surgery: the Navarra experience. J Plast Reconstr Aesthet Surg. 2010; 63(2):289–97.
7. Itoh Y, Arai K. The deep inferior epigastric artery free skin flap: anatomic study and clinical application. Plast Reconstr Surg. 1993;91(5):853–63. discussion 864.
8. Itoh Y, Arai K. Use of recovery-enhanced thermography to localize cutaneous perforators. Ann Plast Surg. 1995;34(5):507–11.
9. Lohman RF, Ozturk CN, Ozturk C, Jayaprakash V, Djohan R. An analysis of current techniques used for intraoperative flap evaluation. Ann Plast Surg. 2014.
10. Tenorio X, Mahajan AL, Wettstein R, Harder Y, Pawlovski M, Pittet B. Early detection of flap failure using a new thermographic device. J Surg Res. 2009;151(1):15–21.
11. Salmi AM, Tukiainen E, Asko-Seljavaara S. Thermographic mapping of perforators and skin blood flow in the free transverse rectus abdominis musculocutaneous flap. Ann Plast Surg. 1995;35(2):159–64.
12. de Weerd L, Mercer JB, Weum S. Dynamic infrared thermography. Clin Plast Surg. 2011;38(2):277–92.
13. Whitaker IS, Lie KH, Rozen WM, Chubb D, Ashton MW. Dynamic infrared thermography for the preoperative planning of microsurgical breast reconstruction: a comparison with CTA. J Plast Reconstr Aesthet Surg. 2012;65(1):130–2.
14. Kalra S, Dancey A, Waters R. Intraoperative selection of dominant perforator vessel in DIEP free flaps based on perfusion strength using digital infrared thermography - a pilot study. J Plast Reconstr Aesthet Surg. 2007;60(12): 1365–8.
15. Giunta RE, Geisweid A, Feller AM. The value of preoperative Doppler sonography for planning free perforator flaps. Plast Reconstr Surg. 2000; 105(7):2381–6.
16. Vandevoort M, Vranckx JJ, Fabre G. Perforator topography of the deep inferior epigastric perforator flap in 100 cases of breast reconstruction. Plast Reconstr Surg. 2002;109(6):1912–8.
17. Mathes D, Keys S, Said H, Louie O, Neligan P. The clinical utility of CT angiography in deep inferior epigastric perforator (DIEP) flap microsurgical breast reconstruction. In: Proceedings world congress reconstructive surgery Helsinki. 2011.
18. Hijjawi JB, Blondeel PN. Advancing deep inferior epigastric artery perforator flap breast reconstruction through multidetector row computed tomography: an evolution in preoperative imaging. J Reconstr Microsurg. 2010;26(1):11–20.
19. de Weerd L, Weum S, Mercer JB. The value of dynamic infrared thermography (DIRT) in perforatorselection and planning of free DIEP flaps. Ann Plast Surg. 2009;63(3):274–9.
20. Chubb D, Rozen WM, Whitaker IS, Ashton MW. Images in plastic surgery: digital thermographic photography ("thermal imaging") for preoperative perforator mapping. Ann Plast Surg. 2011;66(4):324–5.
21. Rozen WM, Ashton MW, Le Roux CM, Pan WR, Corlett RJ. The perforator angiosome: a new concept in the design of deep inferior epigastric artery perforator flaps for breast reconstruction. Microsurgery. 2010;30(1):1–7.
22. Taylor GI, Palmer JH. The vascular territories (angiosomes) of the body: experimental study and clinical applications. Br J Plast Surg. 1987;40(2):113–41.
23. Gill PS, Hunt JP, Guerra AB, Dellacroce FJ, Sullivan SK, Boraski J, Metzinger SE, Dupin CL, Allen RJ. A 10-year retrospective review of 758 DIEP flaps for breast reconstruction. Plast Reconstr Surg. 2004;113(4):1153–60.
24. Carramenha e Costa MA, Carriquiry C, Vasconez LO, Grotting JC, Herrera RH, Windle BH. An anatomic study of the venous drainage of the transverse rectus abdominis musculocutaneous flap. Plast Reconstr Surg. 1987;79(2):208–17.
25. Rozen WM, Pan WR, Le Roux CM, Taylor GI, Ashton MW. The venous anatomy of the anterior abdominal wall: an anatomical and clinical study. Plast Reconstr Surg. 2009;124(3):848–53.
26. Taylor G, Ian AO. Vascular anatomy of the lower anterior abdominal wall: a microdissection study on the deep inferior epigastric vessels and the perforator branches by Hamdy H. El-Mrakby, M.D. Richard H. Milner, M.D. Plast Reconstr Surg. 2002;109(2):544–7.
27. Schaverien M, Saint-Cyr M, Arbique G, Brown SA. Arterial and venous anatomies of the deep inferior epigastric perforator and superficial inferior epigastric artery flaps. Plast Reconstr Surg. 2008;121(6):1909–19.
28. de Weerd L, Miland AO, Mercer JB. Perfusion dynamics of free DIEP and SIEA flaps during the first postoperative week monitored with dynamic infrared thermography. Ann Plast Surg. 2009;62(1):42–7.
29. Gurtner GC, Jones GE, Neligan PC, Newman MI, Phillips BT, Sacks JM, Zenn MR. Intraoperative laser angiography using the SPY system: review of the literature and recommendations for use. Ann Surg Innov Res. 2013;7(1):1.

17

Diagnostic imaging strategy for MDCT- or MRI-detected breast lesions: use of targeted sonography

Satoko Nakano[1*], Masahiko Ohtsuka[1], Akemi Mibu[2], Masato Karikomi[3], Hitomi Sakata[4] and Masahiro Yamamoto[4]

Abstract

Background: Leading-edge technology such as magnetic resonance imaging (MRI) or computed tomography (CT) often reveals mammographically and ultrasonographically occult lesions. MRI is a well-documented, effective tool to evaluate these lesions; however, the detection rate of targeted sonography varies for MRI detected lesions, and its significance is not well established in diagnostic strategy of MRI detected lesions. We assessed the utility of targeted sonography for multidetector-row CT (MDCT)- or MRI-detected lesions in practice.

Methods: We retrospectively reviewed 695 patients with newly diagnosed breast cancer who were candidates for breast conserving surgery and underwent MDCT or MRI in our hospital between January 2004 and March 2011. Targeted sonography was performed in all MDCT- or MRI-detected lesions followed by imaging-guided biopsy. Patient background, histopathology features and the sizes of the lesions were compared among benign, malignant and follow-up groups.

Results: Of the 695 patients, 61 lesions in 56 patients were detected by MDCT or MRI. The MDCT- or MRI-detected lesions were identified by targeted sonography in 58 out of 61 lesions (95.1%). Patients with pathological diagnoses were significantly older and more likely to be postmenopausal than the follow-up patients. Pathological diagnosis proved to be benign in 20 cases and malignant in 25. The remaining 16 lesions have been followed up.
Lesion size and shape were not significantly different among the benign, malignant and follow-up groups.

Conclusions: Approximately 95% of MDCT- or MRI-detected lesions were identified by targeted sonography, and nearly half of these lesions were pathologically proven malignancies in this study. Targeted sonography is a useful modality for MDCT- or MRI-detected breast lesions.

Background

Diagnostic procedures are crucial for the early detection of breast cancer. Advancements in imaging technology now enable us to detect mammographically and ultrasonographically occult lesions on magnetic resonance imaging (MRI) or computed tomography (CT) findings. MRI is well known for effectively detecting ductal spreading before breast-conserving surgery with excellent contrast resolution. The advantage of CT is a shorter single acquisition with extent evaluation. In Japan, CT is used for detecting the intraductal component of breast cancer as an alternative to MRI [1-4].

Multidetector-row CT (MDCT) produces imaging with a wide range and short volume acquisition time, recompounding thin slice imaging, and high-resolution and reconstructed imaging [1,2,5].

Enhancement on MDCT or MRI is due to angiogenesis and increased capillary permeability [6,7]. Enhancement of a lesion is an indication of proliferation regardless of whether it is malignant or benign. These lesions are not palpable, therefore imaging-guided biopsy is required for definitive diagnosis. There are three available ways to perform a biopsy under imaging guidance: stereo-guided, sonographically guided and MRI-guided procedures.

National Comprehensive Cancer Network (NCCN)'s guidelines have recommended the performance of MRI-guided needle sampling and/or wire localization of MRI-

* Correspondence: satokon@m2.gyao.ne.jp
[1]Department of Surgery, Kawaguchi Municipal Medical Center, 180 Nishi-araijyuku, Kawaguchi-city, Saitama 333-0833, Japan
Full list of author information is available at the end of the article

detected findings since 2007 [8]. Consequently, the MRI-guided biopsy is widely available in imaging centers in the United States. Although the MRI-guided biopsy is often used for MRI-detected lesions [9,10], MRI has limitations such as its low specificity, the fact that it is a time-consuming procedure, and the variation in its technical accuracy among institutions [9-12]. The availability of MRI-guided biopsy is limited in Asia, including in Japan [9-12]. On the other hand, CT-guided biopsy for MDCT detected lesions is not practical due to radiation exposure concerns [13-18].

The rationale for further modalities needed to evaluate MDCT- or MRI-detected lesions is latent formation of malignant tumors [19-25]. Since ultrasonography involves no radiation exposure, its repeated use is feasible. A second ultrasonography is performed in MDCT- or MRI-detected lesions. This use of ultrasonography is different from the initial ultrasonography involving the screening of the whole breast, and is known as targeted sonography or second-look sonography. When a lesion is detected on targeted sonography, other options in addition to MRI guidance are available, including sonographically guided biopsy, surgical excision with sonographic marking and follow-up with ultrasonography. Targeted sonography is an important tool as a breakthrough to the further examination; however, the detection rate with targeted sonography has varied in previous reports [19-24].

MDCT has been employed for routine applications in our institution since January 2004, and MRI in addition to MDCT has been employed since 2010. Since 2011, only MRI has been routinely used for the detection of ductal lesions of breast cancer due to administrative reason. In this study, we retrospectively reviewed our data regarding MDCT- or MRI-detected lesions that underwent targeted sonography followed by imaging-guided biopsy, and assessed the utility of targeted sonography in practice.

Methods

Patients and lesions

We retrospectively reviewed the medical records of 695 patients with newly diagnosed breast cancer who consecutively underwent MDCT or MRI for preoperative evaluation in a community hospital in Japan between January 2004 and March 2011. Mammography and ultrasonography failed but MDCT or MRI detected 31 lesions in the contralateral breast and 30 in the ipsilateral breast. An ipsilateral breast lesion is defined as a lesion that is in a different segment or more than 3 cm away from the main tumor.

We performed targeted sonography in all 61 MDCT- or MRI-detected lesions in 56 patients (8.1% in 695 patients). When targeted sonography identified MDCT-

or MRI-detected lesions, we investigated cytologic or pathologic outcomes. We followed up sonographically negative lesions after consultation with the patient. Patient demographics and menopausal status were compared between the pathologically confirmed and follow-up groups. We compared the maximum tumor size and depth:width ratio of lesions detected by targeted sonography among benign, malignant and follow-up groups.

Imaging acquisition and radiation exposure

MDCT was performed using a 16-detector row MDCT scanner (SOMATOM 16, Siemens, Germany) set for 2 mm collimation, 120 kVp, and 180 mA. Scanning was performed at 5 min and 70 seconds after the injection of contrast material (Iopamiron 370 mg/ml, Nihon Schering K.K., Osaka, Japan). Axial, coronal and sagittal images were examined, and multiplanar reconstruction (MPR) and maximum intensity projection (MIP) of the sagittal image and volume-rendering image were performed to detect the ipsilateral ductal component and breast cancer. The contralateral breast was evaluated on an axial image. The weighted CT dose indexes (CTDIw) were 7.8 mGy in plane, 14.04 mGy each in the early and delayed phases and 35.88 mGy in total.

MRI was performed on a 1.5 T scanner (Achieva, Phillips) with the use of a dedicated surface breast coil. The imaging protocol consisted of an axial fat-suppressed T2-weighted sequence in a spectral attenuated inversion-recovery sequence, an axial T1-weighted sequence, an axial diffusion-weighted sequence and an axial dynamic three-dimentional fat-suppressed T1-weighted turbo filed-echo sequence (enhanced T1 high resolution isotropic volume examination). After the injection of contrast media, a sagittal contrast-enhanced high resolution T1-weighted gradient-echo sequence was performed between 2 and 5 minutes of dynamic study. Coronal maximum intensity projection images were reconstructed from a sagital contrast-enhanced high resolution T1-weighted gradient-echo sequence.

Breast imaging interpretation

MDCT and MRI images were independently interpreted by one radiologist with knowledge of the clinical and mammographic findings according to the BI-RADS MRI lexicon. A lesion was considered positive if there were focal and segmental enhancements, while diffuse and multiple lesions in bilateral breasts, suggesting fibrocystic changes, were considered negative.

Sonography

Ultrasonographic examinations were performed on a LOGIQ 500 (GE Healthcare) using an 11-MHz linear transducer.

Breast biopsy technique

We performed vacuum-assisted core needle biopsy under ultrasound guidance using 11-gauge probes (Mammotome Biopsys, Irvine, California) for definitive pathological diagnosis.

Analysis

We used the *t*-test and chi-square test to compare mean values between two groups. For comparisons among malignant, benign and follow-up groups, we used the chi-square test and univariate analysis of variance. For multiple comparisons among the three groups, we used the Scheffé test. A value of p<0.05 was considered significant.

Ethical considerations

This study was approved by the institutional review board of Kawaguchi Municipal Medical Center.

Results

Of all 61 MDCT- or MRI-detected lesions, 58 (95.1%) in 53 patients were identified by targeted sonography. Pathologic diagnoses were obtained in 45 lesions, and we followed up 13 lesions. A status of study lesions is shown in Figure 1.

As for the 53 patients, the age and menopausal status of the pathologically confirmed group and the follow-up group are shown in Table 1. Patients in the pathologically confirmed group were significantly older and more likely to be postmenopausal than those in the follow-up group. There were no significant differences in the follow-up period between the two groups (Table 1).

Example images of MDCT and targeted sonography are shown in Figures 2, 3 and 4. Figure 2 shows a suspicious lesion in the ipsilateral breast, and it is more than

Table 1 Patient characteristics (53 patients, 58 US-identified lesions)

	Pathologically diagnosed	Follow-up	Statistical test
Number of patients	42	11	
Mean age (SD)	59.1 (13.2)	48.4 (13.2)	t = 2.4*
Menopausal status			
Premenopausal	14 (33)	8 (73)	Chi-square = 5.
Postmenopausal	28 (67)	3 (27)	6*

*p < .05, ns: not significant.

3 cm distant from the main lesion. MDCT shows linear enhancement surrounded by fat tissues, while targeted sonography depicts a hypoechoic lesion in the atrophic thin breast with a size of 14 x 2 mm and abundant fat tissues surrounding the lesion. Ductal carcinoma in situ (DCIS) was suspected on the MDCT and ultrasonography image findings. It is often difficult to keep the lesion visible during an ultrasound-guided biopsy. We made an excision after marking on the skin of the lesion under ultrasound. The pathologic finding of this lesion was DCIS.

Figure 3 shows a clustered enhanced lesion in the ipsilateral breast on MDCT. The lesion was 1.5 cm distant from the nipple lower outer quadrant in the breast on the MDCT. Targeted sonography showed a faintly hypoechoic lesion as an enhanced area. We excised it simultaneously with performing a lumpectomy of the known breast cancer after sonographically guided marking because it was located in a difficult place to perform sonographically guided biopsy. The pathologic finding of the lesion was columnar cell hyperplasia.

Figure 4 showed a well-demarcated enhanced tumor in the thin breast tissue which was 1.5 cm distant from

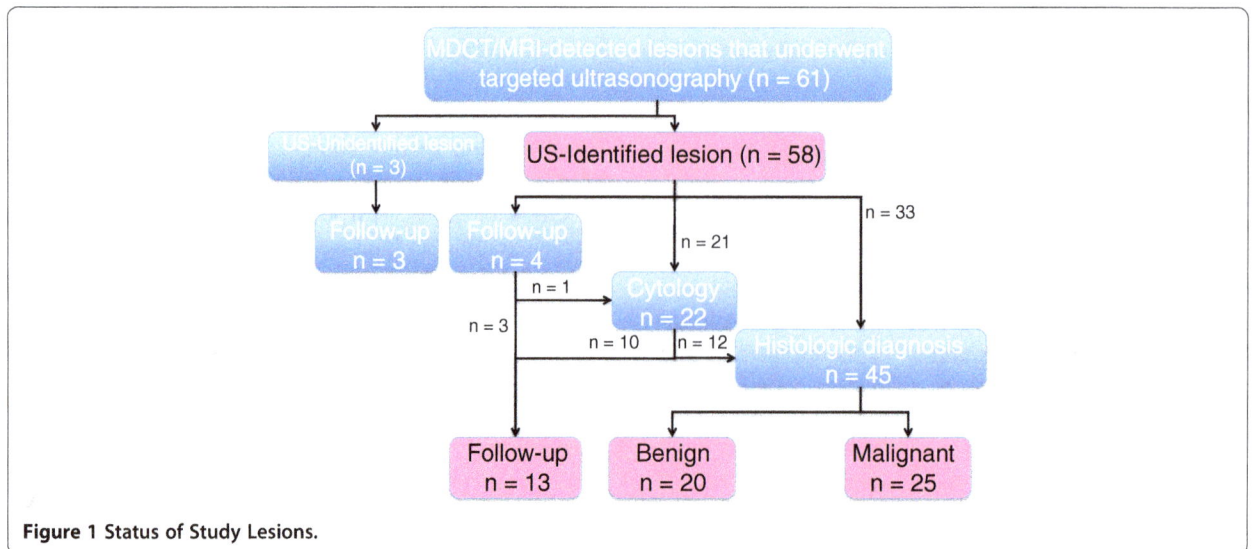

Figure 1 Status of Study Lesions.

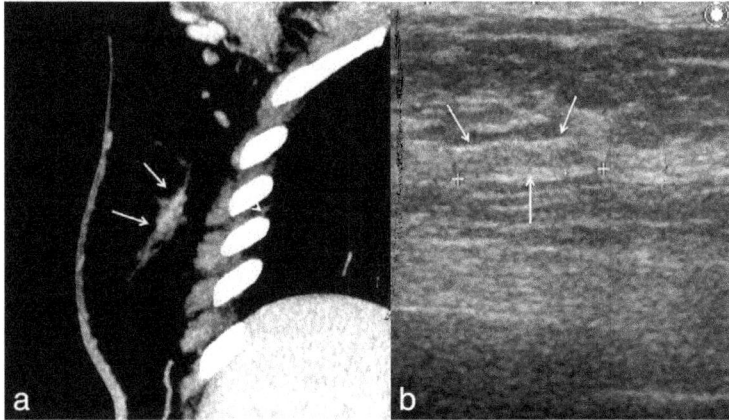

Figure 2 MDCT showed segmental enhancement on the ipsilateral breast. An enhanced lesion was depicted in the thin breast gland. Targeted sonography detected a hypoechoic lesion in the thin breast gland, the size of which was 14x2 mm. Excisional biopsy was performed for definitive diagnosis. Pathological diagnosis was ductal carcinoma in situ.

the nipple on the inner side. The tumor size was 5 × 2 mm. Targeted sonography depicted a hypoechoic mass in the atrophic breast and sonographically guided biopsy was performed under ultrasound guidance. The pathologic finding was hyperplasia.

Sonography-guided fine needle aspiration was performed in 22 lesions, and a pathologic diagnosis was made in 45 lesions. Of the 22 lesions, fine needle aspiration cytology was benign or normal in 7, inadequate in 7, indeterminate in 2, suspicious for malignancy in 1, and malignant in 5. For a pathological diagnosis, 30 lesions underwent sonographically guided biopsy, while 9 lesions underwent surgical biopsy during and before the operation, 5 lesions had extended excisional ranges, and one underwent core needle biopsy.

Pathologic examinations revealed benign in 20 (44%) lesions and malignant in 25 lesions (56%), including one lesion diagnosed as cancer at another hospital. Of the 20 benign tumors pathologically diagnosed in our hospital, 7 were hyperplasia, 5 were intraductal papillomatosis, 3 were fibrocystic change, 2 were fibroadenoma and one was adenoma. Proliferation was not found in 2 lesions with discharge in the dilated duct. Of 25 malignant tumors, DCIS was found in 13 and invasive ductal carcinoma in 12 (Table 2). The mean follow-up period (SD) of 56 patients was 940.2 (553.1) days.

The maximum diameter of the detected lesions as determined by targeted sonography is shown in Table 3. The maximum diameter was under 5.0 mm in 26 lesions, 5.1-10.0 mm in 25 lesions, 10.1-15.0 mm in 6 lesions, and over 15.1 mm in one lesion. The mean (SD) of the maximum tumor size was 6.5 (3.8) mm. As the lesion over 15.1 mm was suspected to be present in the image of one patient, we measured the size of the hypoechoic lesion. There were no significant differences in size among the malignant, benign and follow-up groups (Table 3).

As shown in Table 4, the numbers of lesions with depth:width ratios under and over 0.7 were 45 and 13, respectively. There were no significant differences in the depth:width ratio in the three groups (Table 4).

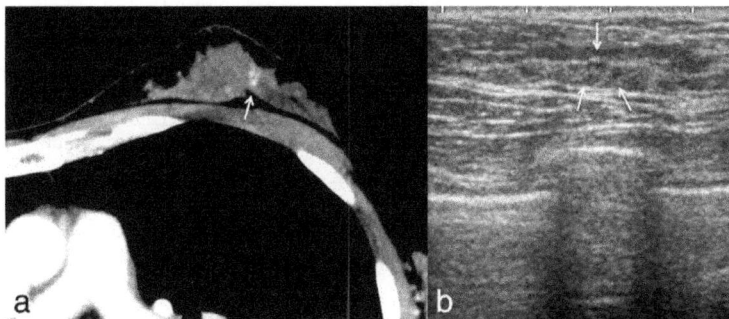

Figure 3 MDCT showed clustered enhancement on the ipsilateral breast. Targeted sonography detected a hypoechoic lesion, but it was difficult to differentiate the surrounding tissue. An excisional biopsy was performed at the same time as breast lumpectomy to obtain a definitive diagnosis. The pathological diagnosis was columnar cell hyperplasia.

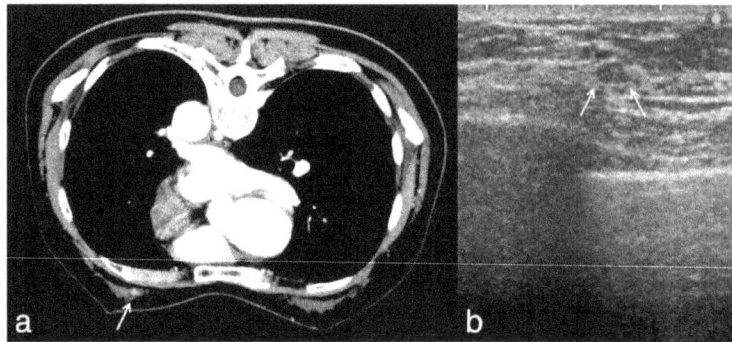

Figure 4 **MDCT showed enhanced focus on the contralateral breast.** Targeted sonography showed a hypoechoic mass connecting to the adjacent ducts, the size of which was 5x2 mm. Sonography-guided vacuum-assisted core needle biopsy was performed to obtain a definitive diagnosis. The pathological diagnosis was hyperplasia.

Based on our experience, we developed a diagnostic imaging strategy for MDCT- or MRI-detected lesions in breast cancer (Figure 5).

Discussion

Approximately 95% of MDCT- or MRI-detected lesions were identified by targeted sonography in this study. The results suggest that targeted sonography, as a diagnostic imaging strategy, is a practical modality for all MDCT- or MRI-detected lesions, allowing more options for further evaluation. In other words, targeted sonography narrows down the number of lesions that really require MRI-guided biopsy.

Pathologic diagnosis is required for MDCT- or MRI-detected lesions because the imaging finding is not the definitive diagnosis. The MDCT- or MRI-detected lesions are not palpable; therefore biopsy is performed under imaging guidance. Regardless of the availability of MRI-guided biopsy, it is practical that targeted sonography is the first procedure to be considered for MDCT- or MRI-detected lesions. The sonographically guided technique provides an advantage. Ultrasonography is the most frequently used and easy-to-use diagnostic tool in daily practice. Once the lesion is depicted on sonography,

targeted sonography provides more options for further evaluation including sonographically guided biopsy, surgical excision after marking under sonography and follow-up with ultrasonography.

The guiding principle in diagnosis depends on whether the lesion is detected with targeted sonography. Because these lesions are difficult to depict by initial mammography or ultrasonography, the detection rate of lesions with targeted sonography varies among institutions [19-24]. There are tips for detecting MDCT- or MRI-detected lesions with targeted sonography. First, the location difference due to the position should be considered. MRI is performed in the prone position, while MDCT is performed in the supine or prone position, depending on the institutions. We performed MDCT in the prone position. The positional difference is larger in the prone position than in the supine position. Attention should be paid to the deviation caused by the arm position even in the supine position. Second, the anatomical positional relation is important. The distance from the nipple, the thickness of the breast gland and the depth of the tumor in the gland should all be referenced. As the nipple is a useful milestone, we use it as a center with the medial or lateral and caudal or cranial directions used to describe locations in reference to it. Breast thickness is

Table 2 Pathologic findings in 45 lesions

Malignant	25
Ductal carcinoma in situ	13
Invasive ductal carcinoma	12
Benign	20
Hyperplasia	7
Intraductal papillomatosis	5
Fibrocystic changes	3
Fibroadenoma	2
Adenoma	1
No malignancy	2

Table 3 Maximum tumor size of the lesion detected by targeted sonography

	Malignant	Benign	Follow-up	Total	p
Maximum diameter (mm)					
~5.0	7 (28)	11 (55)	8 (62)	26 (45)	ns
5.1~10.0	13 (52)	8 (40)	4 (31)	25 (43)	
10.1~15.0	4 (16)	1 (5)	1 (8)	6 (10)	
15.1~	1 (4)	0 (0)	0 (0)	1 (2)	
Total	25 (100)	20 (100)	13 (100)	58 (100)	
Mean (SD)	7.7 (4.8)	5.5 (2.3)	5.4 (2.6)	6.5 (3.8)	

Table 4 Depth:width ratio of the lesion detected by targeted sonography

	Malignant	Benign	Follow-up	Total	P
0.7≧	17 (68)	18 (90)	10 (77)	45 (78)	ns
0.7<	8 (32)	2 (10)	3 (23)	13 (22)	
Total	25 (100)	20 (100)	13 (100)	58 (100)	
Mean (SD)	.58 (.24)	.53 (.16)	.57 (.21)	.56 (.21)	

also helpful. These factors are not affected by positional changes. Third, tumor size, the morphology of the lesion and the structure of the breast gland surrounding the lesion are also useful information for predicting the positional difference. To determine whether the enhanced lesion is nodular, linear or segmental, and whether the breast structure surrounding the lesion is fat or abundant in the breast gland, it is helpful to perform targeted sonography. Also, these attributes are not affected by positional changes. These techniques are helpful to improve the detection rate.

There were no significant differences in the size or the depth:width ratio in the benign, malignant, and follow-up groups in our study. The mean tumor size was 6.5 mm and the mean depth:width ratio was 0.56, suggesting a relatively small and flat lesion. The MDCT or MRI detected lesion, however, has few distinct features; thus it may be found falsely negative on the initial imaging findings. We also performed cytology in 22 lesions in order to obtain a diagnosis. It is often difficult to obtain a large enough sample with fine needle aspiration, and the reliability of this technique is poor if we fail to obtain a sufficient sample. Also, cytology is not sensitive to low-grade tumors. Suspicious lesions warrant pathologic evaluation.

In this study, more than half of the pathologic findings were revealed to be malignant, and half of them were DCIS. The higher probability of malignancy requires preoperative assessment of the extent of the disease because it may alter the surgical management. We reported that MDCT contributed to the detection of occult breast cancer in 2.6% of contralateral breasts [26]. MDCT or MRI in conjunction with targeted sonography is a useful technique for detecting early carcinoma in women who are at increased breast cancer risk.

The pathologic findings revealed that there was no proliferation in 2 out of 45 lesions with discharge in the dilated duct. Because no proven proliferating lesion was found, concern remains that the lesion observed might not be the MDCT- or MRI-detected lesion. La Trenta suggests that it is not unlikely that undetected lesions are malignant [21]. It is difficult to perform core biopsy or small excisional biopsy when the lesion is not detected. At the same time, wide excisional biopsy is rather excessive treatment. A careful follow-up is always necessary to avoid delayed or missed diagnoses. The mean follow-up period for lesions unidentified by targeted sonography was 916 days in this study. So far there are no newly developed lesions or tumor growth.

It has recently been reported that real-time virtual sonography (RVS) can synchronize a sonography image and an MRI or CT image of the same section in real time [12,27]. Accurate comparison of individual positions is a useful technique for confirming a lesion. Ultrasonography greatly depends on the technique, knowledge and experience of the operator. RVS reduces the differences among operators and increases the physician's confidence about the MDCT- or MRI-detected lesion. When the lesion is not detected with targeted

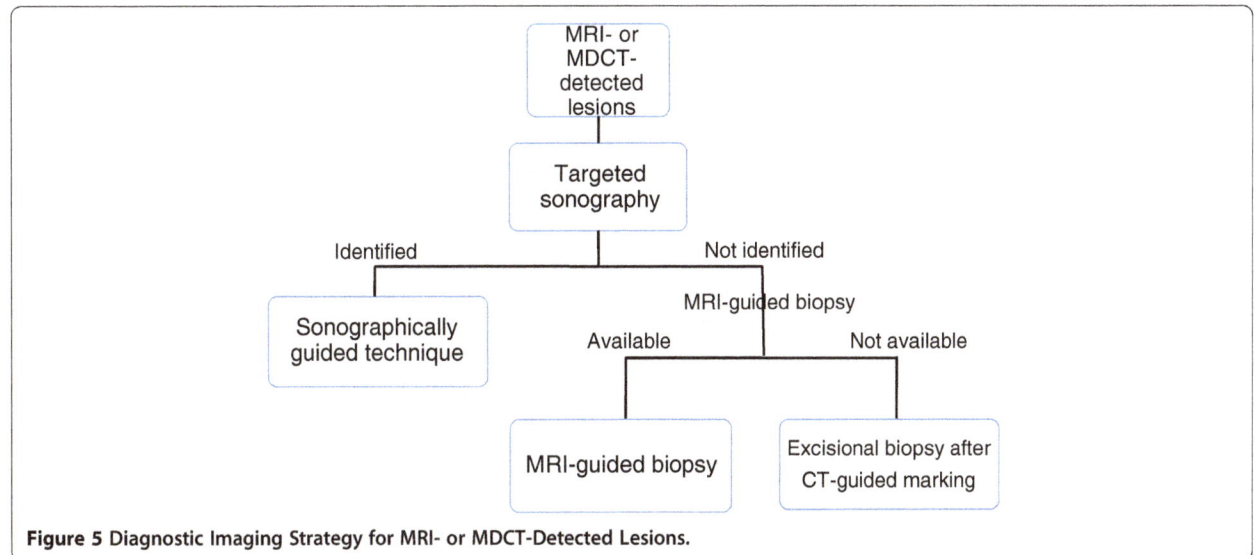

Figure 5 Diagnostic Imaging Strategy for MRI- or MDCT-Detected Lesions.

sonography or RVS, MRI-guided biopsy is indicated; this option or, at the very least, follow-up is required.

We found that significantly more older patients had pathologically confirmed tumors, and they were more likely to be postmenopausal than those in the follow-up group. It is reported that younger patients have higher background parenchymal enhancement and a higher proportion of nodular parenchymal enhancement patterns [28-30]. Since younger and premenopausal groups were suspected to have fibroglandular changes, these patients require follow-up.

Our study has several limitations. It is a retrospective single-center study. Ten lesions with cytological diagnosis were not pathologically evaluated. Although fine needle aspiration cytology has high specificity and positive predictive value for mass lesions [31-33], it is difficult to obtain enough cells for MDCT- or MRI-detected lesions, particularly if it is low-grade or papillary lesion. We used fine needle aspiration as the initial diagnostic modality to provide valuable clues, but the study findings need to be interpreted with caution. We have followed-up with these patients.

Conclusion

Targeted sonography is a useful modality for the evaluation of new unsuspected lesions found on MDCT or MRI in patients with breast cancer. By considering the previous MDCT or MRI findings and the location difference due to the position, the detection rate of targeted sonography can be improved. We achieved a 95% detection rate in this study. As a diagnostic imaging strategy, targeted sonography is a practical consideration for all MDCT- or MRI-detected lesions.

Abbreviations
MRI: Magnetic resonance imaging; CT: Computed tomography; MDCT: Multidetector-row CT; NCCN: National comprehensive cancer network; MPR: Multiplanar reconstruction; MIP: Maximum intensity projection; CTDIw: Weighted CT dose indexes; DCIS: Ductal carcinoma in situ; RVS: Real-time virtual sonography.

Competing interests
The author's declared that they have no competing interests.

Authors' contributions
SN: has made substantial contributions to conception and design, acquisition of data, and analysis and interpretation of data; has written the manuscript. MO: has made substantial contributions to conception and design. AM: has made substantial contributions to conception and design; has performed ultrasonography. MK: has made substantial contributions to conception and design; has interpreted MDCT and MRI images. HS: has participated in the histological diagnosis. MY: has participated in the histological diagnosis. All authors read and approved the final manuscript.

Acknowledgements
Sources of support or individuals requiring acknowledgement: None.

Author details
[1]Department of Surgery, Kawaguchi Municipal Medical Center, 180 Nishi-araijyuku, Kawaguchi-city, Saitama 333-0833, Japan. [2]Department of Laboratory, Kawaguchi Municipal Medical Center, Kawaguchi-city, Japan. [3]Department of Radiology, Kawaguchi Municipal Medical Center, Kawaguchi-city, Japan. [4]Department of Pathology, Kawaguchi Municipal Medical Center, Kawaguchi-city, Japan.

References
1. Doihara H, Fujita T, Takabatake D, Takahashi H, Ogasawara Y, Shimizu N: Clinical significance of multidetector-row computed tomography in breast surgery. Breast J 2006, 12:204–209.
2. Fujita T, Doihara H, Takabatake D, Takahashi H, Yoshitomi S, Ishibe Y, Ogasawara Y, Shimizu N: Multidetector-row computed tomography for diagnosing intraductal extension of breast carcinoma. J Surg Oncol 2005, 91:10–16.
3. Tanaka AS, Fukutomi T, Miyakawa K, Uchiyama N, Tsuda H: Diagnostic value of contrast–enhanced computed tomography for diagnosing the intraductal component of breast cancer. Breast Cancer Res Treat 1998, 49:79–86.
4. Uematsu T: Comparison of magnetic resonance imaging and multidetector computed tomography for evaluating intraductal tumor extension of breast cancer. Jpn J Radiol 2010, 28:563–570.
5. Shimauchi A, Yamada T, Sato A, Takase K, Usami S, Ishida T, Moriya T, Takahashi S: Comparison of MDCT and MRI for evaluating the intraductal component of breast cancer. AJR 2006, 187:322–329.
6. Goh V, Padhani AR: Imaging tumor angiogenesis: functional assessment using MDCT or MRI? Abdom Imaging 2006, 31:194–199.
7. Turetschek K, Huber S, Floyd E, Helbich T, Roberts TP, Shames DM, Tarlo KS, Wendland MF, Brasch RC: MR imaging characterization of microvessels in experimental breast tumors by using a particulate contrast agent with histopathologic correlation. Radiology 2001, 218:562–569.
8. National Comprehensive Cancer Network: NCCN Clinical Practice Guidelines in Oncology v.1, Principles of Dedicated Breast MRI Testing. Fort Washington, PA; 2007. http://www.nccn.org/professionals/physician_gls/f_guidelines.asp.
9. Han BK, Schnall MD, Orei SG, Rosen M: Outcome of MRI-guided breast biopsy. AJR 2008, 191:1798–1804.
10. Tozaki M, Yamashiro N, Suzuki T, Kawano N, Ozaki S, Sakamoto N, Abe S, Ogawa T, Katayama N, Tsunoda Y, Fukuma E: MR-guided vacuum-assisted breast biopsy: is it an essential technique? Breast Cancer 2009, 16:121–125.
11. Lee JM, Kaplan JB, Murray MP, Bartella L, Morris EA, Joo S, Dershaw DD, Liberman L: Imaging-histologic discordance at MRI-guided 9 gauge vacuum-assisted breast biopsy. AJR 2007, 189:852–859.
12. Nakano S, Yoshida M, Fujii K, Yorozuya K, Mouri Y, Kousaka J, Fukutomi T, Kimura J, Ishiguchi T, Ohno K, Mizumto T, Harao M: Fusion of MRI and sonography image for breast cancer evaluation using real-time virtual sonography with magnetic navigation: first experience. Jpn J Clin Oncol 2009, 39:552–559.
13. Brenner DJ, Elliston CD, Hall E, Berdon W: Estimated risks of radiation-induced fatal cancer from pediatric CT. AJR 2001, 176:289–296.
14. Smith-Bindman R, Lipson J, Marcus R, Kim KP, Mahesh M, Gould R, de Berrington González A, Miglioretti DL: Radiation dose associated with common computed tomography examinations and the associated lifetime attributable risk of cancer. Arch Intern Med 2009, 169:2078–2086.
15. Berrington A, Darby S: Risk of cancer from diagnostic X-rays:estimates for the UK and 14 other countries. Lancet 2004, 363:345–351.
16. Einstein AJ, Sanz J, Dellegrottaglie S, Milite M, Sirol M, Henzlova M, Rajagopalan S: Radiation dose and cancer risk estimates in 16-slice computed tomography coronary angiography. J Nucl Cadiol 2008, 15:232–240.
17. Thornton FJ, Paulson EK, Yoshizumi TT, Frush DP, Nelson RC: Single versus multi-detector row CT: comparison of radiation doses and dose profiles. Acad Radiol 2003, 10:379–385.
18. Sardanelli F, Calabrese M, Zandrino F, Melani E, Parodi R, Imperiale A, Massa T, Parodi G, Canavese G: Dynamic helical CT of the breast tumors. J comput Assist Tomogr 1998, 22:398–407.
19. Shin JH, Han BK, Choe YH, Ko K, Choi N: Targeted ultrasound for MR-detected lesions in breast cancer patients. Korean J Radiol 2007, 8:475–483.
20. DeMartini WB, Eby PR, Peacock S, Lehman CD: Utility of targeted sonography for breast lesions that were suspicious on MRI. AJR 2009, 192:1128–1134.

21. LaTrenta LR, Menel JH, Morris EA, Abramson AF, Dershaw DD, Liberman L: **Breast lesions detected with MR imaging: utility and histopathologic importance of identification with US.** *Radiology* 2003, **227**:856–861.

22. Abe H, Schmidt RA, Shah RN, Shimauchi A, Kulkarni K, Sennett CA, Newstead GM: **MR-directed ("Second-Look") ultrasound examination for breast lesions detected initially on MRI: MR and sonographic findings.** *AJR* 2010, **194**:370–377.

23. Trop I, Labelle M, David J, Mayrand MH, Lalonde L: **Second-look targeted studies after breast magnetic resonance imaging: practical tips to improve lesion identification.** *Curr Probl Diagn Radiol* 2010, **39**:200–211.

24. Beran L, Liang W, Nims T, Paquelet J, Sickle-Santanello B: **Correlation of targeted ultrasound with magnetic resonance imaging abnormalities of the breast.** *Am J Surg* 2005, **190**:592–594.

25. Wiener JI, Schilling KJ, Adami C, Obuchowski NA: **Assessment of suspected breast cancer by MRI: a prospective clinical trial using a combined kinetic and morphologic analysis.** *AJR* 2005, **184**:878–886.

26. Nakano S, Sakamoto H, Ohtsuka M, Mibu A, Karikomi M, Sakata H, Yamamoto M: **Successful use of multi-detector row computed tomography for detecting contralateral breast cancer.** *Journal of Computer Assisted Tomography* 2011, **35**:148–152.

27. Inoue T, Tamaki Y, Sato Y, Nakamoto M, Tamura S, Tanji Y, Taguchi T, Noguchi S: **Three-dimentional ultrasound imaging of breast cancer by a real-time intraoperative navigation system.** *Breast Cancer* 2005, **12**:122–129.

28. Jansen SA, Lin VC, Giger ML, Gregory HL, Li H, Karczmar GS, Newstead GM: **Normal parenchymal enhancement pattern in women undergoing MR screening of the breast.** *Eur Radiol* 2011, **21**:1374–1382.

29. Adkisson CD, Vallow LA, Kowalchik K, McNeil R, Hines S, Deperi E, Moreno A, Roy V, Perez EA, McLaughlin SA: **Patient age and preoperative breast MRI in women with breast cancer: biopsy and surgical implications.** *Ann Surg Oncol* 2011, **18**:1678–1683.

30. King V, Brooks JD, Bernstein JL, Reiner AS, Pike MC, Morris EA: **Background Parenchymal Enhancement at Breast MR Imaging and Breast Cancer Risk.** *Radiology* 2011, **260**:50–60.

31. Rosa M, Mohammadi A, Masood S: **The value of fine needle aspiration biopsy in the diagnosis and prognostic assessment of palpable breast lesions.** *Diagn. Cytopathol.* 2012, **40**:26–34.

32. Ishikawa T, Hamaguchi Y, Tanabe M, Momiyama N, Chishima T, Nakatani Y, Nozawa A, Sasaki T, Kitamura H, Shimada H: **False-positive and false negative cases of fine-needle aspiration cytology for palpable breast lesions.** *Breast Cancer* 2007, **14**:388–392.

33. Smith MJ, Heffron CC, Rothwell JR, Loftus BM, Jeffers M, Geraphty JG: **Fine needle aspiration cytology in symptomatic breast lesions: still an important diagnostic modality?** *The Breast J* 2012, **18**:103–110.

18

Is single reading with computer-aided detection (CAD) as good as double reading in mammography screening?

Edward Azavedo[1,4], Sophia Zackrisson[2*], Ingegerd Mejàre[3] and Marianne Heibert Arnlind[3,4]

Abstract

Background: In accordance with European guidelines, mammography screening comprises independent readings by two breast radiologists (double reading). CAD (computer-aided detection) has been suggested to complement or replace one of the two readers (single reading + CAD).
The *aim* of this systematic review is to address the following question: Is the reading of mammographic x-ray images by a single breast radiologist together with CAD at least as accurate as double reading?

Methods: The electronic literature search included the databases Pub Med, EMBASE and The Cochrane Library. Two independent reviewers assessed abstracts and full-text articles.

Results: 1049 abstracts were identified, of which 996 were excluded with reference to inclusion and exclusion criteria; 53 full-text articles were assessed for eligibility. Finally, four articles were included in the qualitative analysis, and one in a GRADE synthesis.

Conclusions: The scientific evidence is insufficient to determine whether the accuracy of *single reading + CAD* is at least equivalent to that obtained in standard practice, i.e. *double reading* where two breast radiologists independently read the mammographic images.

Keywords : CAD, Mammography, Screening, Breast, Cancer, Single reading, Double reading

Background

Following reports from Swedish randomized trials [1-4], breast cancer screening programs with mammography have been established in recent decades in many countries [5]. The age range of women invited to screening varies between countries. The Swedish National Board of Health and Welfare recommends mammography screening at regular intervals to all women between 40 and 74 years. The initial results from the randomized trials, showing a reduction in mortality in breast cancer, have been confirmed by long-term follow-up [6,7] Similar results have been obtained in established population-based service screening programs [8,9]. However, the pros and cons of mammography screening and how the

results should be interpreted [10] are still matters for debate.

Besides the primary aim of detecting breast cancers in screening programs, it is important that recall rates are kept as low as possible without impairing detection rates. In this respect, the recommended recall rate in Sweden and in the rest of Europe should not exceed five per cent [11]. The reasons for recall are several, such as suspicious findings suggesting malignancy, indeterminate findings that need further work-up, and occasionally for technical reasons or if the woman reports clinical symptoms at the time of the screening examination.

As the radiological image of breast tissue is complex, mammograms need to be interpreted by highly specialized radiologists. Figure 1 shows an example of mammography images.

Factors that affect the ability to detect a breast cancer (sensitivity) are e.g. the prevalence of breast cancer in the target population, dense breast tissue, the frequency

* Correspondence: sophia.zackrisson@med.lu.se
[2]Department of Clinical Sciences in Malmö, Diagnostic Radiology, Lund University, Skåne University Hospital Malmö, Malmö SE-205 02, Sweden
Full list of author information is available at the end of the article

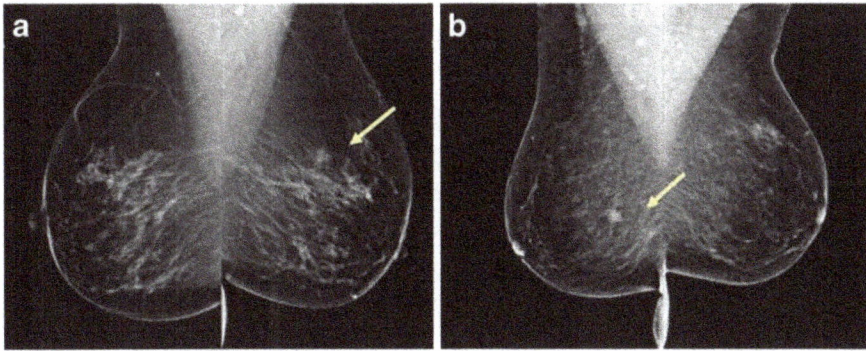

Figure 1 **Figure 1a shows a rather hard to detect breast cancer in the left breast (arrow); the right breast is normal.** Figure 1b shows an easily detected cancer in the right breast (arrow); the left breast is normal.

of tumours with subtle mammographic signs, and suboptimal technical quality. These factors, combined with high daily volumes (each Swedish screening centre usually screens more than 20,000 women annually), makes accurate screening a challenging task. Sensitivity levels of 70–85% and specificity levels of 82–98% at mammography screening have been reported [5]. In order to maintain high sensitivity and specificity, resulting in high cancer detection rates and low false-positive rates, Swedish and European guidelines recommend double reading, i.e. that the breast images are reviewed by two specially trained radiologists (breast radiologists). Double reading has been shown to increase cancer detection rates by 5–17% [12].

Computer-aided detection (CAD) is a computerized method for analysing images in mammography screening. Although the method has existed for approximately 10 years, its contribution to routine screening is still debatable [13-15]. The program used in CAD identifies and marks areas which the software identifies as abnormal breast tissue. The CAD program is not intended to be the sole method for analysing mammography images. Rather, it is designed to alert the radiologist to possibly suspicious areas. Hence, a radiologist must interpret and make a decision to act upon (accept or dismiss) each CAD mark. On average, each screening examination generates two false positive marks; CAD gives 400 false positive marks for each true positive mark [16].

Lack of an adequate number of trained breast radiologists has led to a growing interest in computerized analysis of mammography images. There has been a discussion as to whether CAD in conjunction with mammography screening could replace one of the breast radiologists. A prerequisite would be that diagnostic accuracy and patient benefit are at least equivalent to what is achieved when the mammographic images are read by two breast radiologists. Another important prerequisite is that not too many women need to be recalled for further diagnostic work-up.

The value of CAD in mammography screening has been questioned in earlier reviews [17,18]. The literature is scarce on studies performed in authentic screening situations. As the performance of CAD systems has improved considerably, it was considered appropriate to reassess the performance of CAD in population-based screening programs.

This review is part of a comprehensive systematic review, published in Swedish by SBU (Swedish Council on Health Technology Assessment), of computer-aided detection (CAD) as a diagnostic method in mammography screening [19]. SBU is an independent government agency for the critical evaluation of methods for preventing, diagnosing and treating health problems.

The objective of the present is systematic review is to address the following question: Is the reading of mammographic images by a single breast radiologist plus CAD at least as accurate as readings by two breast radiologists (current practice) in terms of:

- sensitivity (probability that a person with the disease has a positive test result);
- specificity (probability that a healthy person has a negative test result);
- cancer detection rate (number of cancer cases detected per 1,000 women examined);
- recall rate (proportion of women who are recalled for further investigation); and
- cost-effectiveness?

Methods

CAD (Computer-aided detection)

CAD research has been developed over the past two decades. CAD was first applied to digitized (scanned) screen-film mammograms (SFM). The introduction of full-field digital mammography (FFDM) has led to intensified efforts to optimise the method. CAD makes a computerized analysis of mammograms and identifies areas that need to be reviewed. The precise algorithms used by different CAD suppliers are still a commercial secret and are not further reviewed here. Two types of marks are generally used: one for microcalcifications and the other for other mammographic features such as density, mass and distortion. The systems can be adjusted to yield very high sensitivity but at the cost of specificity, generating a high rate of false positive marks.

According to a recent review, the sensitivity of CAD for microcalcifications representing malignancies is 98–99% [16]. However, only 15–20% of detected cancers present as microcalcifications on screening mammograms [20]. The same review reports that the sensitivity of CAD for other mammographic features representing malignancies ranges from 89 to 75%, in some cases down to 50%.

It has been assumed that CAD will be used increasingly with the transition from analogue to digital mammography. The reproducibility of CAD prompts in FFDM is expected to be more consistent than with scanned mammograms. The primary inclusion criterion

in this review was CAD on FFDMs. However, when prospective studies based on FFDM could not be found, scanned analogue images were accepted.

Literature search and selection of articles

The electronic literature search included the databases PubMed, EMBASE, and The Cochrane Library from 1950 to November 2011. All Western European languages were accepted. The Mesh terms were: Breast neoplasms, Breast, Mammography, Breast (TW), Mammography (TW) AND Computer aided detection (TW) AND Computer aided diagnosis (TW) AND Cad (TW), and Economic aspects. The complete search strategy can be provided on request.

The electronic searches yielded 1049 abstracts (Figure 2). Two reviewers (EA and SZ) read the abstracts independently. An article was read in full text if at least one of the two reviewers considered an abstract to be potentially relevant. Hand search and grey literature did not result in any additional articles. The

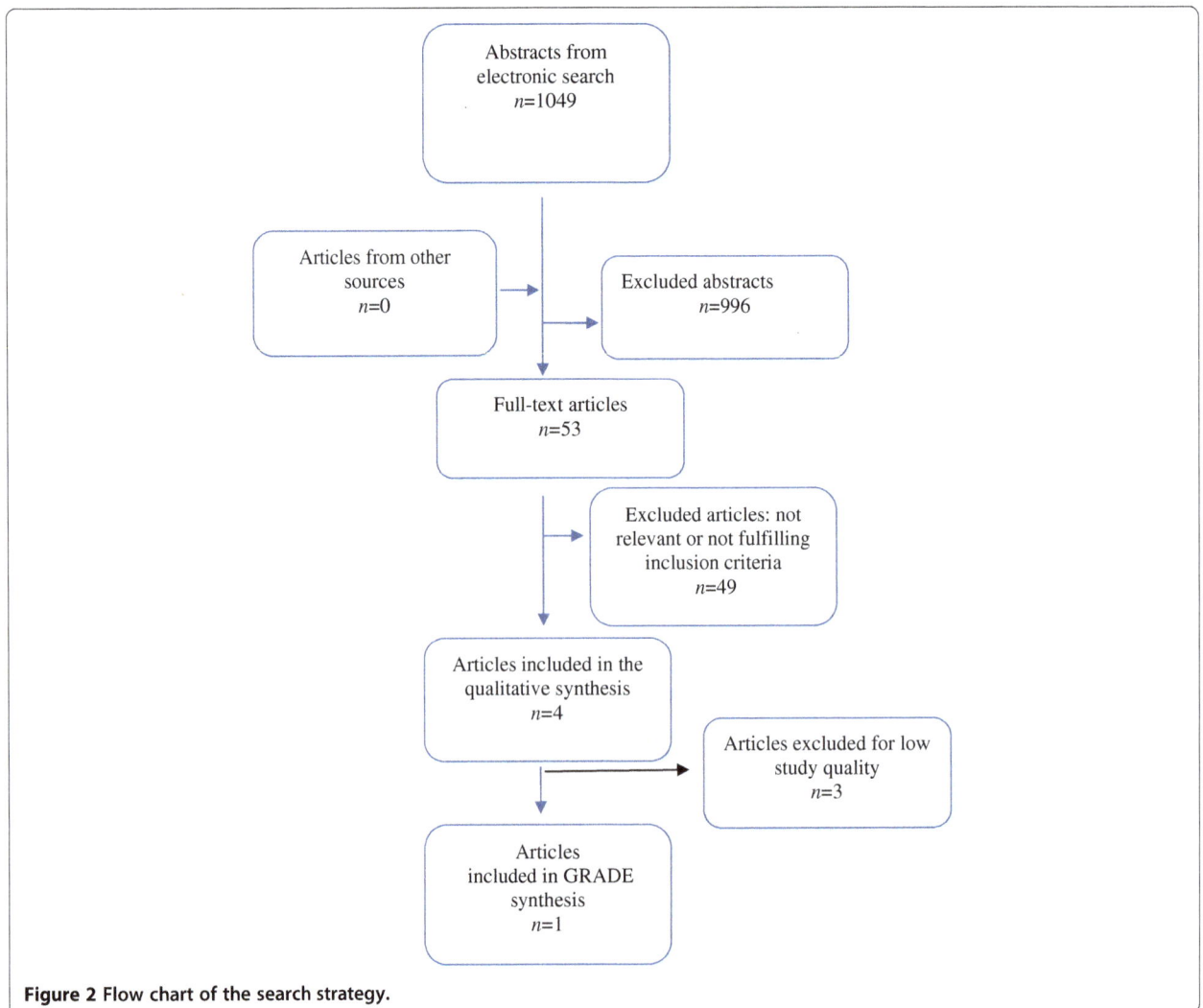

Figure 2 Flow chart of the search strategy.

pre-specified inclusion/exclusion criteria are given below. Altogether, 53 articles were read in full text and assessed independently by the same two reviewers using the QUADAS tool [21]. Of the 53 articles, 49 did not fulfil the inclusion criteria and were excluded from further analysis. A list of excluded articles with the main reason for exclusion is available on request.

PICO elements were used to describe the population, index test, reference test and outcome:

P – Population: women, 40–74 years old, participating in mammography screening
I – Intervention (index test): CAD + one breast radiologist (single reading)
C – Control (reference test): reading by two independent radiologists (double reading)
O – Outcome: sensitivity, specificity, cancer detection rate and recall rate

The inclusion criteria were:

- population-based screening
- ≥5,000 women included
- study setting corresponding to Swedish conditions
- follow-up time ≥ 12 months
- mammography readings with one breast radiologist + CAD compared with readings by two breast radiologists.

Assessment of diagnostic accuracy

The diagnostic accuracy (validity) of a test (index test) requires a reference standard (reference test) for comparison. Two index tests were used here: 1) CAD + single reading, and 2) double reading. The reference standard should reflect the reality as closely as possible and the ideal gold standard is histopathological verification. However, biopsying all individuals is not feasible when screening an asymptomatic population. The reference standard in this review was biopsy of suspected cases or follow-up. The ultimate outcome was survival. Because no randomized controlled trials have been performed to document changes in survival following the use of double reading compared to single reading with CAD, surrogate outcomes such as cancer detection rate and recall rate are used. The main outcome measures are sensitivity and specificity. Sensitivity is the number of true positive tests divided by the total number of true cancer cases. Specificity is the number of true negative tests divided by the total number of healthy breast cases. In addition, cost-effectiveness has been considered.

Rating quality of individual studies

The quality of each included study was rated high, moderate or low according to pre-specified criteria given in Table 1.

Rating evidence across studies

The quality of the evidence of each method's/test's diagnostic accuracy was rated in four levels according to GRADE [22] [23]:

- High (⊕⊕⊕⊕). Based on high or moderate quality studies containing no factors that weaken the overall judgement.
- Moderate (⊕⊕⊕O). Based on high or moderate quality studies containing isolated factors that weaken the overall judgement.
- Limited (⊕⊕OO). Based on high or moderate quality studies containing factors that weaken the overall judgement.
- Insufficient (⊕OOO). The evidence base is insufficient when scientific evidence is lacking, the quality of available studies is low or studies of similar quality are contradictory.

Table 1 Criteria of high, moderate and low study quality, mainly according to QUADAS [21]

High: small risk of bias	Prospective study design. Particular emphasis on the following:
	● adequately described patients constituting a representative and clinically relevant sample (QUADAS items 1, 2).
	● the index test should not form part of the reference standard (item 7).
	● evaluators should be masked to results of index test and reference test (items 10, 11)
	● the tests should be described in sufficient detail to permit replication (items 8, 9).
	● sample size ≥ 5000.
	● diagnostic accuracy presented as sensitivity and specificity.
Moderate: moderate risk of bias	Prospective study design
	Since no prospective studies based on digital mammography could be identified, scanned analogue images were accepted. Otherwise the same criteria as for high quality were required.
Low: high risk of selection and/or verification bias	Retrospective study design. Selected or enriched samples

Table 2 Main characteristics, results and quality rating of four studies on mammography screening

Author, Year (ref)	Study design, Study period, Population, Readers	Index test (I)	Reference test	Results CI= confidence interval Se= sensitivity Sp=specificity	Study quality, Comments
Gilbert et al., 2008 [71]	Prospective, multicentre 2006-2007 *Population:* Initially invited: 68,060 women. Investigated: 28,204. Aged 50-70 years (1 % > 70 years). *Readers:* radiologists (n=17), specially trained staff (n=10). All readers had at least 6 years' experience and >5000 readings/year	I.1: single reading + CAD, n=28,204 I.2: double reading, n=28,204.	Biopsy of suspected cases or follow-up (not all, though; number not reported)	*Cancer detection rate:* Single reading + CAD: 7.02 /1000. Double reading: 7.06/1000. Difference not statistically significant (NS). *Recall rate:* Single reading + CAD: 3.9 %. Double reading: 3.4 %. Difference 0.5 % (95 % CI: 0.3;0.8). *Accuracy:* Single reading + CAD: Se= 87.2 % Sp= 96.9 % Double reading: Se= 87.7 % Sp= 97.4 % Difference in sensitivity: 0.5 % (95 % CI: -7.4;6.6), (NS). Difference in specificity 0.5% (CI not specified but reported NS).	Moderate Restricted generalisability since results were based on single reading +CAD by experienced radiologists. Incomplete follow-up, particularly affecting the estimates of sensitivity. Scanned analogue mammograms.
Gromet et al., 2008 [69]	Retrospective *Population:* 231 221 women 2001-05 *Readers:* Single reading + CAD: specialists in mammography.	I.1: Single reading + CAD n=118,808. I.2: Double reading n=112,413.	Biopsy and follow-up	*Cancer detection rate:* Single reading + CAD: 4.2/1000. Double reading: 4.46/1000 (NS). *Recall rate:* Single reading + CAD: 10.6 %.	Low Retrospective study (controlled for age and time since last screening). Follow-up time unclear. Screening situation not applicable to European conditions

Table 2 Main characteristics, results and quality rating of four studies on mammography screening *(Continued)*

Study	Characteristics	Intervention	Verification / Follow-up	Results	Comments / Quality rating
	Double reading: Specialists in mammography + radiology.			Double reading:11.9%. Difference statistically significant (p=0.001). *Accuracy:* Single reading + CAD: Se= 90.4 % Double reading: Se=88.0 %. Difference statistically significant. Percent of recalled with cancer: Single reading + CAD: 3.9%. Double reading: 3.7%(NS).	(i.e. recall rate higher than accepted in Europe). Invitation procedure and blinded readings unclear. Scanned analogue mammograms.
Georgian-Smith et al., 2007 [68]	Prospective *Study period:* 2001-03 *Population:* 6381 consecutive screening examinations *Readers:* Experienced breast radiologists Single reading + CAD. Double reading: Not independent reading.	I.1: Single reading + CAD n=6381. I.2: Double reading n=6381.	Biopsy and at least 12 months' follow-up to detect false negatives.	*Cancer detection rate:* Single reading +CAD: 2.0/1000. Double reading: 2.4/1000 (NS). *Recall rate:* Single reading +CAD: 7.87%. Double reading: 7.93% (NS). *Accuracy:* Sensitivity and specificity not reported.	Low. Screening situation not applicable to European conditions. Invitation procedure not described. Population, selection criteria, withdrawals unclear. Not independent double reading but blinded to CAD. Number of recalls based on all readings. Scanned analogue radiographs.
Khoo et al., 2005 [70]	Prospective *Study period:* not reported. *Population:* 6,111 women (45-94 years), screening every 3rd year	I.1: Single reading +CAD n= 6111. I.2: Double reading n= 6111.	Biopsy Not reported No follow-up	*Cancer detection rate:* Total for double reading + single reading + symptomatic patients:10/1000. Not reported individually for the groups. *Recall rate:* Single reading + CAD: 6.1%. Double reading: 5.0 %.	Low. A so-called relative sensitivity used since 3-year follow-up not yet achieved. Relatively high screening age and long screening intervals. Unclear whether the readings were blinded. Incomplete follow-up.

Table 2 Main characteristics, results and quality rating of four studies on mammography screening (*Continued*)

Readers:	Difference statistically significant	Scanned analogue radiographs.
Radiologists (n=7) and specially trained staff (n=5).	*Accuracy:* (relative sensitivity)*	
	Single reading + CAD: Se= 91.5%.	
Double reading not always performed by two radiologists.	Double reading: Se= 98.4% (NS).	

* Relative sensitivity= number of detected cancer cases per reader divided by all detected cancer cases (due to lack of follow-up).

Table 3 Quality of evidence of the difference between single reading (radiologist plus CAD) and double reading (two radiologists) related to cancer detection rate and recall rate in mammography screening (GRADE). Data from Gilbert et al. [71]

Outcome	Sample size (no. of studies)	True positive: Single reading + CAD (95% CI)	True positive: Double reading (95% CI)	Absolute difference (95%CI)	Quality of evidence	Rating based on study design/quality, indirectness, consistency, precision and publication bias**
Cancer detection rate	28,204 (1)	0.702% (0.6–0.8)	0.706% (0.6–0.8)	0.004% (NS*)	(⊕OOO) Insufficient	Study quality –1 Indirectness–1
Recall rate	28,204 (1)	3.9% (3,7–4,1)	3.4% (3,2–3,6)	0.5% (0,3–0.8)	(⊕OOO) Insufficient	Study quality –1 Indirectness -1 One study –1

*NS= no statistically significant difference.

** Study quality = Risk of bias, that is, sensitivity probably overestimated due to incomplete follow-up of women with negative test results.

Indirectness = Only breast radiologists with long clinical experience took part in the study.

Lack of precision = The difference in sensitivity between double reading and single reading + CAD has wide confidence intervals.

Applying GRADE serves to obtain answers to the following questions. How much confidence can one have in a particular estimate of effect? Is the result sustainable, or is it likely that new research findings will change the evidence in the foreseeable future? The rating starts at high, but confidence in the evidence may be reduced for several reasons, including limitations in the study design and/or quality, inconsistency or indirectness of results, imprecise estimates and probability of publication bias. Any disagreements on inclusion/exclusion criteria, rating quality of individual studies or quality of evidence of test methods were solved by consensus.

- Sensitivity = probability that a person with a disease has a positive test result.
- Specificity = probability that a healthy person has a negative test result.
- Relative sensitivity = number of detected cancer cases per reader divided by the total number of detected cancer cases.
- Population based mammography screening = all women in certain age groups receive a personal mailed invitation to get a mammogram at regular intervals (1.5 – 3 years)
- Cancer detection rate = the number of cancer cases detected per 1000 women examined.
- Recall rate = the number of women per 1000 woman recalled for further investigation.
- Interval cancer = cancer cases detected between two screening occasions.

Results

The results of the literature search and the outcome of the selection procedures are shown in a flow chart (Figure 2).

Fifty-three articles were reviewed in full text. Nine of them were review articles [12,16-18,24-28]. Many studies had not been performed in screening settings or had selected or enriched populations, sometimes without comparison between single reading + CAD and double reading [14,29-57]. Nine studies had large populations, but compared only single reading + CAD with single reading [58-66]. One study that only described different cancer types was excluded [67].

Four studies were included in the summary results, Table 2 (see Additional file 1). Three of them had methodological shortcomings and were judged to be of low quality [68-70]. Only one study, of moderate quality, was included in the GRADE synthesis, Table 3 [71]. This was a prospective multicentre study based on the UK national screening program and including 28,204 women aged 50–70 years. No statistically significant difference was found between single reading + CAD and double reading for cancer detection rate (7.02/1000 and 7.06/1

000). The overall agreement between the two strategies was 74.9% (170/227). However, single reading with CAD gave a significantly higher recall rate (3.9% versus 3.4%; p = 0.001). Compared to double reading, single reading with CAD gave lower sensitivity (87.2% versus 87.7%) and lower specificity (96.9% versus 97.4%) but the differences were not statistically significant. Due to incomplete follow-up, sensitivity was likely to be overestimated. Overall, there was no statistically significant difference between the two strategies as regards pathological characteristics of the 57 detected cancers. Study results are reported in Tables 2 and 3.

Because of their shortcomings, the remaining three studies were not considered in our conclusions. However they deserve to be described. Two were conducted in the U.S.A. [68,69], where population-based screening programs are not used. The populations are less well described and it is not clear whether the women received a personal invitation or had sought to get for mammography on their own. Moreover, recall rates were 8–12%, notably higher than recommended in Sweden and Europe (<5%). The larger of these two studies was retrospective and included 231,221 women who underwent mammography screening [69]. The other study was prospective with 6381 consecutive screening examinations [68]. Their results showed no statistically significant difference in cancer detection rate and the recall rates were inconsistent.

The third study was conducted within the framework of the United Kingdom National Health Service Screening Programme [70]. It was prospective and included 6111 screening examinations with a relatively high total cancer detection rate; 10/1000 including those detected by double reading and single reading with CAD and because of symptoms. Even women over 64 years of age (the upper limit for screening in the UK) were included, which may partly explain the relatively high prevalence of cancer cases. Another explanation may be that the interval between screening sessions was three years (usually 1.5-2 years in Europe). Due to lack of follow-up, the authors calculated a so-called relative sensitivity, where single reading + CAD gave a lower but not statistically significant different sensitivity of 91.5% compared to 98.4% with double reading. Single reading + CAD had a significantly higher recall rate (6.1%) compared to double reading (5.0%).

To conclude, these three studies show partly conflicting results and it is difficult to draw any conclusions. According to Gilbert et al. [71], the two reading methods resulted in equal numbers of cancer cases. However, this was achieved at the expense of a statistically significantly higher recall rate, implying unnecessary additional examinations. Recall rates in the two studies from the USA [68,69] were two to three times higher than in

Sweden (average 3% [20,72]) and not in accordance with European guidelines (<5% [11]).

Economic aspects

The results of the literature search on economic aspects show that out of 44 abstracts, only one led to the inclusion of the full-text article [14]. The medical scientific evidence was insufficient to study cost-effectiveness and the quality of the study was judged to be low.

Discussion

The results of this systematic review indicate that the scientific evidence is insufficient to determine whether single mammographic reading by one breast radiologist + CAD is as accurate as the current practice of double reading involving two breast radiologists.

CAD has been developed to act as a second reader for two main reasons: to enhance the diagnostic sensitivity of mammography screening and to compensate for the lack of trained breast radiologists. Most of the literature on CAD for mammography comprises studies concerning technical aspects, such as improvements to software, analysis of subtypes of breast cancer, e.g. microcalcifications only, densities only, distortions or combinations of these. The majority of the clinical studies was performed on selected materials enriched with cancer cases, and thus did not represent a true screening situation. Furthermore, comparison with double reading was not a standard procedure in many of the studies. Since the aim of this review was to critically evaluate the scientific evidence of CAD's performance in large population-based screening programs, only four studies met our strict inclusion criteria [68-71]. Of these, only one was considered to have sufficient relevance and quality [71].

Two major shortcomings in study design apply to all four included studies. One is survival rate, which is the most important outcome in mammography screening. None of these studies compared the survival rates with the two strategies, and therefore the present outcome measures (cancer detection rate and recall rate) can be regarded as surrogate outcomes. The other shortcoming is incomplete follow-up. As pointed out in the study by Gilbert et al. [71], sensitivity will be overestimated because of this shortcoming.

Although the study by Gilbert et al. [71] comprised a large population and had an elaborate study set-up, its generalisability is limited since all participating breast radiologists had extensive experience of mammography screening. This is not always the case in an authentic setting. The impact of CAD performance on scanned analogue radiographs as compared to digital mammography is also a matter of concern.

Initially, all CAD studies were performed on scanned analogue mammograms that were analysed with CAD.

Over time there has been a transition from analogue to digital mammography and this process is still ongoing in many parts of the world. The reliability of CAD analysis of scanned films has been questioned [73]. This aspect, together with the fact that modern mammography is performed in a digital environment, implies that new studies are required to fully understand CAD's performance and outcomes in large population-based screening programmes using digital mammography.

Lack of trained radiologists remains a problem even when CAD is used. Using CAD as a first/second reader due to unavailability of a trained breast radiologist could be unsustainable, for instance due to retirement. In any case, new generations of breast radiologists must be secured. Besides, being able to discuss uncertain cases with an experienced colleague is absolutely essential, both for educational purposes and in order to avoid too many false positives/false negatives. When working with CAD, a single radiologist will always have to make the final decision to recall or not to recall a woman for further work-up. This decision may depend on a single CAD mark in an area where the radiologist did not react initially. In our opinion, the single radiologist using CAD needs to be highly experienced, particularly when deciding not to recall a woman for further work-up when a potential cancer might be missed. In conclusion, education and training of new generations of breast radiologists have to be done irrespective of the use of CAD, although it has been suggested that CAD could be used in the training of radiologists [74].

As pointed out earlier, screening policies vary between countries and this review has been performed from a European perspective. However, all screening settings have some features in common, be they population-based, centrally-organized or non-organized ("wild" or "opportunistic" screening) mammographies on asymptomatic women. High throughput is one of these factors that place high demands on smooth screening workflows. Integrating CAD into the workflow would mean that the radiologist would have actively to consider all CAD prompts, which in turn increases the total reading time.

High recall rates imply that more women have to return for additional investigation, involving new mammographic images and often also ultrasound examination. In addition, some have to undergo biopsy and in some cases even surgery. This also means more visits to doctors/hospitals for these women. Overall, additional resources are required and women are worried unnecessarily. Since the medical consequences are not convincingly positive, it is not possible to determine either the cost-effectiveness and/or the socioeconomic consequences of replacing one of the readers with CAD in the context of mammography screening.

Conclusions

The conclusions from this systematic review are:

- The scientific evidence is insufficient to determine whether CAD + *single reading* by one breast radiologist would yield results that are at least equivalent to those obtained in standard practice, i.e. *double reading* where two breast radiologists independently read the mammographic images.
- Since the medical consequences are uncertain, it is not possible to determine the cost-effectiveness or the socioeconomic consequences of replacing one of the readings with CAD in the context of mammography screening.
- Since this literature review, CAD technology has advanced further, thanks to improvements in computer software and digitalization.
- Additional prospective and preferably randomized population-based studies are essential to understand the method's specific benefits, consequences, and costs.

Competing interest
The authors declare that they have no competing interest.

Authors' contributions
EA: Study concept, analysis, interpretation of data and drafting the manuscript. SZ: Study concept, analysis, interpretation of data and drafting the manuscript. IM: Study concept, analysis, interpretation of data and drafting the manuscript. MHA: Study concept, analysis, interpretation of data and drafting the manuscript. All four authors are responsible for the content and writing of the paper and approved the final manuscript.

Authors' information
*First authorship shared by Azavedo E and Zackrisson S.

Author details
[1]Department of Diagnostic Radiology, Karolinska Institutet, Stockholm, Sweden. [2]Department of Clinical Sciences in Malmö, Diagnostic Radiology, Lund University, Skåne University Hospital Malmö, Malmö SE-205 02, Sweden. [3]Swedish Council on Health Technology Assessment (SBU), Stockholm, Sweden. [4]LIME/MMC, Karolinska Institutet, Stockholm, Sweden.

References
1. Tabar L, Fagerberg CJ, Gad A, Baldetorp L, Holmberg LH, Grontoft O, Ljungquist U, Lundstrom B, Manson JC, Eklund G, et al: Reduction in mortality from breast cancer after mass screening with mammography. Randomised trial from the Breast Cancer Screening Working Group of the Swedish National Board of Health and Welfare. Lancet 1985, 1(8433):829–832.
2. Andersson I, Aspregren K, Janzon L, Landberg T, Lindholm K, Linell F, Ljungberg O, Ranstam J, Sigfusson B: Mammographic screening and mortality from breast cancer: the Malmo mammographic screening trial. BMJ 1988, 297(6654):943–948.
3. Bjurstam N, Bjorneld L, Duffy SW, Smith TC, Cahlin E, Eriksson O, Hafstrom LO, Lingaas H, Mattsson J, Persson S, et al: The Gothenburg breast screening trial: first results on mortality, incidence, and mode of detection for women ages 39–49 years at randomization. Cancer 1997, 80(11):2091–2099.
4. Frisell J, Glas U, Hellstrom L, Somell A: Randomized mammographic screening for breast cancer in Stockholm. Design, first round results and comparisons. Breast Cancer Res Treat 1986, 8(1):45–54.
5. Vainio H, Bianchini F: IARC Handbooks of Cancer Prevention- Breast Cancer Screening. Lyon, France: IARCPress; 2002:2002.
6. Nystrom L, Andersson I, Bjurstam N, Frisell J, Nordenskjold B, Rutqvist LE: Long-term effects of mammography screening: updated overview of the Swedish randomised trials. Lancet 2002, 359(9310):909–919.
7. Tabar L, Vitak B, Chen TH, Yen AM, Cohen A, Tot T, Chiu SY, Chen SL, Fann JC, Rosell J, et al: Swedish two-county trial: impact of mammographic screening on breast cancer mortality during 3 decades. Radiology 2011, 260(3):658–663.
8. Hellquist BN, Duffy SW, Abdsaleh S, Bjorneld L, Bordas P, Tabar L, Vitak B, Zackrisson S, Nystrom L, Jonsson H: Effectiveness of population-based service screening with mammography for women ages 40 to 49 years: evaluation of the Swedish Mammography Screening in Young Women (SCRY) cohort. Cancer 2011, 117(4):714–722.
9. SOSSEG SOSSEG: Reduction in breast cancer mortality from organized service screening with mammography: 1. Further confirmation with extended data. Cancer Epidemiol Biomarkers Prev 2006, 15(1):45–51.
10. Gotzsche PC, Nielsen M: Screening for breast cancer with mammography. Cochrane Database Syst Rev 2011, (1):CD001877.
11. Perry N, Broeders M, de Wolf C, Törnberg S, Holland R, von Karsa L: European guidelines for quality assurance in breast cancer screening and diagnosis. 4th edition. Luxembourg: Office for Official Publications of the European Communities; 2006. ISBN 2006 ISBN 92-79-01258-4: EU.
12. Helvie M: Improving mammographic interpretation: double reading and computer-aided diagnosis. Radiol Clin North Am 2007, 45(5):801–811. vi.
13. Guerriero C, Gillan MG, Cairns J, Wallis MG, Gilbert FJ: Is computer aided detection (CAD) cost effective in screening mammography? A model based on the CADET II study. BMC Health Serv Res 2011, 11(1):11.
14. Taylor P, Champness J, Given-Wilson R, Johnston K, Potts H: Impact of computer-aided detection prompts on the sensitivity and specificity of screening mammography. Health Technol Assess 2005, 9(6):1–58. iii.
15. Houssami N, Given-Wilson R: Incorporating new technologies into clinical practice without evidence of effectiveness in prospective studies: computer-aided detection (CAD) in breast screening reinforces the need for better initial evaluation. Breast 2007, 16(3):219–221.
16. Houssami N, Given-Wilson R, Ciatto S: Early detection of breast cancer: overview of the evidence on computer-aided detection in mammography screening. J Med Imaging Radiat Oncol 2009, 53(2):171–176.
17. Taylor P, Potts HW: Computer aids and human second reading as interventions in screening mammography: two systematic reviews to compare effects on cancer detection and recall rate. Eur J Cancer 2008, 44(6):798–807.
18. Bennett RL, Blanks RG, Moss SM: Does the accuracy of single reading with CAD (computer-aided detection) compare with that of double reading?: A review of the literature. Clin Radiol 2006, 61(12):1023–1028.
19. SBU: Computer-Aided Detection (CAD) in Mammography Screening. Stockholm: Statens beredning för medicinsk utvärdering (SBU): SBU; 2011.
20. Azavedo E, Svane G: Radiologic aspects of breast cancers detected through a breast cancer screening program. Eur J Radiol 1991, 13(2):88–90.
21. Whiting P, Rutjes AW, Reitsma JB, Bossuyt PM, Kleijnen J: The development of QUADAS: a tool for the quality assessment of studies of diagnostic accuracy included in systematic reviews. BMC Med Res Methodol 2003, 3:25.
22. Guyatt GH, Oxman AD, Vist GE, Kunz R, Falck-Ytter Y, Alonso-Coello P, Schunemann HJ: GRADE: an emerging consensus on rating quality of evidence and strength of recommendations. BMJ 2008, 336(7650):924–926.
23. Schunemann HJ, Oxman AD, Brozek J, Glasziou P, Bossuyt P, Chang S, Muti P, Jaeschke R, Guyatt GH: GRADE: assessing the quality of evidence for diagnostic recommendations. Evid Based Med 2008, 13(6):162–163.
24. Boyer B, Balleyguier C, Granat O, Pharaboz C: CAD in questions/answers Review of the literature. Eur J Radiol 2009, 69(1):24–33.
25. G-S G, Chersevani R, Ciatto S, Del Favero C, Frigerio A, Giordano L, Giuseppetti G, Naldoni C, Panizza P, Petrella M, Gruppo di studio G-S, Chersevani R, Ciatto S, Del Favero C, Frigerio A, Giordano L, Giuseppetti G, Naldoni C, Panizza P, Petrella M, et al: "CADEAT": considerations on the use of CAD (computer-aided diagnosis) in mammography. La Radiologia medica 2010, 115(4):563–570.

26. Kolb GR: The financial impact of computer-aided detection on the mammography practice. *Applied Radiology* 2001, **30**(11 SUPPL.):21–24.

27. Nishikawa RM: Evaluation of computer-aided detection and computer detection systems. *Applied Radiology* 2001, **30**(11 SUPPL.):14–16.

28. Noble M, Bruening W, Uhl S, Schoelles K: Computer-aided detection mammography for breast cancer screening: systematic review and meta-analysis. *Arch Gynecol Obstet* 2009, **279**(6):881–890.

29. Cawson JN, Nickson C, Amos A, Hill G, Whan AB, Kavanagh AM: Invasive breast cancers detected by screening mammography: a detailed comparison of computer-aided detection-assisted single reading and double reading. *J Med Imaging Radiat Oncol* 2009, **53**(5):442–449.

30. van den Biggelaar FJ, Kessels AG, van Engelshoven JM, Flobbe K: Strategies for digital mammography interpretation in a clinical patient population. *Int J Cancer* 2009, **125**(12):2923–2929.

31. Paquerault S, Samuelson FW, Petrick N, Myers KJ, Smith RC: Investigation of reading mode and relative sensitivity as factors that influence reader performance when using computer-aided detection software. *Acad Radiol* 2009, **16**(9):1095–1107.

32. van den Biggelaar FJ, Kessels AG, van Engelshoven JM, Boetes C, Flobbe K: Computer-aided detection in full-field digital mammography in a clinical population: performance of radiologist and technologists. *Breast Cancer Res Treat* 2010, **120**(2):499–506.

33. James JJ, Cornford EJ: Does computer-aided detection have a role in the arbitration of discordant double-reading opinions in a breast-screening programme? *Clin Radiol* 2009, **64**(1):46–51.

34. Kim SJ, Moon WK, Cho N, Cha JH, Kim SM, Im JG: Computer-aided detection in full-field digital mammography: sensitivity and reproducibility in serial examinations. *Radiology* 2008, **246**(1):71–80.

35. Brancato B, Houssami N, Francesca D, Bianchi S, Risso G, Catarzi S, Taschini R, Rosselli Del Turco M, Ciatto S: Does computer-aided detection (CAD) contribute to the performance of digital mammography in a self-referred population? *Breast Cancer Res Treat* 2008, **111**(2):373–376.

36. Yang SK, Moon WK, Cho N, Park JS, Cha JH, Kim SM, Kim SJ, Im JG: Screening mammography-detected cancers: sensitivity of a computer-aided detection system applied to full-field digital mammograms. *Radiology* 2007, **244**(1):104–111.

37. Skaane P, Kshirsagar A, Stapleton S, Young K, Castellino RA: Effect of computer-aided detection on independent double reading of paired screen-film and full-field digital screening mammograms. *AJR Am J Roentgenol* 2007, **188**(2):377–384.

38. Gilbert FJ, Astley SM, McGee MA, Gillan MG, Boggis CR, Griffiths PM, Duffy SW: Single reading with computer-aided detection and double reading of screening mammograms in the United Kingdom National Breast Screening Program. *Radiology* 2006, **241**(1):47–53.

39. Dean JC, Ilvento CC: Improved cancer detection using computer-aided detection with diagnostic and screening mammography: prospective study of 104 cancers. *AJR Am J Roentgenol* 2006, **187**(1):20–28.

40. Hukkinen K, Vehmas T, Pamilo M, Kivisaari L: Effect of computer-aided detection on mammographic performance: experimental study on readers with different levels of experience. *Acta Radiol* 2006, **47**(3):257–263.

41. Ciatto S, Ambrogetti D, Collini G, Cruciani A, Ercolini E, Risso G, Rosselli Del Turco M: Computer-aided detection (CAD) of cancers detected on double reading by one reader only. *Breast* 2006, **15**(4):528–532.

42. Hukkinen K, Pamilo M: Does computer-aided detection assist in the early detection of breast cancer? *Acta Radiol* 2005, **46**(2):135–139.

43. Destounis SV, DiNitto P, Logan-Young W, Bonaccio E, Zuley ML, Willison KM: Can computer-aided detection with double reading of screening mammograms help decrease the false-negative rate? Initial experience. *Radiology* 2004, **232**(2):578–584.

44. Ciatto S, Rosselli Del Turco M, Burke P, Visioli C, Paci E, Zappa M: Comparison of standard and double reading and computer-aided detection (CAD) of interval cancers at prior negative screening mammograms: blind review. *Br J Cancer* 2003, **89**(9):1645–1649.

45. Ciatto S, Brancato B, Rosselli Del Turco M, Risso G, Catarzi S, Morrone D, Bricolo D, Zappa M: Comparison of standard reading and computer aided diagnosis (CAD) on a proficiency test of screening mammography. *Radiol Med* 2003, **106**(1–2):59–65.

46. Brem RF, Baum J, Lechner M, Kaplan S, Souders S, Naul LG, Hoffmeister J: Improvement in sensitivity of screening mammography with computer-aided detection: a multiinstitutional trial. *AJR Am J Roentgenol* 2003, **181**(3):687–693.

47. Quek ST, Thng CH, Khoo JB, Koh WL: Radiologists' detection of mammographic abnormalities with and without a computer-aided detection system. *Australas Radiol* 2003, **47**(3):257–260.

48. Zheng B, Hardesty LA, Poller WR, Sumkin JH, Golla S: Mammography with computer-aided detection: reproducibility assessment initial experience. *Radiology* 2003, **228**(1):58–62.

49. Karssemeijer N, Otten JD, Verbeek AL, Groenewoud JH, de Koning HJ, Hendriks JH, Holland R: Computer-aided detection versus independent double reading of masses on mammograms. *Radiology* 2003, **227**(1):192–200.

50. Ciatto S, Del Turco MR, Risso G, Catarzi S, Bonardi R, Viterbo V, Gnutti P, Guglielmoni B, Pinelli L, Pandiscia A, *et al*: Comparison of standard reading and computer aided detection (CAD) on a national proficiency test of screening mammography. *Eur J Radiol* 2003, **45**(2):135–138.

51. Malich A, Marx C, Facius M, Boehm T, Fleck M, Kaiser WA: Tumour detection rate of a new commercially available computer-aided detection system. *Eur Radiol* 2001, **11**(12):2454–2459.

52. Moberg K, Bjurstam N, Wilczek B, Rostgard L, Egge E, Muren C: Computed assisted detection of interval breast cancers. *Eur J Radiol* 2001, **39**(2):104–110.

53. Warren Burhenne LJ, Wood SA, D'Orsi CJ, Feig SA, Kopans DB, O'Shaughnessy KF, Sickles EA, Tabar L, Vyborny CJ, Castellino RA: Potential contribution of computer-aided detection to the sensitivity of screening mammography. *Radiology* 2000, **215**(2):554–562.

54. Jiang Y, Nishikawa RM, Schmidt RA, Metz CE, Giger ML, Doi K: Improving breast cancer diagnosis with computer-aided diagnosis. *Acad Radiol* 1999, **6**(1):22–33.

55. Thurfjell E, Thurfjell MG, Egge E, Bjurstam N: Sensitivity and specificity of computer-assisted breast cancer detection in mammography screening. *Acta Radiol* 1998, **39**(4):384–388.

56. Sang KY, Woo KM, Cho N, Jeong SP, Joo HC, Sun MK, Seung JK, Im JG: Screening mammography-detected cancers: Sensitivity of a computer-aided detection system applied to full-field digital mammograms. *Radiology* 2007, **244**(1):104–111.

57. Li JG, Li S, Xu HM, Xu K: Evaluation on the use and results of computer-aided detection for full-field digital mammorgraphy. *Chinese Journal of Radiology* 2006, **40**(7):729–732.

58. Birdwell RL, Bandodkar P, Ikeda DM: Computer-aided detection with screening mammography in a university hospital setting. *Radiology* 2005, **236**(2):451–457.

59. Cupples TE, Cunningham JE, Reynolds JC: Impact of computer-aided detection in a regional screening mammography program. *AJR Am J Roentgenol* 2005, **185**(4):944–950.

60. Fenton JJ, Taplin SH, Carney PA, Abraham L, Sickles EA, D'Orsi C, Berns EA, Cutter G, Hendrick RE, Barlow WE, *et al*: Influence of computer-aided detection on performance of screening mammography. *N Engl J Med* 2007, **356**(14):1399–1409.

61. Freer TW, Ulissey MJ: Screening mammography with computer-aided detection: prospective study of 12,860 patients in a community breast center. *Radiology* 2001, **220**(3):781–786.

62. Gur D, Sumkin JH, Rockette HE, Ganott M, Hakim C, Hardesty L, Poller WR, Shah R, Wallace L: Changes in breast cancer detection and mammography recall rates after the introduction of a computer-aided detection system. *J Natl Cancer Inst* 2004, **96**(3):185–190.

63. Karssemeijer N, Bluekens AM, Beijerinck D, Deurenberg JJ, Beekman M, Visser R, van Engen R, Bartels-Kortland A, Broeders MJ: Breast cancer screening results 5 years after introduction of digital mammography in a population-based screening program. *Radiology* 2009, **253**(2):353–358.

64. Ko JM, Nicholas MJ, Mendel JB, Slanetz PJ: Prospective assessment of computer-aided detection in interpretation of screening mammography. *AJR Am J Roentgenol* 2006, **187**(6):1483–1491.

65. Morton MJ, Whaley DH, Brandt KR, Amrami KK: Screening mammograms: interpretation with computer-aided detection–prospective evaluation. *Radiology* 2006, **239**(2):375–383.

66. Sanchez Gomez S, Torres Tabanera M, Vega Bolivar A, Sainz Miranda M, Baroja Mazo A, Ruiz Diaz M, Martinez Miravete P, Lag Asturiano E, Munoz Cacho P, Delgado Macias T: Impact of a CAD system in a screen-film mammography screening program: A prospective study. *Eur J Radiol* 2010, .

67. James JJ, Gilbert FJ, Wallis MG, Gillan MG, Astley SM, Boggis CR, Agbaje OF, Brentnall AR, Duffy SW: **Mammographic features of breast cancers at single reading with computer-aided detection and at double reading in a large multicenter prospective trial of computer-aided detection: CADET II.** *Radiology* 2010, **256**(2):379–386.

68. Georgian-Smith D, Moore RH, Halpern E, Yeh ED, Rafferty EA, D'Alessandro HA, Staffa M, Hall DA, McCarthy KA, Kopans DB: **Blinded comparison of computer-aided detection with human second reading in screening mammography.** *AJR Am J Roentgenol* 2007, **189**(5):1135–1141.

69. Gromet M: **Comparison of computer-aided detection to double reading of screening mammograms: review of 231,221 mammograms.** *AJR Am J Roentgenol* 2008, **190**(4):854–859.

70. Khoo LA, Taylor P, Given-Wilson RM: **Computer-aided detection in the United Kingdom National Breast Screening Programme: prospective study.** *Radiology* 2005, **237**(2):444–449.

71. Gilbert FJ, Astley SM, Gillan MG, Agbaje OF, Wallis MG, James J, Boggis CR, Duffy SW: **Single reading with computer-aided detection for screening mammography.** *N Engl J Med* 2008, **359**(16):1675–1684.

72. Azavedo E, Svane G: **Radial scars detected mammographically in a breast cancer screening programme.** *Eur J Radiol* 1992, **15**(1):18–21.

73. Malich A, Azhari T, Bohm T, Fleck M, Kaiser WA: **Reproducibility–an important factor determining the quality of computer-aided detection (CAD) systems.** *Eur J Radiol* 2000, **36**(3):170–174.

74. Luo P, Qian W, Romilly P: **CAD-aided mammogram training.** *Acad Radiol* 2005, **12**(8):1039–1048.

Permissions

The contributors of this book come from diverse backgrounds, making this book a truly international effort. This book will bring forth new frontiers with its revolutionizing research information and detailed analysis of the nascent developments around the world.

We would like to thank all the contributing authors for lending their expertise to make the book truly unique. They have played a crucial role in the development of this book. Without their invaluable contributions this book wouldn't have been possible. They have made vital efforts to compile up to date information on the varied aspects of this subject to make this book a valuable addition to the collection of many professionals and students.

This book was conceptualized with the vision of imparting up-to-date information and advanced data in this field. To ensure the same, a matchless editorial board was set up. Every individual on the board went through rigorous rounds of assessment to prove their worth. After which they invested a large part of their time researching and compiling the most relevant data for our readers.

The editorial board has been involved in producing this book since its inception. They have spent rigorous hours researching and exploring the diverse topics which have resulted in the successful publishing of this book. They have passed on their knowledge of decades through this book. To expedite this challenging task, the publisher supported the team at every step. A small team of assistant editors was also appointed to further simplify the editing procedure and attain best results for the readers.

Apart from the editorial board, the designing team has also invested a significant amount of their time in understanding the subject and creating the most relevant covers. They scrutinized every image to scout for the most suitable representation of the subject and create an appropriate cover for the book.

The publishing team has been an ardent support to the editorial, designing and production team. Their endless efforts to recruit the best for this project, has resulted in the accomplishment of this book. They are a veteran in the field of academics and their pool of knowledge is as vast as their experience in printing. Their expertise and guidance has proved useful at every step. Their uncompromising quality standards have made this book an exceptional effort. Their encouragement from time to time has been an inspiration for everyone.

The publisher and the editorial board hope that this book will prove to be a valuable piece of knowledge for researchers, students, practitioners and scholars across the globe.

List of Contributors

Lindsey McKeen-Polizzotti, Kira M Henderson and George E Plopper
Department of Biology, Center for Biotechnology and Interdisciplinary Studies, Rensselaer Polytechnic Institute, Troy, New York, USA

Basak Oztan, C Cagatay Bilgin and Bülent Yener
Department of Computer Science, Rensselaer Polytechnic Institute, Troy, New York, USA

Jimmy Okello, Harriet Kisembo and Sam Bugeza
Department of Radiology and Radiotherapy, Mulago National Referral and University Teaching Hospital, Kampala, Uganda

Moses Galukande
Department of Surgery, College of Health Sciences, Makerere University, Kampala, Uganda

Mohammad Mehrmohammadi and Mostafa Fatemi
Department of Physiology and Biomedical Engineering, Mayo Clinic College of Medicine, 200 First Street SW, Rochester, MN 55905, USA

Azra Alizad
Department of Physiology and Biomedical Engineering, Mayo Clinic College of Medicine, 200 First Street SW, Rochester, MN 55905, USA
Division of General Internal Medicine, Department of Medicine, Mayo Clinic College of Medicine, 200 First Street SW, Rochester, MN 55905, USA

Karthik Ghosh
Division of General Internal Medicine, Department of Medicine, Mayo Clinic College of Medicine, 200 First Street SW, Rochester, MN 55905, USA

Katrina N Glazebrook and Dana H Whaley
Department of Radiology, Mayo Clinic College of Medicine, 200 First Street SW, Rochester, MN 55905, USA

Rickey E Carter
Division of Biomedical Statistics and Informatics, Department of Health Sciences Research Mayo Clinic College of Medicine, 200 First Street SW, Rochester, MN 55905, USA

Leman Gunbery Karaberkmez
Bolu IBD Hospital, Radiology, Sanayi Sitesi 32. Blok Demirciler Ve Nalburcular Odasi Hiz. Binasi Alti, No:1,14100 Bolu, Turkey

Letizia Vivona, Donato Cascio, Francesco Fauci and Giuseppe Raso
Dipartimento di Fisica e Chimica, Università Degli Studi di Palermo, Palermo,Italy

Edward J Kendall
Discipline of Radiology, Janeway Child Health Centre, Memorial University of Newfoundland, Newfoundland A1B 3V6, Canada

Michael G Barnett
Prairie North Health Region, Battlefords Office, 1092 107th Street, North Battleford, Saskatchewan S9A 1Z1, Canada

Krista Chytyk-Praznik
Radiation Oncology Department, Nova Scotia Cancer Centre, 5820 University Avenue, Halifax, Nova Scotia B3H 1V7, Canada

Sebastian Wojcinski and Peter Hillemanns
Hannover Medical School, Department for Obstetrics and Gynecology, OE 6410, Carl-Neuberg-Straße 1, Hannover 30625, Germany

Jennifer Dupont
Main-Taunus-Kreis Hospital, Department for Obstetrics and Gynecology, Bad Soden, Germany

Werner Schmidt
University Hospital of Saarland, Department for Obstetrics and Gynecology, Homburg/Saar, Germany

Michael Cassel
University of Potsdam, Center for Sports Medicine, Recreational and High Performance Sports, Potsdam, Germany

Kazuyoshi Motomura
Departments of Surgery, Osaka Medical Center for Cancer and Cardiovascular Diseases, 1-3-3 Nakamichi, Higashinari-ku 537-8511Osaka, Japan

Hiroshi Sumino, Atsushi Noguchi, Takashi Horinouchi and Katsuyuki Nakanishi
Departments of Radiology, Osaka Medical Center for Cancer and Cardiovascular Diseases, 1-3-3 Nakamichi, Higashinari-ku 537-8511Osaka, Japan

Kazuyoshi Motomura
Department of Surgery, Osaka Medical Center for Cancer and Cardiovascular Diseases, 1-3-3 Nakamichi, Higashinari-ku, Osaka 537-8511, Japan

Tetsuta Izumi, Souichirou Tateishi, Hiroshi Sumino, Atsushi Noguchi, Takashi Horinouchi and Katsuyuki Nakanishi
Department of Radiology, Osaka Medical Center for Cancer and Cardiovascular Diseases, Osaka, Japan

Maria Julia Gregorio Calas
Department of Radiology, Federal University of Rio de Janeiro, Rua Prof. Rodolpho Paulo Rocco 255, Cidade Universitária, Rio de Janeiro, RJ 21941-617, Brazil
Department of Breast Imaging, Clínica de Diagnóstico porImagem (CDPI), Av. Ataulfo de Paiva 669, 2nd floor, Leblon, Rio de Janeiro, RJ 22440-032, Brazil

Fernanda Philadelpho Arantes Pereira
Department of Radiology, Federal University of Rio de Janeiro, Rua Prof. Rodolpho Paulo Rocco 255, Cidade Universitária, Rio de Janeiro, RJ 21941-617, Brazil
Department of Breast Imaging, Clínica de Diagnóstico porImagem (CDPI), Av. Ataulfo de Paiva 669, 2nd floor, Leblon, Rio de Janeiro, RJ 22440-032, Brazil
Department of Magnetic Resonance Imaging, Clínica de Diagnóstico por Imagem (CDPI), Av. Ataulfo de Paiva 669, 2nd floor, Leblon, Rio de Janeiro, RJ 22440-032, Brazil

Emerson Leandro Gasparetto
Department of Radiology, Federal University of Rio de Janeiro, Rua Prof. Rodolpho Paulo Rocco 255, Cidade Universitária, Rio de Janeiro, RJ 21941-617, Brazil
Department of Magnetic Resonance Imaging, Clínica de Diagnóstico por Imagem (CDPI), Av. Ataulfo de Paiva 669, 2nd floor, Leblon, Rio de Janeiro, RJ 22440-032, Brazil

Gabriela Martins
Department of Breast Imaging, Clínica de Diagnóstico porImagem (CDPI), Av. Ataulfo de Paiva 669, 2nd floor, Leblon, Rio de Janeiro, RJ 22440-032, Brazil
Department of Magnetic Resonance Imaging, Clínica de Diagnóstico por Imagem (CDPI), Av. Ataulfo de Paiva 669, 2nd floor, Leblon, Rio de Janeiro, RJ 22440-032, Brazil

Maria Veronica Fonseca Torres de Oliveira and Lea Mirian Barbosa da Fonseca
Department of Nuclear Medicine,Federal University of Rio de Janeiro, Rua Prof. Rodolpho Paulo Rocco 255,Cidade Universitária, Rio de Janeiro, RJ 21941-617, Brazil
Department of Nuclear Medicine, Clínica de Diagnóstico por Imagem (CDPI), Av. Ataulfo de Paiva 669, 2nd floor, Leblon, Rio de Janeiro, RJ 22440-032, Brazil

Sebastian Wojcinski, Philipp Soergel and Peter Hillemanns
Department of OB/GYN, Hannover Medical School, OE 6410, Carl-Neuberg-Straße 1, 30625 Hannover, Germany

Samuel Gyapong, André Farrokh and Friedrich Degenhardt
Department of OB/GYN, Franziskus Hospital, Bielefeld, Germany

Donato Cascio, Francesco Fauci and Giuseppe Raso
Dipartimento di Fisica e Chimica, Università Degli Studi di Palermo, Palermo, Italy

Marius Iacomi
Dipartimento di Fisica e Chimica, Università Degli Studi di Palermo, Palermo, Italy
Institutul de Ştiinţe Spaţiale, Bucharest, Măgurele, Romania

José Sanz-Santos, Pere Serra, Gloria Bonet and Juan Ruiz Manzano
Pulmonology Department, Hospital Universitari Germans Trias Pujol, Planta 8, Carretera del Canyet s/n. 08916, Badalona, Spain

José Antonio Fiz
Pulmonology Department, Hospital Universitari Germans Trias Pujol, Planta 8, Carretera del Canyet s/n. 08916, Badalona, Spain
TALP Research Center, UPC, Barcelona, Spain

Felipe Andreo
Pulmonology Department, Hospital Universitari Germans Trias Pujol, Planta 8, Carretera del Canyet s/n. 08916, Badalona, Spain
Ciber de Enfermedades Respiratorias (CiBERES), Bunyola, Balearic Islands, Spain

Enrique Monte-Moreno
TALP Research Center, UPC, Barcelona, Spain

Santiago José Auteri
Pulmonology Department Hospital de rehabilitación Respiratoria María Ferrer, Buenos Aires, Argentina

Eva Castellà
Pathology Department Hospital Universitari Germans Trias Pujol, Badalona, Spain

H. Preibsch and L. K. Wanner
Department of Diagnostic and Interventional Radiology, University Hospital Tuebingen, Hoppe-Seyler-Str. 3, 72076 Tuebingen, Germany

A. Staebler
Department of Pathology and Neuropathology, University Hospital Tuebingen, Liebermeisterstr. 8, 72076 Tuebingen, Germany

M. Hahn
Department of Obstetrics and Gynecology, University Hospital Tuebingen, Calwerstr. 7, 72076 Tuebingen, Germany

K. C. Siegmann-Luz
Diagnostic Breast Centre and Breast Cancer Screening Brandenburg East, Koepenicker Str. 29, 15711 Koenigs Wusterhausen, Germany

Haim Paran, Ilana Haas and Patricia Malinger
Breast unit, Meir Medical Center, Kfar Saba, Israel

Zvi Kaufman
Breast unit, Meir Medical Center, Kfar Saba, Israel
Department of Surgery, Meir Medical Center, Kfar Sava, Israel

Tania Zehavi
Department of pathology, Meir Medical Center, Kfar Saba, Israel

Tamar Karni and Izhak Pappo
Breast unit, Assaf Harofeh Medical Center, Zrifin, Israel

Judith Sandbank
Department of Pathology, Assaf Harofeh Medical Center, Zrifin, Israel

Judith Diment
Department of Pathology, Kaplan Medical Center, Rehovot, Israel

Tanir Allweis
Breast Unit, Kaplan Medical Center, Rehovot, Israel

Christina Baun, Kirsten Falch, Jeanette Hansen, Tram Nguyen, Poul-Flemming Høilund-Carlsen and Malene G. Hildebrandt
Department of Nuclear Medicine, University Hospital, Sdr. Boulevard 29, 5000 Odense C, Denmark

Oke Gerke
Department of Nuclear Medicine, University Hospital, Sdr. Boulevard 29, 5000 Odense C, Denmark
Centre of Health Economics Research, University of Southern Denmark, Odense, Denmark

Abass Alavi
University of Pennsylvania, Philadelphia, USA

Sven Weum and James B. Mercer
Medical Imaging Research Group, Department of Clinical Medicine, UiT The Arctic University of Norway, 9037 Tromsø, Norway
Department of Radiology, University Hospital of North Norway, Sykehusveien 38, Tromsø, Norway

Louis de Weerd
Medical Imaging Research Group, Department of Clinical Medicine, UiT The Arctic University of Norway, 9037 Tromsø, Norway
Department of Plastic Surgery and Hand Surgery, University Hospital of North Norway, Tromsø, Norway

Satoko Nakano and Masahiko Ohtsuka
Department of Surgery, Kawaguchi Municipal Medical Center, 180 Nishiaraijyuku, Kawaguchi-city, Saitama 333-0833, Japan

Akemi Mibu
Department of Laboratory, Kawaguchi Municipal Medical Center, Kawaguchi-city, Japan

Masato Karikomi
Department of Radiology, Kawaguchi Municipal
Medical Center, Kawaguchi-city, Japan

Hitomi Sakata and Masahiro Yamamoto
Department of Pathology, Kawaguchi Municipal
Medical Center, Kawaguchi-city, Japan

Edward Azavedo
Department of Diagnostic Radiology, Karolinska
Institutet, Stockholm, Sweden
LIME/MMC, Karolinska Institutet, Stockholm,
Sweden

Sophia Zackrisson
Department of Clinical Sciences in Malmö,
Diagnostic Radiology, Lund University, Skåne
University Hospital Malmö, Malmö SE-205 02,
Sweden

Ingegerd Mejàre
Swedish Council on Health Technology Assessment
(SBU), Stockholm, Sweden

Marianne Heibert Arnlind
Swedish Council on Health Technology Assessment
(SBU), Stockholm, Sweden
LIME/MMC, Karolinska Institutet, Stockholm,
Sweden

Index

www.ingramcontent.com/pod-product-compliance
Lightning Source LLC
Chambersburg PA
CBHW082011190326
41458CB00010B/3149